Infectious Diseases and Microbiology

nova
New York

Infectious Diseases and Microbiology

COVID-19 Contracting: Opportunities, Actions and Reimbursements
Eric Neudorf
2022. ISBN: 978-1-68507-710-5 (Hardcover)
2022. ISBN: 978-1-68507-733-4 (eBook)

The Aviation Industry and COVID-19
Stefan Schneider
2022. ISBN: 978-1-68507-712-9 (Hardcover)
2022. ISBN: 978-1-68507-729-7 (eBook)

Diseases Transmitted by Ticks
Hacer İşler (Editor), Metin Özdemir, MD (Editor)
2021. ISBN: 978-1-68507-359-6 (Hardcover)
2021. ISBN: 978-1-68507-383-1 (eBook)

Impacts and Implications of COVID-19: An Analytical and Empirical Study
Anand Sharma (Editor)
Prateek Agrawal (Editor)
Vishu Madaan (Editor)
Anuj Agarwal (Editor)
2021. ISBN: 978-1-53619-670-2 (Hardcover)
2021. ISBN: 978-1-68507-081-6 (eBook)

Understanding the Spread of Infectious Diseases
Andrew J. Hinerman (Editor)
2020. ISBN: 978-1-53618-892-9 (Hardcover)
2020. ISBN: 978-1-53618-917-9 (eBook)

COVID 19
Sujith Ovallath, MBBS, MD, DNB, DM (Editor)
2020. ISBN: 978-1-53618-691-8 (Softcover)
2020. ISBN: 978-1-53618-729-8 (eBook)

More information about this series can be found at https://novapublishers.com/product-category/series/infectious-diseases-and-microbiology/

John Schroder
Editor

COVID-19 Vaccines

Development, Distribution and Mandates

snova
New York

Library of Congress Cataloging-in-Publication Data

ISBN: 979-8-88697-150-7

Published by Nova Science Publishers, Inc. † New York

Contents

Preface

Vaccines protect people from disease by preparing the body to respond to an infection. Vaccinations are a key part of individual and community health, but vaccine development remains complex and costly. Innovative technologies and approaches may enhance the nation's ability to respond to infectious diseases. For example, reverse vaccinology and next-generation platforms—combined with existing research—helped researchers develop some COVID-19 vaccines more quickly and effectively.

Chapter 1 - The CARES Act included a provision for GAO to report on its ongoing monitoring and oversight efforts related to the COVID-19 pandemic. This chapter discusses technologies, approaches, and associated challenges for vaccine (1) research and development, (2) testing, and (3) manufacturing, as well as (4) the economic factors that affect vaccine investment.

GAO conducted literature searches including scholarly articles and government reports relevant to these four areas. GAO interviewed stakeholders and experts with a diverse set of perspectives on the science, administration, and economics of vaccine development. GAO also convened a 3-day meeting of 22 experts with expertise in at least one area related to our four objectives with assistance from the National Academies of Sciences, Engineering, and Medicine. GAO received technical comments on a draft of this chapter from 1 federal agency and 9 participants at its expert meeting, which it incorporated as appropriate.

GAO is identifying policy options in this chapter.

Chapter 2 - This is an edited, reformatted and augmented version of Hearing before the Select Subcommittee on the Coronavirus Crisis of the Committee on Oversight and Reform, House of Representatives, Serial No. 117–34, dated July 1, 2021.

Chapter 3 - This is an edited, reformatted and augmented version of Hearing before the Select Subcommittee on the Coronavirus Crisis of the Committee on Oversight and Reform, House of Representatives, Serial No. 117–51, dated November 10, 2021.

Chapter 4 - This is an edited, reformatted and augmented version of Centers for Disease Control and Prevention Insights Report 25, dated May 12, 2022.

Chapter 5 - Federal efforts to develop, manufacture, purchase, and distribute Coronavirus Disease 2019 (COVID-19) vaccines have involved a number of agencies. Many of these efforts have thus far been funded by appropriations in COVID-19 relief acts, especially funding to the Department of Health and Human Services (HHS) U.S. Public Health Service (PHS) agencies and accounts in FY2020 and FY2021 supplemental appropriations and in the American Rescue Plan Act (ARPA, P.L. 117-2) budget reconciliation measure enacted in March 2021.

The following provides an overview of both (1) appropriations and (2) allocations and obligations for selected domestic COVID-19 vaccine related activities.

(With the exception of the mandatory funding provided by ARPA, all funding amounts discussed below are classified as discretionary.) The followingis meant to informa general understanding of relevant funding, but does not capture every federal account that can be used for vaccine- related activities. This chapter does not address financing for vaccine administration (e.g., health insurance coverage) or global vaccination funding (although some of the funding for research and development [R&D], manufacture, and purchase has flexibility for international uses).

Chapter 6 - This chapter answers frequently asked questions regarding domestic and global vaccine supply and distribution, and U.S. spending on Coronavirus Disease 2019 (COVID-19) vaccines. Unless otherwise stated, information is current as of January 10, 2022.

Chapter 7 - The Coronavirus Disease 2019 (COVID-19) pandemic has led to severe health and economic consequences across the globe, as governments work to contain the spread of the virus and its variants. In late 2020, researchers started identifying several COVID-19 variants, now driving surges in related cases and deaths across Africa and south Asia.

The United States, India, and Brazil have the highest number of confirmed COVID-19 cases, many caused by the Delta variant. Vaccines and other countermeasures play a growing role in COVID-19 control. However, insufficient access to vaccines in many low- and middle-income countries (LMICs) raises questions about how inequities may hinder pandemic control worldwide.

Congress appropriated approximately $15 billion for a range of COVID-19-related responses through supplemental appropriations (P.L. 116-123, P.L. 116-136, P.L. 116-260, and P.L. 117-2), including $4 billion for multilateral COVID-19 vaccine efforts. The Biden Administration has announced that the United States will provide over 500 million vaccine doses worldwide through direct donations and contributions via COVAX—a multilateral effort comprising nearly 200 countries, co-led by the World Health Organization (WHO), the Coalition for Epidemic Preparedness and Innovation (CEPI), and Gavi, the Vaccine Alliance. On May 31, 2021, the International Monetary Fund (IMF), the World Bank Group, WHO, and the World Trade Organization (WTO) established the Task Force on COVID-19 Vaccines, Therapeutics and Diagnostics for Developing Countries (the Task Force). The Task Force is seeking an additional $50 billion in support of COVAX and the Access to COVID-19 Tools Accelerator (ACT-A), so that at least 40% of all people worldwide could be vaccinated by the end of 2021.

Chapter 8 - The ongoing Coronavirus Disease 2019 (COVID-19) pandemic has caused millions of cases and deaths, according to the World Health Organization (WHO). The resources below provide information on tracking the international spread of the virus and global efforts to control it through vaccine distribution, diagnostic supplies, and therapeutics.

These resources are not a comprehensive list of global COVID-19 data sources. They are a starting point that may help congressional staff find resources for frequently requested data. Some links may work best with the internet browsers Chrome and Firefox.

Chapter 9 - Vaccination remains critical in the federal response to the COVID-19 pandemic. Vaccine implementation— prioritizing, allocating, distributing, and administering doses—requires coordination among federal, state, and local levels and other stakeholders.

HHS agencies—including CDC and HRSA—set up federal vaccine distribution programs, such as CDC's retail pharmacy program that sends doses directly to pharmacies. The federal government also sends vaccine doses to states for further distribution.

The CARES Act includes a provision for GAO to report on its ongoing monitoring and oversight efforts related to the COVID-19 pandemic. This chapter examines (1) stakeholder perspectives on federal programs to distribute and administer COVID-19 vaccines, (2) efforts to inform health officials, providers, and the public about vaccination, and (3) actions HHS agencies are taking to evaluate their vaccine implementation efforts.

GAO reviewed data and documents from HHS, CDC, and HRSA, and reviewed information from and interviewed state and local health officials in four states and one city selected, in part, for geographic variation. GAO also interviewed other stakeholders, including 12 national associations representing health care providers and others.

Chapter 10 - Vaccines have played a crucial role in battling the COVID-19 pandemic. The CAG worked with vaccine companies to develop COVID-19 vaccines, and made available a sufficient supply for all eligible people in the nation. An April 2021 memorandum of understanding between HHS and DOD called for the transfer of remaining CAG responsibilities to HHS and for identification of lessons learned.

The CARES Act includes a provision for GAO to report on its ongoing monitoring and oversight efforts related to the COVID-19 pandemic. This report examines, among other things, the CAG's progress on (1) transitioning its responsibilities to HHS, and (2) developing a process for a joint interagency lessons learned review.

GAO reviewed CAG transition and contracting documents and interviewed or received written responses from CAG officials, federal agencies, and representatives from the six vaccine companies that worked with the CAG.

Chapter 11 - The sources below can help congressional staff track the progress of the U.S. Coronavirus Disease 2019 (COVID-19) vaccination campaign at the national, state, and local levels.

Chapter 12 - On June 21, 2021, the Occupational Safety and Health Administration (OSHA) promulgated an Emergency Temporary Standard (ETS) for the prevention of the transmission of SARS-CoV-2, the virus that causes COVID-19 in health care employment settings. On December 27, 2021, OSHA announced that it was withdrawing all provisions of this ETS, with the exception of certain COVID-19 reporting requirements.

On November 5, 2021, OSHA promulgated a separate ETS that requires employers with 100 or more employees to require that all employees either be fully vaccinated against COVID-19 by January 4, 2022, or test negative for COVID-19 weekly in order to work onsite. After earlier actions by the U.S. Courts of Appeals for the Fifth and Sixth Circuits, on January 13, 2022, the U.S. Supreme Court granted a stay of the OSHA COVID-19 vaccination and testing ETS pending additional judicial review by the U.S. Court of Appeals for the Sixth Circuit. On January 25, 2022, OSHA announced that it was withdrawing all provisions of this ETS. The ETS will continue to serve as a proposed permanent standard subject to normal rulemaking.

The Occupational Safety and Health Act of 1970 (OSH Act) gives OSHA the ability to promulgate an ETS that would remain in effect for up to six months without going through the normal review and comment process of rulemaking. OSHA, however, has rarely used this authority prior to the COVID-19 pandemic—not since the courts struck down its ETS on asbestos in 1983.

All employers are required to comply with the general duty clause of the OSH Act as well as existing OSHA standards on respiratory protection and recordkeeping that may apply to the current COVID-19 pandemic. Pursuant to guidance issued by OSHA on May 22, 2021, employers are not required to record or report any injuries or illnesses caused by the COVID-19 vaccine. This guidance supersedes earlier OSHA guidance that had required employers to record and report adverse reactions to the vaccine if vaccination was a condition of employment.

The California Division of Occupational Safety and Health (Cal/OSHA), which operates California's state occupational safety and health plan, has had an aerosol transmissible disease (ATD) standard since 2009. This standard includes, among other provisions, the requirement that employers provide covered employees with respirators, rather than surgical masks, when these workers interact with ATDs, such as known or suspected COVID-19 cases. In addition, according to the Cal/OSHA ATD standard, certain procedures require the use of powered air purifying respirators (PAPR). Cal/OSHA has also promulgated an ETS to specifically address COVID-19 exposure in the workplace. The agency that operates the state occupational safety health plan in Michigan (MIOSHA) has promulgated an ETS, which was later rescinded and replaced with the OSHA COVID-19 ETS for health care employers, to specifically address COVID-19 in workplaces. In January 2021, the Virginia state plan (VOSH) promulgated a permanent standard to supersede its ETS, and in May 2021, the Oregon state plan (Oregon OSHA) replaced its ETS with a permanent standard.

Chapter 13 - The Coronavirus Disease 2019 (COVID-19) vaccines licensed or authorized by the U.S. Food and Drug Administration (FDA) are a critical tool to reduce the spread and severity of COVID-19. FDA initially authorized the vaccines, between December 2020 and February 2021, under Section 564 of the Federal Food, Drug, and Cosmetic Act (FD&C Act), a regulatory pathway that allows certain medical products to be made available in the market prior to full FDA approval under specified circumstances, including during a public health emergency. In August 2021, FDA licensed the first COVID- 19 vaccine, Pfizer's Comirnaty, for the prevention of COVID-19 in individuals 16 years of age and older, after determining that the vaccine, for the licensed use, meets the standards for safety, purity, and potency (i.e., effectiveness) under the Public Health Service Act.

Given the data supporting the safety and efficacy of the licensed and authorized COVID-19 vaccines, many public health experts view promoting high COVID-19 vaccination rates—along with continued engagement in community mitigation activities that prevent transmission, such as mask wearing in certain settings—as key components of the United States' pandemic response.

One available legal tool for increasing vaccination rates is for governments to require vaccination. In 2021, various state, local, and federal governmental entities instituted COVID-19 vaccination requirements to address the pandemic, particularly as the Delta variant—a highly contagious strain of SARS-CoV-2 (the virus that causes COVID-19)—spread in the United States. Under the United States' federalist system, states and the federal government share regulatory authority over public health matters, with states traditionally exercising the bulk of the authority in this area pursuant to their general police power. That power authorizes states, within constitutional limits, to enact laws "to provide for the public health, safety, and morals" of the states' inhabitants. In contrast to this general power, the federal government's powers are confined to those enumerated in the Constitution.

This chapter provides an overview of state and federal authority to mandate vaccination. The first part of the report provides background on state and local authority to mandate vaccination under the states' general police power. It discusses the Supreme Court's long-standing recognition of state and local authority to mandate vaccination as an exercise of their police power, and modern courts' analyses of more recent challenges to state vaccination mandates based on the First Amendment's Free Exercise Clause. The report then analyzes the Supreme Court's evolving free exercise jurisprudence and the questions it raises regarding whether and when governments must provide for or grant religious exemptions to vaccination requirements. It then looks at how courts have addressed challenges to COVID-19 vaccination requirements imposed by states and state entities.

The second part of the report provides an overview of federal authority to mandate vaccination. It discusses several sources of existing federal statutory authority that could serve, or have been invoked, as the basis for federal COVID-19 vaccination mandates. It then provides an overview of four employment-based civilian mandates issued by the executive branch to date directed at (1) federal executive agency civilian employees; (2) federal contractors for executive departments, agencies, and offices; (3) most Medicare- and Medicaid-certified providers and suppliers; and (4) employers with 100 or more employees. The report then discusses the state of litigation challenging these mandates. This part also reviews the extent of Congress's constitutional authority under the Constitution's Spending and Commerce Clauses to mandate vaccination.

The report concludes with a brief discussion of a legal issue specific to COVID-19 vaccination mandates, particularly before FDA's licensure of Comirnaty. Namely, it reviews how courts have addressed some litigants' argument that the Emergency Use Authorization status of COVID-19 vaccines preclude entities from mandating COVID-19 vaccination.

Chapter 14 - In 2021, various federal, state, and private entities instituted Coronavirus Disease 2019 (COVID-19) vaccination requirements to address the pandemic, particularly as the Delta variant—a highly contagious strain of SARS-CoV-2 (the virus that causes COVID-19)—spread in the United States. The federal COVID-19 vaccination requirements issued to date by the President or executive agencies include those directed at (1) federal executive agency civilian employees (federal employee mandate); (2) federal contractors for executive departments, agencies, and offices (federal contractor mandate); (3) most Medicare- and Medicaid-certified providers and suppliers (Centers for Medicare and Medicaid Services' [CMS's] Medicare/Medicaid provider mandate); and (4) employers with 100 or more employees (Occupational Safety and Health Administration's [OSHA's] large employer vaccination and testing mandate). These employment- or workforce-based mandates—subject to accommodations required by federal law—either directly require certain employees to receive COVID-19 vaccinations or direct certain employers to impose a vaccination or vaccination-and-testing requirement on their employees or staff.

These federal vaccination mandates have generated numerous legal challenges that have moved quickly through the courts. To date, some of these mandates have been enjoined by courts either on a nationwide basis or only in certain states. Table 1 below provides a summary of the mandates and their statuses.

Chapter 15 - In March 2021, the United States announced efforts to donate Coronavirus Disease 2019 (COVID-19) vaccines abroad. In many high-income countries, vaccines and other medical countermeasures are playing a critical role in controlling the spread of COVID-19. Vaccine distribution efforts in low- and middle-income countries (LMICs) have been comparatively slow for a variety of reasons, raising concerns about how inequities may hinder pandemic control. Some vaccine manufacturers and others willing to donate COVID-19 vaccines are concerned about legal exposure should there be adverse health events arising from COVID-19 vaccination outside of the United States.

For example, U.S. government vaccine donations to India reportedly remain in a Delhi warehouse because the Indian government has not agreed to indemnify vaccine manufacturers for vaccine-related injuries. Only a relatively small percentage of the Indian population is fully vaccinated against COVID-19; donated doses could potentially increase vaccination rates in the country. This chapter discusses potential liability issues that vaccine manufacturers and donors may face and options Congress might consider while deliberating vaccine distribution and liability issues.

Chapter 16 - More than 200 million Americans, and billions of people worldwide, have received one or more doses of a vaccine to protect against Coronavirus Disease 2019 (COVID-19). Most common side effects to COVID-19 vaccines are mild and generally resolve in a few days. However, in rare instances, COVID-19 vaccines can cause serious adverse events. For example, roughly one person out of every 200,000 who receives an mRNA-based COVID-19 vaccine experiences a severe allergic reaction. Other reported serious adverse events, such as myocarditis and Guillain- Barré Syndrome, are rare but may be associated with some COVID-19 vaccines.

Individuals who believe they are injured by COVID-19 vaccines may seek compensation for those injuries and other associated harms or costs. Absent an applicable federal law, individuals allegedly injured by a vaccine might seek redress by filing a state tort law claim against the vaccine manufacturer. However, federal law has two distinct compensation regimes that limit legal liability for vaccine manufacturers and provide potential compensation—without requiring a showing of fault—for individuals harmed by adverse reactions to vaccines. For injuries and deaths associated with most vaccines recommended by the Centers for Disease Control and Prevention (CDC) for routine administration in the United States (such as pediatric and seasonal influenza vaccines), the National Vaccine Injury Compensation Program (VICP) may provide compensation. During public health emergencies declared under the Public Readiness and Emergency Preparedness Act (PREP Act), the Countermeasures Injury Compensation Program (CICP) may provide compensation for injuries and deaths resulting from the administration of "covered countermeasures," which may include vaccines.

The VICP and CICP regimes are similar but distinct. Compensation through CICP is generally somewhat more limited than through VICP. CICP is a regulatory process administered by the Health Resources and Services Administration (HRSA), an agency within the U.S. Department of Health and Human Services (HHS). CICP compensation is available only for death or serious injuries resulting from a covered countermeasure that warrant hospitalization or lead to a significant loss of function or disability. A claimant must generally file a request form and associated documentation with HRSA within one year of the date that the covered countermeasure was administered. For injuries not listed by the Secretary of HHS on a Countermeasure Injury Table, the claimant must demonstrate that the injury was a direct result of the countermeasure's administration based on compelling medical and scientific evidence. Eligibility and compensation decisions are made by HRSA; judicial review is not available. CICP compensation is limited to reasonable medical expenses, loss of employment income, and a death benefit in cases where the claimant's death is a direct result of the administration or use of a covered countermeasure.

Under the Secretary of HHS's current PREP Act Declaration for COVID-19, FDA-authorized or -approved COVID-19 vaccines are covered countermeasures. While a PREP Act declaration is in effect, CICP is the sole remedy available for injuries related to covered countermeasures, including any covered vaccines. As a result, CICP—and not VICP—will apply to injuries resulting from COVID-19 vaccinations while the public health emergency persists and the Declaration remains in force. After the termination of the PREP Act public health emergency for COVID-19, COVID-19 vaccine injuries may be compensated through VICP, contingent on additional regulatory and statutory changes. In order for VICP to apply to a COVID-19 vaccine, (1) the vaccine must be recommended by the CDC for routine administration to children or pregnant women; (2) the vaccine must be made subject by act of Congress to the excise tax that funds VICP; and (3) the Secretary of HHS must add the vaccine to the Vaccine Injury Table, which lists injuries and conditions associated with covered vaccines.

Presuming all of those changes occur, VICP would apply to COVID-19 vaccine injuries. To receive compensation through VICP for a vaccine-related injury or death, the injured person must file a petition with the U.S. Court of Federal Claims, generally within three years of the first symptom or significant aggravation of the injury, or within two years of a death or four years of the first symptom resulting in death. To receive compensation, the injured party must show either that he or she experienced an injury listed for the vaccine in the Vaccine Injury Table within the time frame specified in the Table, or directly prove that the vaccine caused the injury. Eligibility and compensation determinations are made by a special master in a trial-like proceeding, which may be appealed to the U.S. Court of Federal Claims and the U.S. Court of Appeals for the Federal Circuit. Successful petitioners may receive medical expenses, lost income, a set death benefit, and reasonable attorneys' fees. Petitioners who are dissatisfied with the compensation they receive, or whose claims are delayed, may opt to pursue civil actions in court, subject to certain limitations on vaccine manufacturer liability.

Chapter 1

Vaccine Development: Capabilities and Challenges for Addressing Infectious Diseases*

United States Government Accountability Office

Why GAO Did This Study

The CARES Act included a provision for GAO to report on its ongoing monitoring and oversight efforts related to the COVID-19 pandemic. This chapter discusses technologies, approaches, and associated challenges for vaccine (1) research and development, (2) testing, and (3) manufacturing, as well as (4) the economic factors that affect vaccine investment.

GAO conducted literature searches including scholarly articles and government reports relevant to these four areas. GAO interviewed stakeholders and experts with a diverse set of perspectives on the science, administration, and economics of vaccine development. GAO also convened a 3-day meeting of 22 experts with expertise in at least one area related to our four objectives with assistance from the National Academies of Sciences, Engineering, and Medicine. GAO received technical comments on a draft of this chapter from 1 federal agency and 9 participants at its expert meeting, which it incorporated as appropriate.

GAO is identifying policy options in this chapter.

What GAO Found

Vaccines protect people from disease by preparing the body to respond to an infection. Vaccinations are a key part of individual and community health, but vaccine development remains complex and costly. Innovative technologies and approaches, such as those identified in this chapter, may enhance the nation's ability to respond to infectious diseases. For example, reverse vaccinology and next-generation platforms—combined with existing research—helped researchers develop some COVID-19 vaccines more quickly and effectively.

However, key challenges may hinder the adoption of these innovative technologies and approaches. Some promising technologies face issues and challenges such as inherent technical

* This is an edited, reformatted and augmented version of United States Government Accountability Office, Report to Congressional Committees, Technology Assessment, Publication No. GAO-22-104371, dated November 2021.

In: COVID-19 Vaccines
Editor: John Schroder
ISBN: 979-8-88697-150-7

limitations and high cost. For example, organ chips may facilitate testing, but they are not yet able to replicate many of the complex functions of the human immune system. Similarly, single-use systems may increase the flexibility of vaccine manufacturing facilities, but may require extensive testing to ensure that they do not negatively affect the resulting vaccine. Further, economic challenges may hinder vaccine development. Experts attribute underinvestment in vaccines to market failures (i.e., market interactions that fall short of what would have been socially beneficial). For example, vaccines benefit those who are vaccinated, and, to some degree, those who are not. This additional benefit is not captured in the price, which reduces return on vaccine investment.

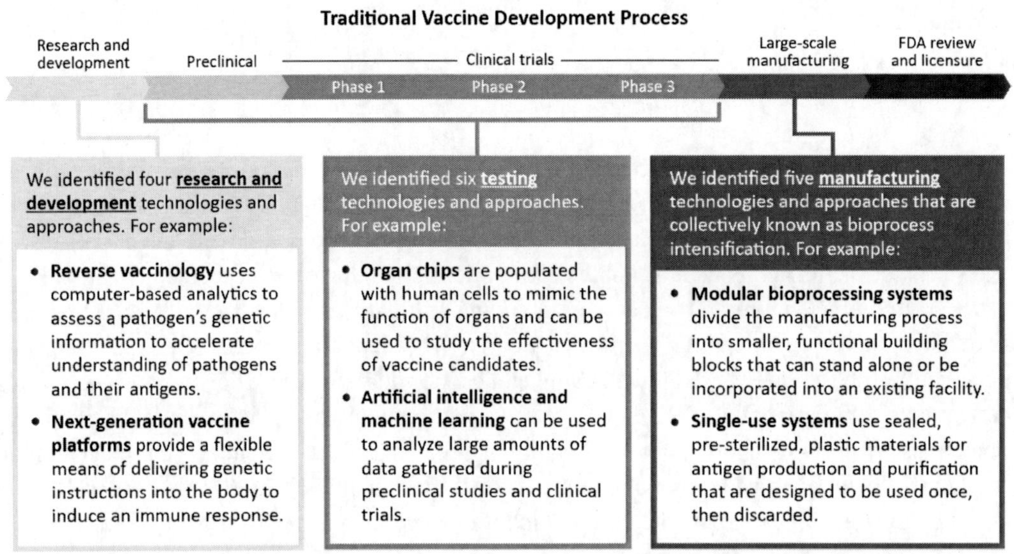

Source: GAO analysis. | GAO-22-104371.

GAO identified 9 policy options that may help address challenges hindering the adoption of vaccine development technologies and approaches or economic challenges. These policy options involve possible new actions by policymakers, who may include Congress, federal agencies, state and local governments, academic and research institutions, and industry. See below for details for some of the policy options and relevant opportunities and considerations.

Selected policy options to address challenges in vaccine development

	Opportunities	Considerations
Prioritize infectious disease pathogens (report page 21) Policymakers could collaborate across sectors (e.g., government, academia, researchers, industry, and nonprofit organizations) to prioritize infectious disease pathogens with pandemic potential for vaccine R&D.	• Prioritizing pathogens with pandemic potential could improve strategic vaccine R&D decision-making and help focus resources on developing and adopting key technologies and approaches that most effectively address those pathogens.	• As new threats are identified, priorities may change, which may cause uncertainty for vaccine developers. • Policymakers may have different priorities based on their respective missions.

	Opportunities	Considerations
For example, policymakers could develop a working group to prioritize pathogens with pandemic potential and work more closely with international organizations to prioritize vaccine development as well as develop monoclonal antibodies.	• With greater leadership and strategic partnerships, policymakers could more quickly address threats to the U.S. population. • Appropriately matching the technologies and approaches to the prioritized potential pandemic pathogens then leveraging technologies may help address certain technical limitations and cost.	There may be disagreements as to which key technologies should be prioritized and used, resulting in the need for policymakers to weigh the potential advantages and disadvantages associated with various options.
Improve preparedness (report page 21) Policymakers could provide support for public-private partnerships to strategically address potential pandemic pathogens identified as priorities. These partnerships could, for example, develop and test vaccine candidates that may provide protection from pathogens with pandemic potential.	• This early development could provide a coordinated foundation that can be mobilized in an emergency. Such an approach could speed vaccine development as well as potentially reduce risk for vaccine researchers and developers concerning questions of safety, efficacy, and manufacturability.	• The lack of certainty of the commercial market and government funding for vaccines against pathogens with pandemic potential may be too risky for the private sector to undertake.
Further support development of data standards (report page 32) Policymakers could further support coordinated efforts to obtain the views of all stakeholders and to develop standards for health data and their use in clinical trials.	• Integrating researchers' needs into the standards development process could better ensure the necessary data are available. • Access to high-quality data in a standardized format may allow streamlined patient recruitment for clinical trials.	• Expanding access to patient heath data requires attention to ensure privacy. • Developing and implementing standardized data formats and IT infrastructure is time-consuming and costly.
Improve preparedness (report page 41) Policymakers could provide support for public/private partnerships to strategically develop manufacturing capacity to respond to surge requirements. To maintain this capacity, partnerships could manufacture prototype vaccine candidates against high-priority pathogens.	• Manufacturing, testing, and stockpiling vaccines could be mobilized in an emergency and more rapidly mitigate future pandemics. • By leveraging strategic partnerships, policymakers could take steps to increase the availability of vaccines to more quickly address threats to the U.S. population.	• May require new resources or reallocation of resources from other efforts. • There may be a risk that the vaccines manufactured, tested, and stockpiled against prioritized pathogen classes miss certain pandemic pathogens. • The stockpiled vaccines would need to be regularly replenished prior to expiration.
Evaluate factors that inhibit vaccine investment and mechanisms to increase it (report page 54) Policymakers could collaborate across sectors, such as government, academia, and industry, to conduct a systematic evaluation of factors that inhibit developers from investing in new vaccines.	• A clear understanding of the range of factors discouraging vaccine investment would provide the basis for effectively addressing those factors.	• Collaboration between policymakers and other stakeholders to obtain all relevant viewpoints can be time-consuming and it may be hard to reach a consensus.

Source: GAO. \| GAO-22-104371.

Abbreviations

AI	artificial intelligence
BARDA	Biomedical Advanced Research and Development Authority
CDC	Centers for Disease Control and Prevention
COVID-19	Coronavirus Disease 2019
DOD	Department of Defense
EHR	electronic health record
EUA	emergency use authorization
FDA	Food and Drug Administration
HHS	Department of Health and Human Services
MERS	middle east respiratory syndrome
ML	machine learning
mRNA	messenger RNA
NIAID	National Institute of Allergy and Infectious Diseases
NIH	National Institutes of Health
R&D	research and development
SARS	severe acute respiratory syndrome
WHO	World Health Organization

Introduction

November 16, 2021
Congressional Committees

Vaccinations are an important tool for individual and public health, and have saved millions of lives. For example, between 1900 and 1980, smallpox killed approximately 300 million people and disfigured millions more. However, by 1980, a successful vaccination campaign eliminated smallpox worldwide. Similarly, in 1988, at the onset of a global campaign to end polio, there were 350,000 polio cases worldwide. According to the World Health Organization (WHO), the number of polio cases has since declined by over 99 percent worldwide.

Infectious diseases carry a high price tag for society. According to the World Bank, the economic losses from six major outbreaks of highly fatal infectious diseases that occurred between 1997 and 2009 amounted to at least $80 billion globally.[1] According to the National Foundation for Infectious Diseases, in the U.S., an average influenza illness can last up to 15 days, typically resulting in 5 or 6 missed work or school days. Adults who contract hepatitis A lose an average of one month of work. Further, when people are not vaccinated, they may be vulnerable to serious infections, such as human papillomavirus and hepatitis B (both can cause cancer), which have significant personal and economic burdens.

---

[1] The infectious diseases included in this study were Nipah Virus (Malaysia), West Nile Fever (U.S.), severe acute respiratory syndrome (Asia, Canada, other), highly pathogenic avian Influenza (Asia, Europe), bovine spongiform encephalopathy (U.S., U.K.), Rift Valley Fever (Tanzania, Kenya, Somalia). See World Bank People, Pathogens and our Planet: The Economics of One Health. 2012, Washington, DC. https://openknowledge.worldbank.org/handle/10986/11892.

Providing the public with safe and effective vaccines is also crucial to mitigating global pandemics. The Coronavirus Disease 2019 (COVID-19) pandemic has highlighted the devastating impact new infectious diseases can have. As of November 1, 2021, the Centers for Disease Control and Prevention (CDC) reported that over 745,000 people in the U.S. had died of COVID-19. An October 2020 study estimated the total economic cost of the at more than $16 trillion, or approximately 90 percent of the annual U.S. gross domestic product.[2] In December 2020, the U.S. took an important step to protect the public against COVID-19, as the first COVID-19 vaccines—developed in a shorter time than any previous vaccine—were authorized for emergency use and administered.[3] As of November 2021, three COVID-19 vaccines were available in the United States. One vaccine was licensed by the Food and Drug Administration (FDA) for individuals 16 and older, and was also available for individuals aged 5-15 years under an emergency use authorization (EUA).[4] Since implementation of the COVID-19 vaccine program in December of 2020, the number of new daily cases has declined.[5] For example, the number of COVID-19 cases in the U.S. reached a high of over 290,000 new daily cases on January 8, 2021, but declined to about 75,000 new daily cases as of November 2, 2021.[6]

While the National Institutes of Health (NIH) conducts and supports research that contributes to relevant technological advances, vaccine development overall continues to be a difficult, complex, and costly endeavor, and from an investment standpoint remains highly risky for those who pursue it. Economists we spoke to stated that the benefits that vaccines provide are not necessarily commensurate with the return on investment from developing or manufacturing them and vaccine development from discovery to licensure can cost billions of dollars and can take over 10 years to complete.[7] Vaccine developers face numerous technical challenges related to the biological complexity of some infectious diseases and the maturity of new vaccine technologies. Other challenges include long development time frames, high rates of clinical trial failure, and the lack of incentives to invest in vaccines.

---

[2] D.M. Cutler and L. Summers "The COVID-19 Pandemic and the $16 Trillion Virus," *Journal of the American Medical Association*, Oct. 20, 2020.

[3] The Secretary of Health and Human Services (HHS) may declare that circumstances, prescribed by statute, justify the emergency use of certain medical products, such as vaccines. Once a declaration of an emergency has been made, the Food and Drug Administration (FDA) may temporarily allow use of unlicensed vaccines through an emergency use authorization (EUA). For FDA to issue an EUA for a vaccine, it must be reasonable to believe that the vaccine may be effective and that the known and potential benefits of the vaccine outweigh the known and potential risks, among other statutory criteria. See 21 U.S.C. § 360bbb-3. See also HHS, FDA, Center for Biologics Evaluation and Research, Emergency Use Authorization for Vaccines to Prevent COVID-19, Guidance for Industry, (Washington, D.C.: May 2021).

[4] FDA licenses biological products, such as vaccines, through review and approval of a biologics license application. See 42 U.S.C. § 262. FDA guidance indicates that licensure is the goal for COVID-19 vaccines, including those that first receive an EUA.

[5] COVID-19 vaccine implementation involves the prioritization, allocation, distribution, and administration of vaccine doses.

[6] For more information on the accelerated COVID-19 vaccine development process, see GAO, *COVID-19: Efforts to Increase Vaccine Availability and Perspectives on Initial Implementation*, GAO-21-443, (Washington, D.C.: April 14, 2021), GAO, *Operation Warp Speed: Accelerated COVID-19 Vaccine Development Status and Efforts to Address Manufacturing Challenges*, GAO-21-319, (Washington, D.C.: Feb. 11, 2021), and GAO, *COVID-19: Federal Efforts Accelerate Vaccine and Therapeutic Development, but More Transparency Needed on Emergency Use Authorizations*, GAO-21-207 (Washington, D.C.: Nov. 17, 2020). GAO has also produced an interactive dashboard that integrates multiple data sources to visualize the status of vaccine development, which may be found at https://ows.gaoinnovations.gov/.

[7] D. Gouglas et al., "Estimating the Cost of Vaccine Development against Epidemic Infectious Diseases: a Cost Minimisation Study." *The Lancet Global Health*, vol. 6, no. 12 (2018): pp. e1386-e1396.

Given the public health consequences of infectious disease, policymakers have a vital interest in developing and maintaining modern, flexible, rapid, and robust vaccine development and manufacturing capabilities.[8] These capabilities will allow for better response to endemic levels of infectious disease, as well as better preparation for potential future epidemics and pandemics.[9] This urgent need comes at a time marked by rapid growth in basic scientific understanding—in areas such as genomics and structural biology that are supporting a new era in vaccine development—as well as ongoing challenges.

The CARES Act includes a provision for GAO to report on its ongoing monitoring and oversight efforts related to the COVID-19 pandemic.[10] This technology assessment is part of our body of work in response to the CARES Act and describes various technologies and approaches applicable to developing vaccines for infectious diseases. Specifically, in this technology assessment, we describe

- technologies and approaches for vaccine research and development (R&D) and challenges that affect their use,
- technologies and approaches for vaccine testing and challenges that affect their use,
- technologies and approaches for vaccine manufacturing and challenges that affect their use, and
- economic factors that affect vaccine investment and preparedness for future pandemics.

To address our all of our objectives, we conducted literature searches including scholarly articles and government reports describing current and emerging technologies and approaches for vaccine R&D, testing, and manufacturing.[11] We used the results of our literature review to address our objectives as well as identify experts to interview and invite to participate in our expert meeting. Additionally, we interviewed stakeholders and experts with a diverse set of perspectives on the science, administration, and economics of vaccine development. To address all of our objectives, we held an expert meeting from January 25-28, 2021. This meeting was held in collaboration with the National Academies of Sciences, Engineering, and Medicine, and was divided into six sessions on technologies and approaches for vaccine: (1) research and development; (2) manufacturing, (3) preclinical and clinical trials, (4) pathogen scenarios, (5) economics factors, and (6) lessons learned.

Based on the information we obtained, we developed a series of policy options intended to represent possible options that policymakers can take to address a policy objective. Consistent with our quality assurance framework, we provided the relevant agencies and experts with a

---

[8] Policymakers is a broad term including, for example, Congress, federal agencies, state and local governments, academic and research institutions, and industry.

[9] Endemic refers to the constant presence or usual prevalence of disease in a population within a geographic area. An epidemic refers to an increase, often sudden, in the number of cases of a disease above what is normally expected in a population and area. A pandemic refers to an epidemic that has spread over several countries or continents, usually affecting a large number of people.

[10] Pub. L. No. 116-136, § 19010, 134 Stat. 281, 579-81 (2020). We regularly issue government-wide reports on the federal response to the COVID-19 pandemic. For our 8th comprehensive report on the ongoing federal pandemic response, see GAO, *COVID-19: Additional Actions Needed to Improve Accountability and Program Effectiveness of Federal Response*, GAO-22-105051, (Washington, D.C.: Oct. 27, 2021). Our next government-wide report will be issued in January 2022 and can be found on GAO's website at https://www.gao.gov/coronavirus.

[11] For purposes of this report, vaccine testing refers to preclinical studies, clinical trials, and post-marketing surveillance studies.

draft of our report and solicited their feedback, which we incorporated as appropriate. See appendix I for additional information on our scope and methodology.

We conducted our work from June 2020 through November 2021 in accordance with all sections of GAO's Quality Assurance Framework that are relevant to technology assessments. The framework requires that we plan and perform the engagement to obtain sufficient and appropriate evidence to meet our stated objectives and to discuss any limitations to our work.

We believe the information and data obtained, and the analysis conducted, provide a reasonable basis for any findings and conclusions in this chapter.

1. Background

1.1. How Vaccines Work

Vaccines protect people from disease by triggering the immune system to produce antibodies that will fight a pathogen attacking the body. A pathogen is a bacterium, virus, or other microorganism that can cause disease. Preparing the immune system through vaccination allows the body to respond more quickly if that pathogen infects the individual in the future.

During an infection, the immune system responds to specific parts of a pathogen called antigens by producing antibodies—proteins that help bind to and neutralize specific pathogens—to fight the pathogen and in some cases prevent future infections (see Figure 1). The immune system also produces specific cells—such as T-lymphocytes—that assist in neutralizing pathogens in a process known as cell-mediated immunity. When the human body is exposed to an antigen for the first time, it takes time for the immune system to respond and produce antibodies specific to that antigen. During that period of time, the individual is susceptible to becoming ill from the disease caused by the pathogen. Once antigen-specific antibodies are produced, they work with the rest of the immune system to destroy the pathogen.

Vaccines mimic this natural process by introducing antigens without necessarily introducing the disease-causing pathogen itself; for example, vaccines can use a weakened or inactive pathogen, a microorganism that is closely related to the pathogen but does not cause disease in humans, or a molecule derived from the pathogen.[12] Vaccines may include a variety of ingredients such as stabilizers, adjuvants, and preservatives to enhance the effectiveness of the vaccine or offer other benefits.[13]

Once an immune response has been generated, if the person is exposed later to the pathogen, their immune system will 'remember' seeing that pathogen and respond more quickly, increasing their chances of fighting off the infection. Additionally, vaccines that protect against one pathogen may also protect against similar pathogens. Vaccines may also reduce the spread of infectious disease, which can convey some level of protection to those who are not vaccinated. For example, the bacille Calmette–Guérin vaccine, which contains

---

[12] For example, the smallpox vaccine uses a related poxvirus, the vaccinia virus, which is unlikely to cause significant disease in healthy human recipients, but elicits an immune response that is protective for smallpox.

[13] Stabilizers are substances such as amino acids and other substances that help the antigen maintain its effectiveness during storage. Adjuvants are compounds such as aluminum salts that help to enhance the immune response. Preservatives are chemical substances that help to protect against bacterial and fungal growth during storage. (https://www.fda.gov/vaccines-blood-biologics/safety-availability-biologics/common-ingredients-us-licensed-vaccines).

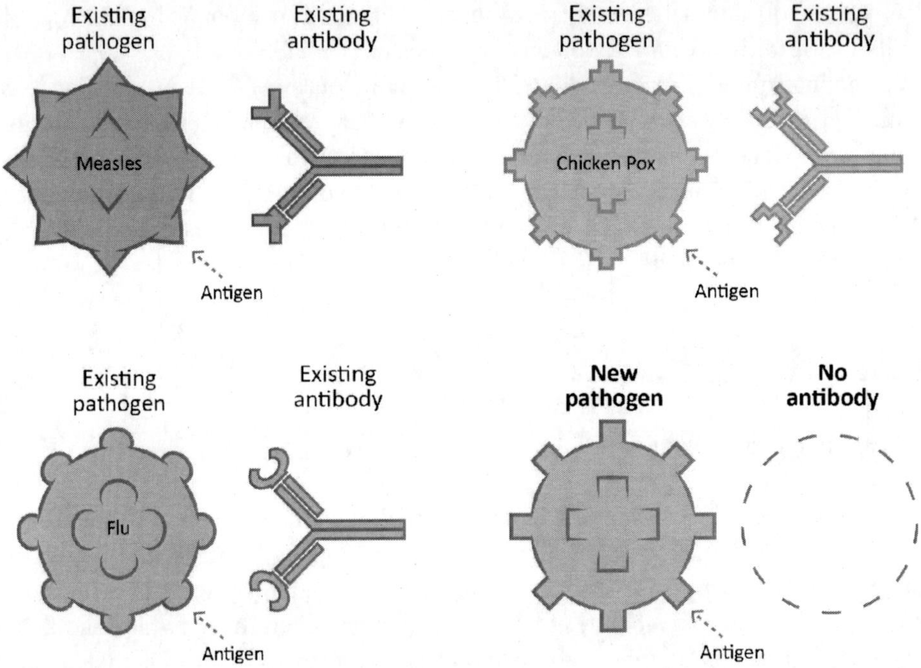

Source: World Health Organization (WHO), https://www.who.int/news-room/feature-stories/detail/how-do-vaccines-work (accessed June 30, 2021). | GAO-22-104371.

Figure 1. How antibodies fight invading pathogens.

weakened *Mycobacterium bovis*—a bacterium that causes tuberculosis in cattle—is used to protect humans from *Mycobacterium tuberculosis*—a bacterium that causes tuberculosis in humans. Further, this vaccine may also provide some protection against *Mycobacterium leprae*—a bacterium that causes leprosy in humans.

1.2. Vaccine Development

The traditional process for developing a new vaccine is well established and tends to be sequential (see Figure 2), although stages sometimes overlap.[14] The purpose of this sequential approach is, in part, to reduce financial risk because each stage is costly— with later stages being especially costly— and each stage improves the understanding of whether the next stage might be successful. However, one expert told us that this is not guaranteed. At any stage, the process can be terminated for a variety of reasons, including detection of adverse events, such as serious side effects or if the evidence suggests that the vaccine is unlikely to be protective.

Sections 2 through 4 of this chapter discuss technologies and approaches to enhance overall response to endemic infectious diseases, as well as improve capabilities to respond to potential future epidemics or pandemics. Specifically, section 2 discusses the vaccine R&D stage; section 3 focuses on vaccine testing, including preclinical testing, clinical trials, and post-marketing surveillance; and section 4 discusses vaccine manufacturing. Section 5 of this

[14] We have previously reported on the traditional vaccine development timeline compared to a potential timeline for COVID-19 vaccine development. See GAO-21-319.

chapter discusses economic challenges that may result in fewer vaccines being developed and tools to incentivize additional vaccine investment to enhance overall response to endemic infectious disease, as well as improve capabilities to respond to potential future epidemics and pandemics.

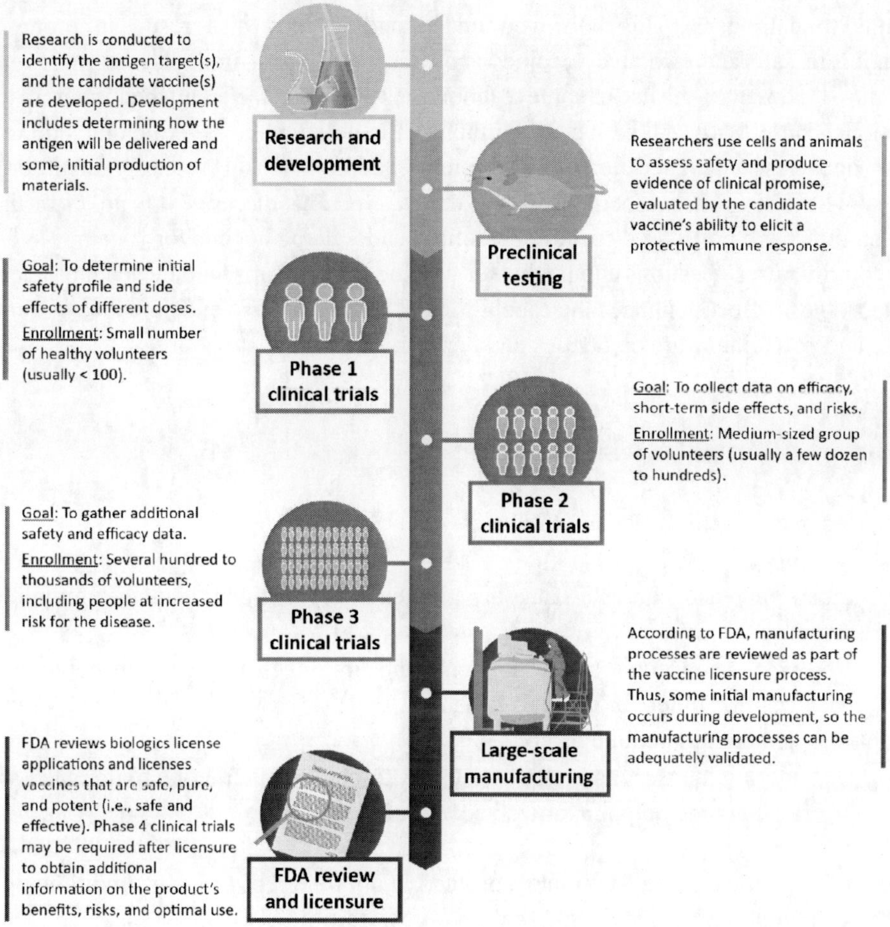

Source: GAO analysis of information from the Food and Drug Administration (FDA) and literature. | GAO-22-104371.

Note: The steps shown in the timeline are not drawn to scale, and the specific development steps for a given vaccine may vary. For example, the federal government accelerated this process for the development of a COVID-19 vaccine under the HHS-DOD COVID-19 Countermeasures Acceleration Group (formerly known as Operation Warp Speed) by overlapping certain phases to speed up the process so the vaccines could be used as quickly as possible to control the pandemic. No trial phases were skipped.

In this chapter, we use the term "efficacy" to refer to the results of adequate and controlled clinical trial studies that evaluate clinical disease endpoints, and "effectiveness" to refer to the results of studies carried out under field conditions. For regulatory purposes, FDA determines whether a vaccine is safe and effective, and effectiveness is generally based on the results of adequate and well controlled studies evaluating a clinical disease endpoint (efficacy studies) or a well-accepted immune endpoint (effectiveness studies).

Figure 2. Traditional vaccine development process.

2. Technologies and Approaches for Vaccine R&D

Technologies and approaches for vaccine R&D may help researchers, developers, or other scientists better identify and characterize pathogens and their antigens—the components of the pathogen that stimulate an immune response—and determine how the human immune system responds to pathogens. This improved understanding may also result in more efficient generation of safe and effective vaccines and other biological products, such as monoclonal antibodies.[15] However, the use of some technologies may be affected by their inherent technical limitations, complexity, and high cost. Further, while policymakers—which include Congress, federal agencies, state and local governments, academic and research institutions, and industry—have supported vaccine R&D for many infectious diseases, it is not clear the extent to which they have prioritized specific potential pandemic pathogens for vaccine R&D.[16] This lack of clarity raises questions about whether vaccine R&D efforts, and the technologies needed to support those efforts, enhance the capabilities to best respond to endemic levels of infectious disease and potential future epidemics and pandemics.

2.1. Factors Affecting Vaccine R&D

Key factors in conducting vaccine R&D are:

- Identifying and characterizing a pathogen's key antigens and the immune system response
- Applying knowledge about antigens and immune responses to rapidly develop vaccines or other biological products that safely and effectively stimulate or complement an immune response
- Considering the various routes of delivery, including alternative routes such as dermal or oral, that may help maximize vaccination rates

Identifying antigens that stimulate a protective immune response has, traditionally, been a slow process done largely through trial-and-error testing. Any given pathogen may have thousands of potential antigens, and the human immune system includes many different types of cells with different functions, not all of which are fully understood. To identify the antigens that most effectively stimulate a protective response in the human immune system, researchers typically select and test potential antigens one or a few at a time. Researchers then run

---

[15] Biological products, which include a wide range of products—including vaccines, blood and blood components, allergenics, somatic cells, gene therapy, and tissues, among other things—are derived from living sources such as humans, animals, and microorganisms. See 42 U.S.C. § 262(i)(1) and 21 C.F.R. § 600.3(h) (2020).

[16] NIH conducts and supports basic, translational, and applied clinical research that contributes to technological advances relevant for vaccine development. For example, NIH officials noted the National Institute of Allergy and Infectious Diseases' (NIAID) role in funding research on SARS and Middle East Respiratory Syndrome (MERS) contributed to the successful development of vaccines for COVID-19. However, we note that no commercial vaccines for SARS or MERS exist. This was partly attributed to lack of continued investments in a vaccine for SARS, for which cases ceased to be reported, and for MERS, which resulted in relatively few and geographically isolated cases. One expert who had developed a SARS vaccine candidate stated that had that vaccine been able to proceed through phase 1 clinical trials and stockpiled, it could have been beneficial for COVID-19 and accelerated vaccine development.

laboratory tests or conduct animal studies to see if any of the antigens they selected produces a protective immune response. (See text box for one example of how antigens were identified).

It is also difficult to quickly develop vaccines that safely and effectively stimulate an immune response. There are many reasons for this, but two key factors are the time needed to produce antigens and a lack of adaptability. First, traditional vaccine development often requires the growth of pathogens or the use of other cells, such as bacteria, yeast, or insect cells, containing the antigen(s) of interest from the pathogen. Viral pathogens can be grown in eggs or other cells—known as cell cultures. These methods can take months to years to develop. Second, traditional methods of vaccine development may be not highly adaptable for multiple pathogens or diverse antigens. This may limit the ability to quickly develop vaccines when new pathogens emerge or change a vaccine when variants arise.[17]

Finally, administering vaccines by injection using a needle and syringe—the traditional method of delivering vaccines—may affect, for example, some individuals' willingness to get a vaccination due to a fear of needles. Additionally, the need for trained personnel and the costs and potential scarcity of vaccination supplies (e.g., vials, syringes, and needles), particularly during pandemics, can make administration of vaccines using traditional injections difficult.

Coronavirus research

In the case of COVID-19, identifying and characterizing the spike protein antigen was the result of decades of previous research dating back to human coronavirus research begun in the 1960s, the Severe Acute Respiratory Syndrome (SARS) epidemic in 2003-2005, and the Middle Eastern Respiratory Syndrome (MERS) outbreak of 2012. If earlier research on SARS and MERS had not been funded, development of a COVID-19 vaccine may have taken significantly longer.

Source: GAO analysis of information from literature and an expert meeting. | GAO-22-104371.

2.2. Technologies and Approaches for Vaccine R&D

Drawing on information from experts, stakeholders, and related literature, we identified four technologies and approaches that may improve vaccine R&D (see Table 1). Appendix II provides additional information on these technologies and approaches.

The technologies and approaches we identified can be applied at different stages of vaccine R&D. For example, in early exploration and research, omics and reverse vaccinology can help researchers to more rapidly identify antigens and how they stimulate an immune response. For later stages of vaccine R&D, genetic code for the identified antigens can be quickly incorporated into delivery vehicles, such as lipid nanoparticles or viral vectors, accelerating vaccine testing (see Figure 3).

---

[17] A variant is a new form of the same pathogen that arises from distinct changes—also known as mutations—in the genetic sequence of the pathogen.

Table 1. Selected technologies and approaches for vaccine research and development (R&D)

Name	Description
Omics	Omics refers to the combined analyses of DNA (genomics and epigenomics), RNA (transcriptomics), proteins (proteomics), other small molecules (metabolomics), and other biological components. In vaccine R&D, omics is meant to improve the understanding of pathogens and host immune responses.
Reverse vaccinology	Reverse vaccinology uses computer-based analytics to assess a pathogen's genetic code and identify potential antigens. Reverse vaccinology allows researchers to identify potential vaccine antigen candidates without the need to grow the pathogens and develop vaccines that were previously difficult or impossible to make.
Next-generation vaccine platforms	Next-generation vaccine platforms incorporate the genetic information that codes for a pathogen's antigen into a delivery vehicle. A delivery vehicle can be another virus (viral vector), a microparticle, or a lipid nanoparticle. The delivery vehicle protects the genetic information until it is administered into an individual, where the immune response is triggered. The platform may also be able to be used in a plug-and-play fashion to pair a delivery vehicle with different genetic sequences to create new or updated vaccines. Vaccine platforms may have uniform, predictable characteristics, such as safety effects; however, each antigen in a specific platform will have different immune response characteristics.[a]
Routes of vaccination	Traditional vaccinations are delivered by injection either under the skin (subcutaneous) or into muscle (intramuscular). The identification and use of nontraditional vaccine delivery routes, such as dermal (skin) and mucosal (oral, nasal) may offer the potential for better immune responses, increased public acceptance, and lower dosages.

Source: GAO. | GAO-22-104371.

[a]According to National Institutes of Health (NIH), vaccine platform technologies are approaches, delivery systems, and other tools that serve as the basis for delivering those vaccine antigen designs and for the development of candidate vaccines. Vaccine prototype design is the research and development that results in a candidate antigen design as the basis of a vaccine.

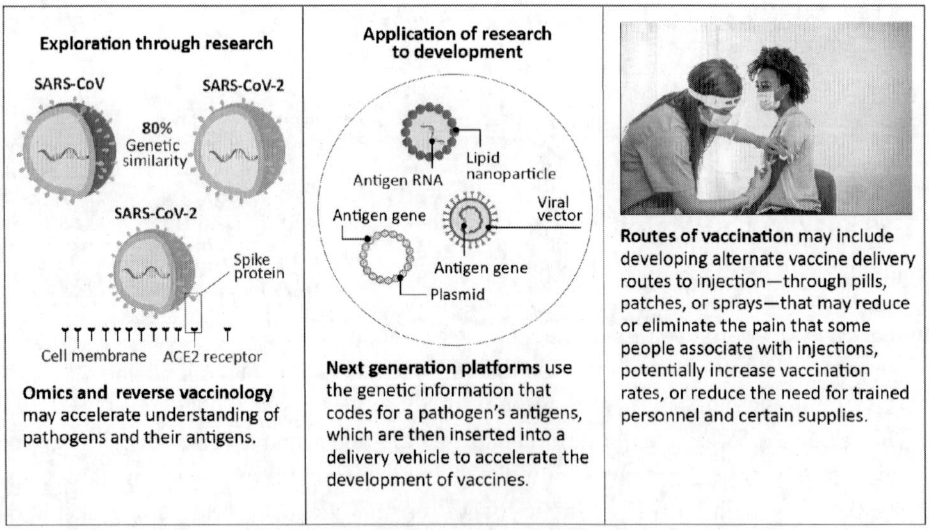

Source: GAO analysis of scientific literature and narstudio/Dragana Gordic/stock.adobe.com. | GAO-22-104371.

Figure 3. Selected application of technologies and approaches used during vaccine research and development.

Omics and reverse vaccinology aid in the early exploration process by helping researchers to more quickly identify antigens that stimulate a protective immune response by analyzing the pathogen's DNA, RNA, proteins, or other biological molecules. Then, researchers can apply computer simulations to predict more quickly which of the potential antigens may stimulate an immune response and which modifications to the antigens may enhance the immune response. As a result, researchers can more quickly begin testing those antigens that are most likely to work. (See text box for an example of how reverse vaccinology has been used).

Reverse vaccinology and the COVID-19 vaccine

Researchers used reverse vaccinology to accelerate development of some COVID-19 vaccines. When the genetic code of SARS-CoV-2—the virus that causes COVID-19— became available, researchers quickly identified it as a coronavirus similar to the Severe Acute Respiratory Syndrome (SARS) coronavirus. According to the National Institutes of Health (NIH), this enabled researchers to use information gained from prior National Institute of Allergy and Infectious Diseases (NIAID)-funded studies, among others, that used reverse vaccinology and protein structure analysis to characterize the SARS and Middle East Respiratory Syndrome (MERS) spike protein antigens and their human cell receptors. This then helped researchers more quickly identify, assess, and stabilize the spike protein from SARS-CoV-2, which, in turn, allowed for the quick development of potential COVID-19 messenger RNA (mRNA) vaccine candidates, according to NIH. Researchers were able to test mRNA vaccines in a phase 1 clinical trial within 90 days of the SARS-CoV-2 genetic code release. In comparison, the vaccine candidates for MERS and SARS reached clinical trials within about 22 months and 25 months, respectively, after their outbreaks. Dengue, Chikungunya, and Zika vaccine candidates took even longer to reach clinical trials: approximately 52 years, 19 years, and 9 years, respectively, after declaration of major outbreaks. According to Food and Drug Administration (FDA) officials, other differences, including the nature of the pathogens and funding levels, also contributed to the extended development timeframes.

Source: GAO analysis of literature. | GAO-22-104371.

Omics can also help researchers characterize the human immune system by allowing researchers to understand which cells provide protection. Omics analysis of the immune system may also enable researchers to predict how individuals may react to vaccines and could allow for tailored vaccines for certain populations.[18]

Next-generation vaccine platforms, such as nucleic acid (e.g., mRNA and DNA) and viral vector platforms, also aid in the development of a vaccine. Specifically, next-generation platforms can help speed development, particularly when new pathogens emerge, because they rely on the pathogen's genetic information that codes for antigens. This eliminates the need to grow the pathogen or purify antigens. These platforms are also highly adaptable to multiple pathogens, allowing the development of many different vaccines to address a diverse range of pathogens on a single platform. They also have the potential to be used to develop universal vaccines which protect against multiple pathogens from the same or closely related families. However, next-generation platforms may not be practical for certain pathogens or developing countries, according to one expert we spoke to.

[18] For example, researchers used omics analysis to characterize the differences in the immune system to the hepatitis B vaccine in two groups of older adults, one that quickly produces high levels of antibodies and another that does not produce any response. The results of these studies may enable researchers to better predict vaccination outcomes—whether a strong, weak, or no immune response occurs—in individuals and help researchers increase vaccine effectiveness.

Three nontraditional routes of vaccination— dermal, nasal, and oral—are an important consideration in vaccine development. Using nontraditional routes of vaccination can reduce or eliminate the pain that some people associate with injections, potentially increasing vaccination rates or reducing the need for trained personnel and certain supplies.

- *Dermal delivery.* Delivering vaccines through the skin can produce strong immune responses at much lower doses than intramuscular and subcutaneous vaccines, making it a good route for vaccination. Microneedles, which can be nearly pain-free, are small structures designed to pierce the skin and deliver vaccines in the epidermis or dermis layers.[19] FDA has licensed one influenza vaccine that uses dermal delivery.
- *Nasal delivery.* Nasal vaccines can induce immunity even at distant sites of the body. The antigens are taken up by cells in the nasal cavity, stimulating a potent antibody in the respiratory tract that prevents the pathogen from entering the body. The antigens also stimulate the body's overall immune response, which may increase the general effectiveness of the vaccine. There are FDA-licensed nasal vaccines for seasonal influenza; however, in the past, one was less effective than an injected vaccine.[20]
- *Oral delivery.* The intestine contains 70 to 80 percent of all antibody-producing cells in the body. Oral vaccination—delivered in a pill or liquid form—can induce a broad protective immune response in the body (including the intestine), which can be difficult to achieve using injections with needles and syringes. However, oral vaccines must be formulated to protect against degradation in the gastrointestinal tract, while still stimulating an effective immune response. Examples of oral vaccines in use today include those for polio, rotavirus, and cholera.[21]

Additionally, experts we spoke with emphasized that monoclonal antibodies are emerging as a potential approach to preventing infections. Monoclonal antibodies are laboratory-produced antibodies that act to mimic the immune system's ability to fight off pathogens. They are not vaccines and have traditionally been used as treatments for individuals that are already infected. However, many of the same types of technologies—for example, omics and delivery platforms—used for vaccine development could also be used for monoclonal antibodies. Unlike vaccines, which can stimulate an individual's immune system to produce protective antibodies for years, monoclonal antibodies may provide shorter protection against infectious diseases, usually for weeks to months. If able to be developed and used early in a pandemic, monoclonal antibodies may potentially provide some initial benefit. It is for this reason that we include monoclonal antibodies as an approach that could be considered alongside traditional vaccine

---

[19] The epidermis is the outermost layer of skin, which provides a waterproof barrier and contributes to skin tone. The dermis lies just beneath the epidermis and contains tough connective tissue, hair follicles, and sweat glands.

[20] After the 2009 H1N1 influenza pandemic, several U.S. studies among 2 through 17-year-olds found that the live attenuated influenza vaccine administered intranasally was as effective against influenza B viruses and influenza A (H3N2) viruses as the traditional injectable vaccine, but it was less effective than the injectable vaccines against the 2009 pandemic H1N1 viruses. These data led CDC to recommend against use of this specific vaccine for the 2016-2017 and 2017-2018 influenza seasons. For more information on the flu mist nasal vaccine, see https://www.fda.gov/vaccines-blood-biologics/vaccines/fda-information-regarding-flumist-quadrivalent-vaccine.

[21] Oral poliovirus vaccine is no longer used in the U.S., but it is used in other countries. The U.S. no longer uses the oral poliovirus vaccine due to the risk of vaccine-derived poliovirus disease in certain individuals. However, other oral vaccines have been shown to be safe when not contraindicated.

R&D. Appendix II provides additional information on monoclonal antibodies. (See text box for examples of COVID-19 monoclonal antibodies).

COVID-19 monoclonal antibodies

During the COVID-19 pandemic, the Food and Drug Administration (FDA) issued four emergency use authorizations (EUA) for monoclonal antibodies to treat COVID-19. Two of these four treatments consist of a mixture of two monoclonal antibodies, while the remaining two treatments each consist of a single monoclonal antibody. Additionally, researchers are investigating using monoclonal antibodies to protect against COVID-19 before someone is infected or for individuals with compromised immune systems. For example, one developer recently published clinical trial data showing that a mixture of two monoclonal antibodies reduced the risk of people developing any COVID-19 symptoms by 77 percent.

Source: GAO analysis of literature. | GAO-22-104371.

2.3. Challenges Affecting the Adoption of R&D Technologies and Approaches

Drawing on information from experts, stakeholders, and related literature, we identified three key challenges affecting the adoption of technologies and approaches for vaccine R&D:

- Inherent technological limitations
- Complex, costly instruments
- The need for highly trained personnel

2.3.1. Inherent Technological Limitations

The extent to which the following technologies and approaches are adopted may depend on their technological limits.

- *Omics and reverse vaccinology.* Reverse vaccinology cannot predict some antigens—such as sugar-based (polysaccharides) or fat-based (lipids and glycolipids) antigens found in bacteria and parasites—so more traditional approaches are used. Also, individual immune system responses among people vary widely, which may limit the ability to identify common immune responses to antigens even with the use of omics.
- *Next-generation vaccine platforms.* To ensure the effectiveness of next-generation vaccine platforms, vaccine researchers need to carefully consider the selected genetic sequences from pathogens that code for antigens. If they do not, the result can be ineffective vaccine candidates. For example, while the first two mRNA COVID-19 vaccines authorized for emergency use were highly effective at preventing disease, a different mRNA vaccine candidate was not as efficacious in clinical trials.[22] Vaccine

[22] In this report, we use the term efficacy to refer to the results of adequate and controlled clinical trial studies that evaluate clinical disease endpoints, and effectiveness to refer to the results of studies carried out under field conditions. For regulatory purposes, FDA determines whether a vaccine is safe and effective, and effectiveness is generally based on the results of adequate and well controlled studies evaluating a clinical disease endpoint (efficacy studies) or a well-accepted immune endpoint (effectiveness studies). For more information on the mRNA

researchers stated that this was partly due to the fact that this vaccine candidate lacked key structural modifications to the mRNA that were made in the first two mRNA vaccines.

The cold storage requirements for some vaccines being developed using next-generation vaccine platforms are also a challenge because they require specialized shipping containers and laboratory refrigerators and freezers not readily available at all health care facilities. Vaccines become less effective or completely ineffective if stored at the incorrect temperature. While most vaccines require refrigerated storage at between 2 and 8°C, some mRNA vaccines require storage in freezers at ultra-low temperatures as cold as -80°C.[23] Challenges associated with cold storage requirements and scaling up the production of vaccines developed using next-generation platforms may affect the ability to use vaccines worldwide. One expert we spoke with noted that these challenges largely impact low and middle income countries.

- *Routes of vaccination.* Nontraditional routes of vaccination require researchers to ensure that the antigen remains capable of producing the required immune response. Some antigens may not be amenable to administration by nontraditional routes. For example, oral vaccines must be developed in such a way that the formulation can survive the harsh gastrointestinal environment. Vaccines that are administered via nontraditional routes may also require investment in manufacturing capability to accommodate new delivery mechanisms. For example, while various vaccines may be able to be delivered via dermal patches, concerns about costs and mass production have been raised.
- *Monoclonal antibodies.* Monoclonal antibodies differ from vaccines in several ways. For example, they are made of proteins that can degrade over time, do not stimulate the human immune system the same way that vaccines do, and do not provide the long-term protection that vaccines may provide. Also, monoclonal antibodies have traditionally been administered intravenously at a medical facility. However, modifications to specific parts of these proteins can extend the period of protection and may allow for delivery by intramuscular or subcutaneous injection rather than intravenously. Monoclonal antibodies have traditionally been developed for use as therapeutics against non-infectious diseases such as various cancers and autoimmune diseases. Careful assessment, development, and evaluation of safety and effectiveness are important for monoclonal antibodies as for vaccines. More than 100 monoclonal antibodies have been licensed for use by FDA, but only seven are indicated to treat or prevent infectious diseases.[24]

---

vaccine candidate that was not as efficacious in clinical trials, see CureVac, *CureVac Provides Update on Phase 2b/3 Trial of First-Generation COVID-19 Vaccine Candidate, CVnCoV* (Tübingen, Germany / Boston, USA, June 16, 2021).

[23] Some vaccines that require freezer storage, such as the two COVID-19 mRNA vaccines authorized for emergency use in the U.S., can be safely stored for a limited time between 2°C and 8°C. See https://www.fda.gov/news-events/press-announcements/fda-brief-fda-authorizes-longer-time-refrigerator-storage-thawed-pfizer-biontech-covid-19-vaccine.

[24] The seven licensed monoclonal antibodies indicated to treat or prevent infectious disease include those for Ebola virus, HIV, *Clostridium difficile, Bacillus anthracis* (the organism that causes anthrax), and respiratory syncytial virus. FDA has also issued four EUAs for monoclonal antibodies to treat COVID-19. Two of these four treatments consist of a mixture of two monoclonal antibodies, while the remaining two treatments each consist of a single monoclonal antibody. Most licensed monoclonal antibodies are used as therapeutics for cancer and other non-infectious diseases, such as rheumatoid arthritis.

2.3.2. Complex, Costly Instruments

The extent to which the following technologies and approaches are adopted may also depend on their complexity and cost.

- *Omics and reverse vaccinology.* The high cost of omics-based instruments, such as massively parallel sequencing instruments and their reagents, and the complexity of the resulting data may prevent use by some researchers.
- *Routes of vaccination.* Developing vaccines for different routes of vaccination may be expensive due to complex technologies used in formulation development, according to one expert we spoke to.
- *Monoclonal antibodies.* Traditionally, development and manufacturing of monoclonal antibodies has been complex, expensive, and time consuming. However, new techniques for easier identification, selection, and optimization of monoclonal antibodies have reduced the complexity and time for development from years to weeks. Further, improvements in manufacturing may decrease production costs.

These potentially high costs and complexity may be exacerbated by the lack of defined or profitable markets, such as vaccines for pathogens with pandemic potential or that primarily affect developing countries. These economic challenges may inhibit new vaccine development.[25]

2.3.3. The Need for Highly Trained Personnel

The extent to which the following technologies and approaches are adopted may also depend on a highly-trained workforce to operate the complex instruments and processes.

- *Omics and reverse vaccinology.* Because the instruments and techniques, such as massively parallel sequencing instruments and bioinformatics tools, needed for omics analyses are complex, highly-trained personnel may also be needed.
- *Monoclonal antibodies.* The complexity of the technology and approaches for monoclonal antibody development and manufacturing require a specialized workforce. For example, a manufacturing run may require up to two weeks with as many as 10 distinct steps.
- *Next-Generation Vaccine Platforms.* The complexity of platform technologies requires a highly skilled workforce, according to an expert we spoke to. For example, for platform technologies, execution of the biological processes is important for consistency of manufactured doses.

2.4. Infectious Disease Prioritization

The federal government supports R&D for infectious disease vaccine development, which is guided, in part, by the Department of Health and Human Services' *Vaccines National Strategic*

---

[25] For additional discussion of economics issues that inhibit vaccine development see Chapter 5.

Plan 2021–2025, among other strategies.[26] This plan provides a strategy to promote vaccine R&D and other areas for the U.S. vaccine and immunization enterprise. Further, the Public Health Emergency Medical Countermeasures Enterprise, which makes recommendations to the Secretary of Health and Human Services, has a list of high-priority biological threats.[27] While this list includes emerging infectious diseases, it does not identify which diseases or disease families have pandemic potential— with the exception of pandemic influenza— for researchers to target development of vaccines against.[28] The Department of Health and Human Services (HHS) also noted that NIAID publishes a list of priority pathogens.[29] However, this list also does not explicitly prioritize specific potential pandemic pathogens that researchers should consider developing vaccines against, and—as noted on the website—it appears the content has not been reviewed since July 2018. As a result, we have not found evidence that a list which prioritizes specific potential pandemic pathogens for vaccine development exists.

While infectious disease prioritization cannot address potential pandemic pathogens yet to be identified, a strategy for vaccine development against families of known pathogens with pandemic potential could help with preparedness.[30] As discussed earlier, the speed of COVID-19 vaccine development was unprecedented. Had it not been for two previous coronavirus outbreaks— Severe Acute Respiratory Syndrome (SARS) and Middle East Respiratory Syndrome (MERS)—and NIH investments in coronavirus research, along with investments in new vaccine platform technologies, the development of a COVID-19 vaccine would have taken significantly longer.

Other countries and international entities, such as the United Kingdom, the WHO, and the Coalition for Epidemic Preparedness Innovations, have lists that prioritize pandemic potential pathogens.[31] These lists assist vaccine researchers and developers in prioritizing their vaccine R&D efforts. (See text box for one approach to prioritization.)

---

[26] NIAID has supported and conducted research for vaccines against viral, bacterial, fungal, and parasitic diseases. *The National Health Security Strategy 2019-2022* "provides a vision for strengthening our nation's ability to prevent, detect, assess, prepare for, mitigate, respond to, and recover from 21st century health security threats." The *National Influenza Vaccine Modernization Strategy 2020-2030* outlines a vision for the U.S. influenza vaccine enterprise to reduce the impact of seasonal and pandemic influenza viruses.

[27] The *2017-2018 Public Health Emergency Medical Countermeasures Enterprise Strategy* lists high-priority threats. The Public Health Emergency Medical Countermeasures Enterprise also developed a risk assessment framework to assess whether specific emerging pathogens should be included on the list of high-priority threats. These pathogens may be included if Public Health Emergency Medical Countermeasures Enterprise leadership determines they have the potential to affect national health security.

[28] Some of the functions of the Public Health Emergency Medical Countermeasures Enterprise have been paused since 2018-2020, and only minimal operations have occurred. We previously reported on recent efforts to restructure the Public Health Emergency Medical Countermeasures Enterprise. See GAO, *COVID-19: Continued Attention Needed to Enhance Federal Preparedness, Response, Service Delivery, and Program Integrity*, GAO-21-551 (Washington, D.C.: July 19, 2021).

[29] This list is available at https://www.niaid.nih.gov/research/emerging-infectious-diseases-pathogens.

[30] According to researchers from the Johns Hopkins University Center for Health Security, of the 24 families of viruses capable of infecting humans, six families have characteristics that will likely result in one of them being the source of the next pandemic. Those characteristics include no existing immunity in the world's population, respiratory transmission, transmissible by infected people who have no symptoms, and the lack of any existing, effective therapeutics or vaccines. Such pathogens constitute a global catastrophic biological risk, according to Johns Hopkins University Center for Health Security researchers. The researchers also noted that RNA viruses merit special concern because of their higher tendency to mutate, and they recommended that vaccines against viruses with these characteristics be pursued due to their higher probability to produce global catastrophic biological risk events.

[31] The Coalition for Epidemic Preparedness Innovations is a global partnership launched in 2017 to develop vaccines to stop future epidemics. Its mission is to accelerate the development of vaccines against emerging infectious diseases and enable equitable access to these vaccines during outbreaks. According to the HHS, NIAID's public

Prioritization of infectious disease

Experts told us that one way of prioritizing infectious disease could be to use a "stock index fund" approach whereby policymakers select a group of about 100 infectious diseases and work toward making incremental progress on each infectious disease. The experts stated that the rapid development of a vaccine for COVID-19 was largely the result of incremental progress that had been made on developing vaccines for Severe Acute Respiratory Syndrome (SARS) and Middle East Respiratory Syndrome (MERS). Using an index fund approach could provide a similar foundation for the development of new vaccines to respond to future epidemics and pandemics. One basis for selecting diseases to include in the "fund" could be by pathogen family so as to leverage progress on one pathogen to others. For example, families of viruses include paramyxoviridae, which include the Nipah virus; orthomyxoviridae, which include influenza viruses; and coronaviridae, which include SARS-CoV-2 that causes COVID-19.

Source: GAO analysis of information from scientific literature and an expert meeting. | GAO-22-104371.

NIH officials noted that potential pandemic pathogen prioritization for vaccine development may stifle innovation. HHS officials also noted that such prioritization would not fully address pathogens that are yet to be identified or pathogens that emerge unexpectedly.[32] However, any prioritized list of pandemic potential infectious diseases or disease families used to guide or direct vaccine R&D efforts could be updated periodically to include newly identified threats.[33]

2.5. Policy Options That May Help Address Challenges Related to Vaccine R&D

We identified two policy options that may help address challenges related to the adoption of vaccine R&D technologies and approaches. We define policymakers in this chapter as a broad term including, for example, Congress, federal agencies, state and local governments, academic and research institutions, and industry.

---

list of priority pathogens includes some of the same pathogens that have been prioritized by the WHO and the Coalition for Epidemic Preparedness Innovations.

[32] As previously noted, the Coalition for Epidemic Preparedness Innovations and the WHO have prioritized pathogen lists for vaccine development that include pathogens that have yet to be identified—termed disease "X." Johns Hopkins University's Center for Health Security states that disease X includes those viral families that are likely to cause future catastrophic outbreaks.

[33] The Department of Homeland Security, in coordination with CDC, the Department of Defense (DOD), and the U.S. Department of Agriculture, has created a tiered list of biological terrorism agents that is regularly updated. As part of this effort, these entities conduct a biological threat risk assessment every two years to address shifting priorities or newly identified threats. This bi-annual risk assessment assists in prioritizing R&D of basic biological threat agent research, biosurveillance methods, and the development of countermeasures. This methodology could be likewise used to regularly update a prioritized list of potential pandemic pathogens.

Policy options that may help address challenges with developing vaccines for infectious diseases

Policy option	Opportunities	Considerations
Prioritize infectious disease pathogens *Policymakers could collaborate across sectors (e.g., government, academia, researchers, industry, and nonprofit organizations) to prioritize infectious disease pathogens with pandemic potential for vaccine R&D.* For example, policymakers could develop a working group to prioritize pathogens with pandemic potential and work more closely with international organizations to prioritize vaccine development as well as develop monoclonal antibodies as prophylactics and therapeutics. The working group could also periodically revisit the prioritized list and update as appropriate to ensure newly identified threats are addressed. This could help address the challenges we identified related to appropriately prioritizing potential pandemic pathogen vaccine R&D efforts and the technologies and approaches needed to support those efforts, address technological limitations, and focus the use of costly instruments and personnel.	Prioritizing pathogens with pandemic potential could improve strategic vaccine R&D decision-making and help focus resources on developing and adopting key technologies and approaches that most effectively address those pathogens. Appropriately matching the technologies and approaches to the prioritized potential pandemic pathogen, then leveraging technologies and expertise held by various entities—such as government, private sector, and academic laboratories—may help address certain technological limitations and costs. With greater leadership and strategic partnerships, policymakers could take steps to increase preparedness to more quickly address threats to the U.S. population.	As new threats are identified, priorities may change, which may cause uncertainty for vaccine developers. Policymakers may have different priorities based on their respective missions; for example, private sector priorities may differ from government priorities. There may be disagreements as to which key technologies should be prioritized and used, resulting in the need for policymakers to weigh the potential advantages and disadvantages associated with various options.
Improve preparedness *Policymakers could provide funding and other support for public/private partnerships to strategically address potential pandemic pathogens identified as priorities.* These partnerships could, for example, develop and test vaccine candidates and monoclonal antibodies that may provide protection from high impact pathogens and pathogens with pandemic potential. Leveraging relationships with the private sector may allow for sharing of highly trained personnel and costs of the complex instruments that are critical parts of the pandemic preparedness infrastructure.	This early development of vaccine candidates and monoclonal antibodies could provide a coordinated foundation that can be mobilized in an emergency. Such an approach could speed vaccine development as well as potentially reduce risk for vaccine researchers and developers concerning questions of safety, efficacy, and manufacturability. Assessing the likelihood of outbreaks from known pathogens, and developing vaccines through at least phase 1 clinical trials may make it easier to more rapidly mitigate future pandemics.	The lack of certainty of the commercial market and government procurement for vaccines against pathogens with pandemic potential may be too risky for the private sector to undertake.

Source: GAO. \| GAO-22-104371.

3. Technologies and Approaches for Vaccine Testing

Innovative technologies and approaches may enhance vaccine testing, which includes preclinical studies, clinical trials, and post-marketing surveillance studies, allowing vaccine developers to more quickly or effectively test for vaccine safety, identify and recruit clinical trial participants, and analyze clinical trial data. However, challenges, including technological maturity, patient privacy, developing data standards, and the need for stakeholder collaboration, may affect widespread adoption.

3.1. Factors Affecting Vaccine Testing

Numerous factors affect developers' ability to test vaccines, including obtaining animals needed for preclinical studies, recruiting a sufficient number of participants for clinical trials, and managing costs for this portion of development. The mean cost of developing a vaccine from preclinical studies through early clinical safety and efficacy testing (phase 2a) is $31 million to $68 million.[34] Further, according to research, about 67 percent of vaccine clinical trials are estimated to fail.[35] Clinical trials may fail for several reasons including failure to demonstrate that a product produces the desired result (57 percent of failures are for this reason); failure to demonstrate that the product is safe (17 percent); failure to address business challenges, such as keeping costs within budget (22 percent); and failure due to unknown reasons (5 percent).[36]

Developers may also struggle to enroll enough participants. According to a 2015 study, 19 percent of all initiated phase 2 and 3 intervention clinical trials in the National Library of Medicine clinical trial registry either failed to enroll enough participants or completed with less than 85 percent of their expected enrollment, thus reducing the sample size from that planned at trial initiation.[37] For randomized control trials (i.e., those that include both a treatment group and a control group, the typical approach for vaccines), one study from the United Kingdom found that 56 percent of trials between 2004 and 2016 achieved the target number of participants.[38]

3.2. Technologies and Approaches That May Enhance Vaccine Testing

Drawing on information from experts, stakeholders, and the scientific literature, we identified six technologies and approaches that may improve vaccine testing and provide additional methods for assessing data gathered during clinical trials (see Table 2). See appendix III for additional information on technologies and approaches related to vaccine testing.

---

[34] D. Gouglas et al., "Estimating the Cost of Vaccine Development Against Epidemic Infectious Diseases: A Cost Minimisation Study." *The Lancet Global Health,* vol. 6, no. 12 (2018): pp. e1386-e1396.

[35] C. Wong et al., "Estimation of Clinical Trial Success Rates and Related Parameters." *Biostatistics,* vol. 20, no. 2 (2019): pp. 273-286.

[36] These statistics are drawn from a study of trials for new drugs, therapeutic biologics, and vaccines. T. Hwang et al., "Failure of Investigational Drugs in Late-Stage Clinical Development and Publication of Trial Results," *JAMA Intern Med,* vol. 176, no. 12 (2016): pp. 1826-1833.

[37] B. Carlisle et al., "Unsuccessful Trial Accrual and Human Subjects Protections: An Empirical Analysis of Recently Closed Trials." *Clin Trials,* vol. 12, no. 1 (2015): pp. 77-83.

[38] S. J. Walters et al., "Recruitment and Retention of Participants in Randomised Controlled Trials: A Review of Trials Funded and Published by the United Kingdom Health Technology Assessment Programme," *BMJ Open,* vol.7, no.3 (2017).

Table 2. Selected technologies and approaches for vaccine testing

Name	Description
Organ chips	Populated with cells and used in preclinical studies, organ chips mimic the function of human organs and can be used to study the effect of a vaccine candidate.
Artificial intelligence (AI) and machine learning (ML)	AI and ML systems can analyze large amounts of data gathered during preclinical studies and clinical trials.
Electronic health records (EHR)	An EHR is a digital record of a patient's medical information that can be used to support trials for patient recruitment, clinical data analysis, and post-trial follow-up.
Common control groups	A common control group allows multiple groups of participants in preclinical studies or clinical trials to be compared with a single control group, reducing the number of participants needed or enabling comparison among vaccine candidates.
Standardized assays	Standardized assays are standardized tests or investigative procedures that can potentially be used by different vaccine developers to determine the immune response induced by a vaccine candidate. For example, standardized assays could measure the presence of antibodies in clinical trial participants who have received different vaccines candidates.
Virtual clinical trials and wearable devices	Virtual clinical trials, also referred to as decentralized trials, extend the reach of clinical investigations to where patients live and work. Data for virtual trials can be collected remotely via wearable digital health technologies including watches, bracelets, patches, textiles, and clothing.

Source: GAO. | GAO-22-104371.

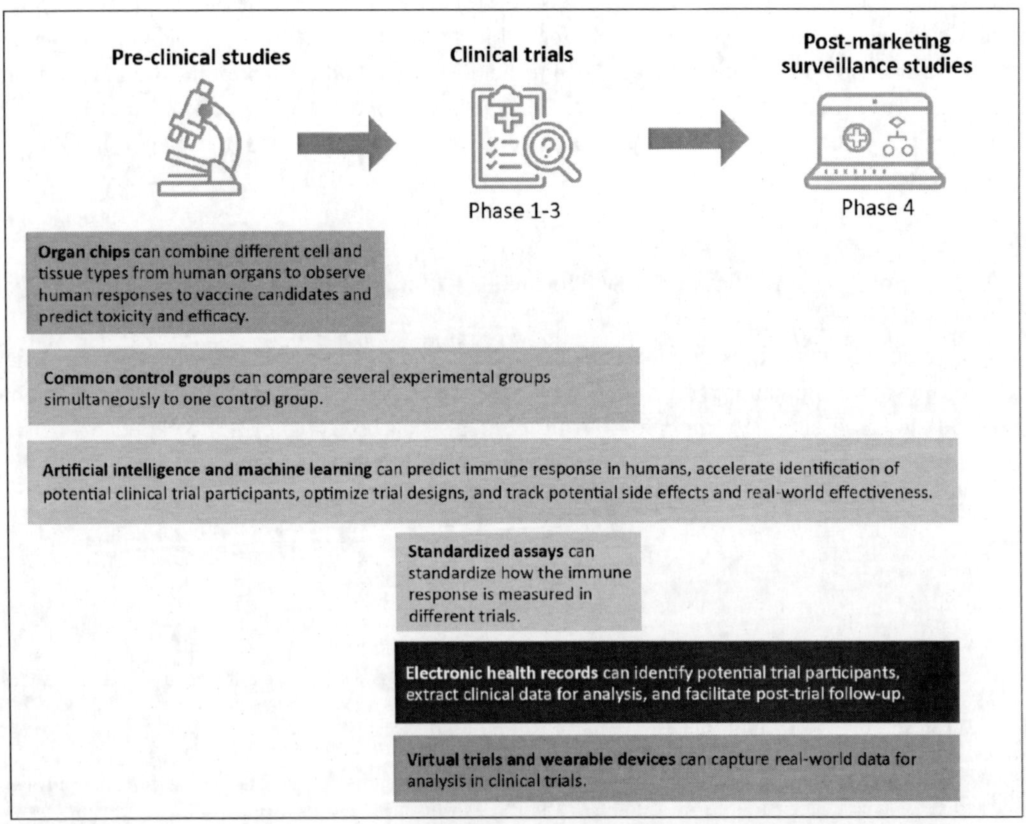

Source: GAO analysis and Sir.Vector/blankstock/stock.adobe.com. | GAO-22-104371.

Figure 4. Selected applications of vaccine testing technologies and approaches.

The technologies and approaches we identified can be applied at different phases of vaccine testing. For example, in the preclinical phase organ chips may be used to determine whether vaccine ingredients have any toxic effects on human cells, which may complement the information gleaned from testing in animals or reduce the need for such testing. Artificial intelligence (AI) and machine learning (ML) may be used for a number of purposes. For example, AI and ML could be used during each phase to predict toxicity in preclinical studies, identify suitable participants for clinical trials, and track long-term side effects during post-marketing surveillance studies (see Figure 4), among other things.[39]

The technologies and approaches we identified may help address factors that affect clinical trials by enabling developers to better collect and analyze safety and efficacy data for various vaccine candidates and more successfully recruit and retain clinical trial participants, among other things (see Figure 5).

Technology /approach	Safety monitoring	Recruiting and retaining participants	Costs	Demonstrating efficacy
	Although safety is monitored in each phase of a clinical trial, issues may only become apparent once larger populations participate in phase 3 trials.	A trial that does not enroll enough participants can result in a sample that is too small to yield valid results.	Clinical trials require extensive funding, time, and resources that increase at each successive phase as increasingly larger numbers of volunteers participate.	The primary reason for clinical trial failure is an inability to demon-strate efficacy.
Organ chips	May complement animal testing to predict a vaccine candidate's toxicity in humans prior to clinical trial testing in humans.	N/A	May reduce the number of animals needed for preclinical studies.	N/A
Artificial intelligence and machine learning	May predict whether a vaccine candidate may cause a low or high number of adverse side effects and may identify rare adverse events from safety reports.	May identify potential participants by assessing suitability from health records and other patient data.	May save money by identifying design efficiencies, such as the ideal number of participants to enroll and the optimal dosage.	May analyze clinical and immunological data from trials and predict antibody response in humans, thereby identifying the immune protection a vaccine candidate may provide.
Common control groups	May allow for evaluating safety data across multiple vaccine candidates.	May increase a patient's chance of receiving a vaccine candidate, which could help with recruiting patients to clinical trials.	May save money since fewer participants are needed when comparing experimental groups to a single control group.	May allow for evaluating efficacy data across multiple vaccine candidates.
Standardized assays	N/A	N/A	N/A	May establish a standard measurement approach that allows for head-to-head vaccine candidate comparisons.
Electronic health records	May be used in safety surveillance to answer specific safety questions about vaccine candidates.	May help identify which individuals receiving care in a health system meet study criteria as eligible participants.	May save money and time by centralizing data collection with an electronic clinical trial management system.	May provide data that can be analyzed for clinical trials.
Virtual trials and wearable devices	May allow for continuous safety monitoring of vaccine candidate side effects.	May expand the pool of potential participants and enable remote data capture, which reduces barriers to participation.	May save money after the initial expense of adopting the technology.	May collect data continuously, potentially providing a more complete picture of participants' health during the trial.

Source: GAO analysis and SergeyCherednichenko/dzm1try/kornkun/blankstock/stock.adobe.com. | GAO-22-104371.

Figure 5. Technologies and approaches that may improve vaccine clinical trials.

---

39 Post-marketing surveillance studies, also referred to as phase 4 clinical trials, may be required after licensure to obtain additional information on the product's benefits, risks, and optimal use.

3.3. Challenges Affecting the Adoption of Vaccine Testing Technologies and Approaches

Based on information from experts, stakeholders, and the scientific literature, we identified four challenges affecting the adoption of technologies and approaches for vaccine testing:

- Limited technological maturity
- Difficulty protecting patient data
- Ongoing data standards development
- Limited stakeholder collaboration and agreement on common approaches to testing

These challenges may affect vaccine developers, researchers who conduct clinical trials, and patients who participate.

3.3.1. Limited Technological Maturity

The extent to which the following technologies and approaches are adopted will depend on their technological maturity or ability to demonstrate validity.

- *Organ chips.* Organ chips are not yet mature enough to replicate many of the complex functions and responses of the human immune system, limiting their applicability. Specifically, according to NIH, organ chips replicate the innate immune response, but the ability to replicate the adaptive immune response is still being developed.[40] While organ chips can be used for some aspects of toxicity testing, further maturity may be needed to demonstrate that they do not produce false negative results.
- *Virtual trials and wearable devices.* To conduct fully virtual trials, many organizations will need to develop new technical capabilities. For example, they will need to integrate wearable technologies and develop ways to capture and analyze potentially large volumes of data. Many wearable devices are in early development and will need to demonstrate analytical and clinical validation to support data submitted for vaccine licensure.

3.3.2. Challenges Protecting Patient Data

When patients consent to allow data from their health records and other sources to be made available for use in trials, more people gain access to this information, and the challenge of protecting data privacy increases.[41] Researchers conducting clinical trials must adhere to

---

[40] The innate immune system is the body's first line of defense against germs entering the body. It consists of protection offered by the skin, mucous membranes, immune system cells, and proteins. The adaptive immune system responds if the innate immune system is not able to destroy the germs. It is made up of T-lymphocytes, B-lymphocytes, and antibodies.

[41] The Health Insurance Portability and Accountability Act Privacy Rule establishes the conditions under which protected health information may be used or disclosed for research purposes. Researchers may obtain an individual authorization from the patient that meets the requirements set out in the Privacy Rule or they may seek an institutional review board or privacy board waiver of the Privacy Rule's authorization requirement. 45 C.F.R. §§ 164.508, 164.512(i)(1)(i).

federal privacy laws and regulations, such as the Health Insurance Portability and Accountability Act Privacy Rule and other relevant requirements.[42]

Technologies and approaches directly affected by the need to protect patient data include:

- *Electronic health records (EHR).* EHRs contain a wealth of sensitive information including patients' social security numbers, addresses, and health diagnoses.
- *AI and ML.* AI and ML systems that are deployed in clinical settings contribute to privacy risks, and there are concerns that the use of increasingly sophisticated computer techniques could make it easier to re-identify data from patient records and other sources.
- *Virtual trials and wearable devices.* Virtual trials collect data outside the traditional clinical care setting. There is a need for security in the transmission of data. Researchers must maintain protections in accordance with the Privacy Rule.

3.3.3. Ongoing Data Standards Development

In 2020, the HHS Office of the National Coordinator for Health Information Technology and the Centers for Medicare & Medicaid Services issued final rules that require data exchange and data element standards for use in EHRs in order to promote interoperability—generally defined as the ability of a system to exchange electronic health information with, and use electronic health information from other systems, without special effort on the part of the user.[43] This includes the use of technical standards for transmitting EHR data and vocabulary standards for the content of EHR data.[44]

HHS has identified the need for securely available electronic health information since 2015, and has stated that it expects improved interoperability to benefit researchers. Specifically, due to a lack of data standards and interoperability in the past, researchers have been hindered in their ability to use EHRs for research including clinical trials. The new rules may help address the following challenges to the use of EHRs in clinical trials:

- *Lack of consistency in health record data.* For some kinds of clinical data, standards either have not been previously developed or have not been universally adopted. This

[42] A HIPAA-covered entity may also "de-identify" patient data in accordance with the Privacy Rule prior to sharing it for research purposes. 45 C.F.R. §§ 164.502(d), 164.514. This is typically done by removing data fields such as names, social security numbers, account numbers, and full faced photographs. However, studies have shown that even properly de-identified data may retain some risk of re-identification.

[43] 21st Century Cures Act: Interoperability, Information Blocking, and the Office of the National Coordinator for Health Information Technology Health IT Certification Program, 85 Fed. Reg. 25,642 (May 1, 2020). Interoperability and Patient Access Final Rule, and 85 Fed. Reg. 25,510 (May 1, 2020). The Office of the National Coordinator for Health Information Technology's final rule establishes new rules to prevent "information blocking" practices by healthcare providers, developers of certified health information technology, and other entities as required by the 21st Century Cures Act. Pub. L. No. 114-255, § 4004, 130 Stat. 1034, 1176 (2016). The Centers for Medicare & Medicaid Services' final rule requires, among other things, that health plans in Medicare Advantage, Medicaid, the Children's Health Insurance Program, and the federal exchanges make certain data available to patients through an application programming interface.

[44] Key requirements of the Office of the National Coordinator for Health Information Technology and the Centers for Medicare & Medicaid Services rules are (1) the adoption of the Health Level 7 (HL7®) Fast Healthcare Interoperability Resources application programming interface standard, which enables health information technology systems and applications to receive and exchange information from EHRs and (2) adoption of the United States Core Data for Interoperability standard, which is a common set of data elements, organized by data classes, that use a standardized content and format.

inconsistency has hindered the ability to use criteria to identify eligible patients and analyze data from EHRs.

- *Lack of EHR interoperability.* EHR data have in the past been based on different data standards that cannot be exchanged easily. A lack of widely adopted data standards has hindered the exchange of data between EHRs and electronic data capture systems, which researchers use to collect and manage clinical trial data.[45]

While improved interoperability is expected to benefit researchers who use EHRs, new data standards may affect how researchers are able to use data. The Office of the National Coordinator for Health Information Technology stated that while standardized data elements successfully gather general structured information, these data are limited and often insufficient for clinical trials, which require data that can answer specific research questions. It also stated that researchers may need to supplement these data from sources outside the EHR, such as genomic data, but these data are not currently available using the adopted standard. Additionally, data standards are still being developed, which may affect the availability of data elements for research, including for clinical trials.[46]

Expanding and implementing standards for electronic health data requires cooperation between health care providers, government, and industry. Industry representatives told us there's a need to develop implementation guidance collaboratively and that even with data standards in place, it will be difficult for researchers to use EHR data in clinical trials without additional guidance. If efforts to develop standards and advance interoperability do not continue to incorporate the specific needs of the research and clinical trial communities, researchers may be unable to optimize the potential for electronic health data to be used in clinical trials.

3.3.4. Limited Stakeholder Collaboration and Agreement on Common Approaches to Vaccine Testing

Using common approaches, such as standardized assays and common control groups, allows for direct comparisons among multiple vaccine candidates. However, vaccine developers traditionally test their vaccines candidates using their own assays and recruit their own participants for clinical trials because companies tend to operate independently. Also, the tasks involved to develop assays and plan trials are often closely integrated, and the timing of clinical trials for different vaccines would need to align in order to use a common control group. Using developer-specific approaches to vaccine testing makes it more difficult to compare data from clinical trials of more than one vaccine candidate and determine the relative efficacy of each. While experts said it is important for different kinds of vaccines to be developed during a pandemic, they also said it is important to be able to directly compare the results to better understand the potential differences in protection provided by each vaccine candidate. Stakeholders, including vaccine developers and government decision-makers, would need to

[45] Food and Drug Administration, *Use of Electronic Health Record Data in Clinical Investigations* (Silver Spring, Md.: July 2018).

[46] For example, the Office of the National Coordinator for Health Information Technology's final rule states that clinical notes would be included within the United States Core Data for Interoperability standard and it adopts eight types of clinical notes as standard data elements. Version 2 of the United States Core Data for Interoperability standard was released in July 2021 and it includes only five data elements within the clinical notes data class: consultation note, discharge summary note, history & physical, procedure note, and progress note.

collaborate to use standardized assays and common control groups in order to benefit from the advantages they may provide.

According to experts we met with, it may be feasible and advantageous to use standardized assays and common control groups in some scenarios. For example, when government invests in developing a vaccine, it has an opportunity to work with industry stakeholders to design clinical trials that include these features. Experts said master protocols, also known as common protocols (a common set of processes that govern a set of studies), could be developed that include the use of standardized assays and common control groups that vaccine developers could agree to follow in vaccine testing.[47] The protocols would ideally be developed prior to the onset of a pandemic event, according to experts, but the approach might also be possible in an emergency.

The master protocol approach has been used previously with therapeutics, including for COVID-19, but HHS officials told us COVID-19 vaccine developers maintained control over their own trial protocols. However, it may be possible to incentivize developers to agree to master protocols by completing formative work such as the difficult process of developing assays, or by tying government funding for vaccine development to the use of master protocols. One expert told us that expanding inventories of available assays for pathogens and families of pathogens could expedite the development and testing of new vaccine candidates. Another expert told us that developing standardized assays to measure cellular response to vaccine candidates could streamline the evaluation of vaccine efficacy during clinical trials.

According to NIH officials, however, developing meaningful master protocols for using standardized assays and common control groups in advance of a pandemic outbreak from a novel pathogen would be challenging. According to officials, the development of assays can require substantial investment of time and resources to ensure their safety, validity, and reproducibility, and this would likely need to be done for each individual pathogen. Furthermore, officials said adopting common control groups across multiple vaccine developers' vaccine trials also requires care, particularly if there are differences in the doses required or the timing of when different vaccine companies are ready to begin clinical trials. NIH officials said there may be ways to address these challenges, however. They said NIH's Rapid Acceleration of Diagnostics program is an example of early-stage government investment to jump-start diagnostic development when a new infectious agent threatens public health, and NIH's clinical trial evaluating mixed COVID-19 vaccine schedules serves as a model for addressing these challenges.

One expert stated that even if standardized assays are not ready at the start of a clinical trial, once the assays are available they can be used on stored samples from trials. The expert said that this approach could be part of the protocols and could help in making comparisons across vaccine candidates. Furthermore, according to the expert, when the federal government is contributing funding it could also encourage companies to share biological samples and establish common definitions of infection and disease, which would help improve the ability to compare results across vaccine candidates.

As part of the response to the COVID-19 pandemic, NIH's Accelerating COVID-19 Therapeutic Interventions and Vaccines partnership initiative used some common protocols,

---

[47] FDA guidance defines a master protocol as a protocol designed with multiple sub-studies, which may have different objectives and involve coordinated efforts to evaluate one or more investigational drugs in one or more disease subtypes within the overall trial structure. FDA, *COVID-19: Master Protocols Evaluating Drugs and Biological Products for Treatment or Prevention* (Silver Spring, Md.: May 2021).

including standardized assays, to guide phase 3 clinical trials of certain COVID-19 vaccines (see text box for an example of how harmonized protocols have been used).[48]

Experts said that the Accelerating COVID-19 Therapeutic Interventions and Vaccines partnership could provide a model for using master protocols for vaccine clinical trials. Following this approach, stakeholders could collaborate to develop protocols and could follow the protocols to advance vaccine candidates to phase 1 clinical trials. Once a pandemic event occurs, the protocols could be modified as necessary, according to experts. Such protocols could also guide phase 3 clinical trials as was done for COVID-19 vaccine candidates.

Harmonized protocols for COVID-19 vaccine candidates

The National Institutes of Health (NIH)-led Accelerating COVID-19 Therapeutic Interventions and Vaccines is a public-private partnership that was formed to speed development of the most promising treatments and vaccines for COVID-19 by coordinating activities by federal agencies, vaccine developers, and other stakeholders. The partnership advised on protocol designs to harmonize the approach to phase 3 clinical trials for COVID-19 vaccines conducted through the National Institute of Allergy and Infectious Diseases' (NIAID) COVID-19 Prevention Network.[49]

Features of the harmonized protocols included:

- Standardized assays. Standardized assays were developed collaboratively and were used to evaluate the efficacy of COVID-19 vaccine candidates in phase 3 clinical trials.
- Shared data and safety monitoring board. Clinical trials were overseen by a single shared independent data safety monitoring board, established by NIAID.
- Separate control groups. Phase 3 clinical trials for COVID-19 vaccine candidates maintained separate control groups for each vaccine trial.

According to NIH, clinical trials of COVID-19 vaccines conducted through NIAID's COVID-19 Prevention Network used these standardized assays. The Accelerating COVID-19 Therapeutic Interventions and Vaccines partnership coordinated efforts helped address challenges related to enrolling enough participants for trials and interpreting and comparing trial results.

Source: GAO analysis of information from scientific literature and an expert meeting. | GAO-22-104371.

Although the Accelerating COVID-19 Therapeutic Interventions and Vaccines partnership did not use common control groups—and they may not be applicable in every scenario—experts told us that doing so has the potential to improve trial recruitment and might enable adaptive designs that could speed up clinical trials involving multiple vaccine candidates.[50] Along with the adoption of data standards, which may improve the readiness of EHRs for use in clinical trials, these potentially allow for more efficient means to enhance the response to endemic levels of infectious disease as well as better respond to potential future epidemics and pandemics.

---

[48] The Accelerating COVID-19 Therapeutic Interventions and Vaccines public-private partnership is coordinated by the Foundation for the National Institutes of Health and brings together NIH, the Biomedical Advanced Research and Development Authority (BARDA), CDC, FDA, DOD, the Department of Veterans Affairs, the HHS-DOD COVID-19 Countermeasures Acceleration Group (formerly known as Operation Warp Speed), the European Medicines Agency, and representatives from academia, philanthropic organizations, and numerous biopharmaceutical companies.

[49] According to NIH, the harmonized approach was intended to guide vaccine developers. However, developers still designed their own specific clinical trial protocols.

[50] FDA defines an adaptive design as a clinical trial design that allows for prospectively planned modifications to one or more aspects of the design based on accumulating data from subjects in the trial. FDA, *Adaptive Designs for Clinical Trials of Drugs and Biologics* (Silver Spring, Md.: Nov. 2019).

3.4. Policy Options That May Help Address Challenges Related to Vaccine Testing

We identified two policy options that may help address challenges related to the adoption of testing technologies and approaches. As mentioned previously, policymakers include Congress, federal agencies, state and local governments, academic and research institutions, and industry.

Policy options that may help address challenges related to vaccine testing

Policy option	Opportunities	Considerations
Further support development of data standards *Policymakers could further support coordinated efforts to obtain the views of all stakeholders and to develop standards for health data and their use in clinical trials.* This support could help address the challenge we identified related to ongoing data standards development.	• Integrating researchers' needs into the standards development process could better ensure the necessary data are available. • Data standards could more easily allow researchers to combine different data sets, enabling better transmission of data for analysis in trials. • Interoperable systems may eliminate the manual transcription of data, reducing data entry errors. • Access to high-quality data in a standardized format may allow streamlined patient recruitment for clinical trials. • Improving standards may facilitate identification of differences in clinical trial efficacy across population subgroups (e.g., differences by age, race, and gender) by broadening the pool of patient records available for research.	• Expanding access to patient heath data requires attention to ensure privacy. If patient data have been de-identified, combining data from multiple sources may make it easier to re-identify. • Data from different sources, such as wearable devices and clinical notes, may vary in quality and reliability, making it difficult to use them in combination. • Developing and implementing standardized data formats and IT infrastructure is time-consuming and costly. • Disparities in access to health care, particularly among some population groups, may limit the pool of patient records available for research.
Study feasibility of using common control groups and standardized assays *Policymakers could study the feasibility of collaborating with industry for use of standardized assays and common control groups during pandemic and non-pandemic scenarios.* This option could help address the challenge we identified related to limited stakeholder collaboration and agreement on common approaches to testing.	• Trial logistics could be streamlined, and cost-sharing could produce savings. • Meeting recruitment goals could be faster, which can be important during pandemics. • Trial participants are more likely to receive a vaccine candidate, which may boost recruitment. • Incorporating adaptive trial designs in planned protocols may lessen regulatory review requirements when modifications need to be made. • A head-to-head comparison of vaccine candidates, enabled by following master protocols, improves understanding of efficacy. The master protocol approach may also facilitate the implementation of clinical research across successive outbreaks of a disease since protocols will already be in place.	• Vaccine developers may be unwilling to give up control of designing trials and use of proprietary assays, and may resist having head-to-head comparisons with other vaccine candidates. • If not agreed to in advance, stakeholder coordination, infrastructure requirements, and complex trial design elements could make the start-up time for a master protocol longer than that of a single-purpose trial. • Determining the timing and predicting the required funding level could be difficult if new vaccine candidates will be added to a trial design on an ongoing basis. • Developing assays requires significant effort. Harmonizing results across vaccine candidates, as was done for COVID-19 phase 3 clinical trials, may be more achievable than requiring developers to use a standardized method to measure immune response.

Source: GAO. | GAO-22-104371.

4. Technologies and Approaches for Vaccine Manufacturing

Certain technologies and approaches for vaccine manufacturing may have the potential to enhance the U.S.'s ability to address infectious diseases and prepare for future epidemics and pandemics. These technologies and approaches may allow for an increase in manufacturing flexibility—the ability to quickly switch from manufacturing one vaccine to another—and an increase in manufacturing productivity. However, challenges such as technical limitations, costs, and the need for highly trained personnel affect vaccine manufacturers' ability to adopt new technologies and approaches. Further, private manufacturers may be reluctant to establish and maintain costly excess manufacturing capacity to address surges in vaccine demand during pandemics. The federal government has attempted to address these issues; however, challenges remain.

4.1. Factors Affecting Vaccine Manufacturing

Factors that affect vaccine manufacturing include:[51]

- A lack of flexibility to rapidly switch manufacturing lines from one vaccine to another
- An inability to rapidly scale up manufacturing to meet surges in new vaccine demand
- An inability to use available capacity to manufacture new vaccines without impacting the manufacture of other licensed vaccines

Vaccine manufacturing is traditionally inflexible, with many manufacturers producing single vaccines products in centrally located, dedicated facilities. As a result, new vaccines cannot be easily incorporated into existing facilities, and different vaccines cannot be manufactured simultaneously, in quick succession, or closer to the geographic point of need. Further, centrally located, dedicated product manufacturing facilities can be a single point of failure—a risk that can negatively impact vaccine supply.

Besides influenza vaccine manufacturing, the U.S. lacks the infrastructure—known as surge capacity—needed to quickly scale up the manufacture of new vaccines to address outbreaks, including pandemics. The lack of surge capacity is caused partially by the reluctance of vaccine manufacturers in the private sector to invest in the high cost of maintaining excess, idle capacity in anticipation of unknown future vaccine needs. As a result, U.S. manufacturing capacity is generally focused on meeting market demand for vaccines listed on the child and adolescent immunization schedule (e.g., measles, mumps, rubella, and polio) and those on the adult immunization schedule for which profitable markets exist (e.g., shingles and pneumonia).[52]

---

[51] As noted in GAO-21-207, vaccine manufacturing supply chains may be strained by disruptions caused by the COVID-19 pandemic, including changes in the labor market, increases or decreases in the demand for certain goods, or export restrictions implemented by some countries. For example, obtaining manufacturing materials, such as disposable reactor bags, reagents, and certain chemicals, may be a challenge. Further, the supply of materials used in fill-finish manufacturing, such as glass vials and pre-filled syringes, may be limited.

[52] The child and adolescent immunization schedule includes recommended vaccines for children from birth through age 18. The adult immunization schedule includes recommended vaccines for ages 19 years and older.

To increase U.S. surge capacity, the Biomedical Advanced Research and Development Authority (BARDA), within HHS's Office of the Assistant Secretary for Preparedness and Response, established three Centers for Innovation in Advanced Development and Manufacturing in June 2012.[53] Among other capabilities, these centers were designed to provide technical assistance and to support additional surge capacity that would be capable of delivering finished doses of pandemic vaccine within 12 weeks of the declaration of a pandemic.[54] However, as noted by representatives from these centers that we spoke with, these facilities had difficulties in maintaining operational readiness. Further, in congressional testimony, a representative from another center noted the challenge of maintaining operational readiness.[55] These centers' facilities also needed retrofitting, such as equipment and facility upgrades, to be able to sufficiently and timely manufacture the vaccines needed to respond to the COVID-19 pandemic.

4.2. Technologies and Approaches for Vaccine Manufacturing

Drawing on information from experts, stakeholders, and the scientific literature, we identified five selected technologies and approaches that may improve vaccine manufacturing—collectively known as bioprocess intensification (see Table 3). These selected technologies and approaches are not necessarily new: some have been used for years in other industries, including chemical and pharmaceutical manufacturing, and some have already been applied in vaccine manufacturing processes. These technologies and approaches may help vaccine manufacturers increase flexibility and capacity by allowing for rapid switching between different vaccines within the same facility, increasing productivity to help manage surge demand, and potentially distributing manufacturing closer to points of need. See appendix IV for additional information on technologies and approaches related to vaccine manufacturing.

The technologies and approaches we identified can be applied at different stages of vaccine manufacturing. For example, modular bioprocessing systems may replace fixed, inflexible infrastructure, potentially allowing for rapid switching between vaccines, scale up, and customization. Process optimization can enable vaccine manufacturers to increase antigen yields and use smaller production volumes through, for example, the use of specific cell lines and growth ingredients (see Figure 6).

---

[53] Created as public-private partnerships, the three Centers for Innovation in Advanced Development and Manufacturing were established to address influenza pandemic vaccine availability, which fell short in 2009 because of an outdated egg-based manufacturing process and bottlenecks in the fill-finish step. The term fill-finish refers to the process of filling sterile containers with vaccine and finishing the process of packaging filled containers for distribution. To address the fill-finish bottlenecks, the federal government established the Fill Finish Manufacturing Network, a group of pre-qualified facilities that fill and finish vaccines for manufacturers in a public health emergency. See GAO, "*National Preparedness: HHS Has Funded Flexible Manufacturing Activities for Medical Countermeasures, but It Is Too Soon to Assess Their Effect*," GAO-14-329 (Washington, D.C.: March 31, 2014).

[54] While the 12-week goal is specific to an influenza pandemic, the capacity and capabilities developed for pandemic influenza preparedness could enable HHS to respond more effectively to other emerging infectious diseases. HHS's Office of the Assistant Secretary for Preparedness and Response's goal is to provide 600 million doses of pandemic vaccine for the U.S. within 6 months or less after a pandemic is declared.

[55] Transcript from "Examining Emergent Biosolutions' Failure to Protect Public Health and Public Funds Hearing Before the Select Subcommittee On The Coronavirus Crisis of the Committee on Oversight and Reform House of Representatives One Hundred Seventeenth Congress First Session May 19, 2021".

Table 3. Selected technologies and approaches for vaccine manufacturing

Name	Description
Single-use systems	Single-use systems refer to bioprocessing equipment that is designed to be used once and then discarded. Such equipment is generally composed of sealed, pre-sterilized, plastic components.
Modular bioprocessing systems	These systems divide the manufacturing process into smaller functional building blocks known as modules, suites, or pods that can stand alone or be incorporated into an existing facility. For example, new modules can be added to quickly expand capacity or switched to rapidly change processes, according to an expert we spoke to.
Cell-free synthesis	Biological enzymes—proteins that cause biochemical reactions—are used to generate antigens, which are then combined with other materials to create vaccines.
Process optimization	This approach improves the cells and growth ingredients—known as medium—and other processing steps. According to an expert we interviewed, this technology may increase productivity and allow manufactures to get more out of the same equipment or facility.
Continuous manufacturing systems	These systems use automated, high-throughput, small-footprint production and purification equipment to manufacture vaccines. In contrast to existing batch processing methods, which use separate tanks for each step in the process, continuous manufacturing allows all steps of vaccine production to continue without interruption as the materials flow through the system.

Source: GAO. | GAO-22-104371.

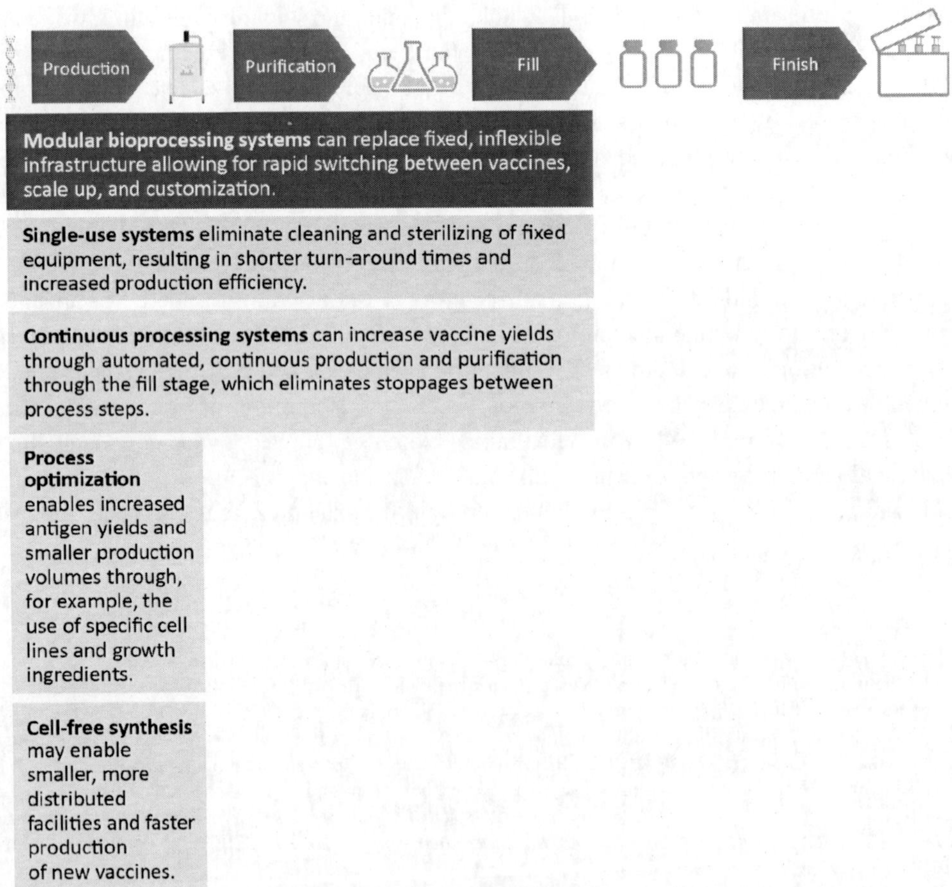

Source: GAO analysis of scientific literature and rashadshurov/tutti_frutti/StockBURIN/divstock/stock.adobe.com. | GAO-22-104371.

Figure 6. Selected applications of vaccine manufacturing technologies and approaches.

Single-use systems may help vaccine manufacturers increase the flexibility of their vaccine manufacturing facilities. For example, manufacturers can replace traditional stainless-steel vessels—known as bioreactors—that are used to grow the cells that produce antigens with disposable plastic bioreactor bags. Single-use systems eliminate the need for cleaning and sterilizing fixed equipment between vaccine manufacturing runs—also known as batches—resulting in shorter turn-around times and increased efficiency. Since they are discarded after each use, single-use systems may also reduce the potential for contamination caused by inadequate cleaning or sterilization.

Modular bioprocessing systems may also help vaccine manufacturers increase the flexibility of their facilities. For example, a vaccine facility's fixed infrastructure, such as rooms and areas dedicated to specific bioprocessing steps, can be replaced with modular components. These modular components can allow manufacturers to rapidly switch from manufacturing one vaccine to another, scale up manufacturing, or add a new facility in a new location more quickly, according to an expert we spoke to. Modular bioprocessing systems also allow vaccine manufacturers to continuously customize and reconfigure their equipment to accommodate new vaccines or processes more quickly—changes that are traditionally difficult and costly. This ability to customize bioprocesses could allow vaccine manufacturers to establish smaller vaccine manufacturing facilities at sites closer to infectious disease outbreaks.

For some vaccines, cell-free synthesis may eliminate the need to grow living cells to produce the antigen of interest, potentially resulting in smaller, more distributed facilities, and faster manufacture of new vaccines in existing facilities. Cell-free synthesis combines purified biological molecules to produce antigens, which are then purified and formulated into vaccines.[56] Additionally, while the first step in mRNA vaccine manufacturing involves traditional growth of cells to generate a key component—DNA—needed to make the vaccine, the subsequent step to manufacture the mRNA uses cell-free synthesis. The flexibility of cell-free synthesis reduces the single point of failure risk that may be associated with centrally located, dedicated product facilities. Further, cell-free synthesis may allow for the simultaneous manufacture of different vaccine antigens within the same facility, which cannot be done in most existing facilities.

Process optimization allows manufacturers to increase antigen yields through, for example, the use of cells specifically developed to increase antigen productivity, known as optimized cell lines, matched with specific growth ingredients, known as growth medium. Antigen productivity can be increased by growing cells at higher densities.[57] High-cell density can be achieved by selecting for or artificially modifying cells that grow to high densities or by changing how the cells are grown. For example, cells that freely grow in liquid medium—called suspension cultures, typically result in higher cell densities and antigen yields than cells that have been adapted to grow attached to a surface, called adherent cultures.

Continuous manufacturing systems may also increase vaccine yields through automated, continuous antigen production and purification. Continuous manufacturing systems may run for weeks or even months, reducing, for example, the requirement to start new cell cultures for antigen production, stoppages between production and purification steps, and the potential for contamination. For example, one manufacturer we spoke with has tested its closed-production

[56] Cell-free synthesis uses a number of purified biological molecules, including enzymes and nucleic acids.
[57] Cell density describes the number of cells in a specific volume of growth medium.

systems with continuous downstream processing technology to produce vaccines for clinical trials.[58]

4.3. Challenges Affecting the Adoption of Vaccine Manufacturing Technologies

Drawing on information from experts, stakeholders, and the scientific literature, we identified three key challenges that affect the adoption of technologies for vaccine manufacturing:

- Inherent technological limitations
- High costs and the need for highly trained personnel
- Business risk

4.3.1. Inherent Technological Limitations

The extent to which some technologies and approaches are adopted for vaccine manufacturing will depend on their technological limits.

- *Single-use systems.* Some of the plastic materials used in single-use systems may leach unwanted substances into the process, and disposable bioreactor bags may leak.[59] Also, limitations in disposable bioreactor scale require scale out versus scale up, according to an expert we spoke to. Further, there are concerns about the environmental impact of the waste plastic materials used in single-use systems after disposal.
- *Cell-free synthesis.* Cell-free systems may be unable to synthesize some proteins, such as sugar-based (polysaccharide) antigens, or to produce properly folded or modified proteins.
- *Continuous manufacturing.* Continuous manufacturing cannot be used for all types of vaccines. For example, vaccines produced in eggs, such as most seasonal influenza vaccines, cannot use continuous manufacturing processes. Additionally, continuous manufacturing processes cannot be used for some vaccines because the biochemical processes by which cells produce the antigens are not well defined and the ability to control the production process is limited.
  Changing from batch to continuous manufacturing also presents challenges because depending on the circumstances, vaccine companies also may be required to seek and obtain FDA approval of manufacturing changes prior to vaccine distribution to ensure the safety and effectiveness of the vaccine have not been adversely affected.[60]

---

[58] A closed-production system uses equipment designed and operated in such a way that the product is not exposed to the room environment. Materials may be introduced to a closed system, but exposure of the product to the room environment must be avoided.

[59] Because these leachable substances may be present, manufacturers perform extensive testing to ensure that single-use systems do not negatively impact the vaccine and so that batches do not need to be discarded, according to an expert we spoke to.

[60] A sponsor may be required to seek and obtain FDA approval of certain changes to an existing biologics license application to ensure the safety and effectiveness of the biologic has not been adversely affected. This may include changes to the product, production process, quality controls, equipment, facilities, or responsible personnel. See 21 C.F.R. § 601.12 (2020).

4.3.2. High Costs and the Need for Highly Trained Personnel

The extent to which some technologies and approaches are adopted will also depend on their cost and need for specialized personnel. For example, these technologies require upfront capital expenditures by manufacturers that may be prohibitively expensive. Further, manufacturers may be reluctant to replace equipment for which they have already made significant capital expenditures.

- *Single-use and modular bioprocessing systems.* Modular bioprocessing systems may involve significant capital expenditures to implement. However, once implemented, single-use and modular bioprocessing systems may reduce operational costs and increase efficiencies that offset upfront expenses. Further, building an integrated modular facility requires more skill and expertise, including technical construction and qualified, experienced personnel to get a facility fully operational.
- *Continuous bioprocessing.* The costs involved in developing new infrastructure and adding new equipment and automation for continuous processing may discourage the use of this technology. Further, the skill set and capabilities required to design, develop, validate, and operate a continuous flow process are different from those required for conventional batch processing.[61]

4.3.3. Business Risk

The extent to which some technologies and approaches are adopted may also depend on how manufacturers perceive the business risk. Manufacturers may face uncertainty in how regulators will evaluate a new vaccine manufacturing technology and how that could affect its financial viability. According to a National Academies of Sciences, Engineering, and Medicine report that was sponsored by FDA, if introducing an innovative technology might result in additional activities, costs, and time to support product approval, it often makes business sense for a manufacturer to use more conventional technology for the product.[62] Furthermore, different requirements in other countries pose additional challenges to manufactures that aspire to market a product internationally. While the National Academies of Sciences, Engineering, and Medicine report focused on pharmaceutical manufacturing, one expert we spoke to said the same principles apply to manufacturing for vaccines.

4.4. Challenges Affecting Scaling up Manufacturing to Meet Surges in Demand

Two key challenges impact the ability to meet surges in vaccine demand, including surges caused by epidemics or global pandemics. The first is the capability of private sector manufacturers to meet new demand without negatively impacting their ability to manufacture other licensed vaccines. The second is the ability of the federal government to ensure that manufacturing capacity to respond to pandemics is available and operational.

---

[61] Baxendale, I. R., R.D. Braatz, B. K.Hodnett, K. F. Jensen, M. D. Johnson, P. Sharratt, J-P. Sherlock, and A. J. Florence, “Achieving Continuous Manufacturing: Technologies and Approaches for Synthesis, Workup, and Isolation of Drug Substance,” *Journal of Pharmaceutical Sciences*, vol. 104, no. 3, (2015): 781-791.

[62] National Academies of Sciences, Engineering, and Medicine, Innovations in Pharmaceutical Manufacturing on the Horizon, Consensus Study Report Highlights, National Academies Press (2021).

According to experts we spoke with, vaccine manufacturers cannot fully address novel threats from different categories of pathogens because they do not create excess, unused capacity for emergency events, and using existing infrastructure to manufacture pandemic vaccines could negatively impact the production of current vaccines for diseases such as measles, mumps, and rubella.

The federal government has attempted to address private sector capacity gaps by establishing manufacturing capacity and flexibility across a range of vaccine platforms to respond to infectious disease outbreaks. However, these attempts have not created adequate capacity to address real-world pandemic manufacturing needs.[63] For example, the Centers for Innovation in Advanced Development and Manufacturing have not been effectively maintained, updated, or made operationally ready to meet the new COVID-19 vaccine surge in manufacturing during the pandemic as noted by representatives from one center we spoke with and in congressional testimony.[64] Two key barriers inhibit scaling up manufacturing to meet such surges in demand.

- *Sufficiently trained personnel are limited.* For example, the COVID-19 vaccine cross contamination problems at the Maryland center appeared to be due, in part, to inadequately trained personnel. Similarly, the Texas center found it challenging to fill open mid- and upper-management positions during COVID-19 vaccine ramp up.
- *Technologies and approaches that enhance flexibility or increase productivity are not supported.* For example, facility retrofitting and technology transfer of new manufacturing processes for COVID-19 vaccines required for the Texas and Maryland centers were done during the pandemic rather than in advance.

4.5. Policy Options That May Help Address Challenges Related to Vaccine Manufacturing

We identified two options for policymakers that may help address challenges related to the adoption of technologies and the improvement of vaccine manufacturing capacity and operational readiness. As mentioned previously, policymakers include Congress, federal agencies, state and local governments, academic and research institutions, and industry.

---

[63] While the approximately 10.5 months it took to develop a COVID-19 vaccine was unprecedented, innovations and new approaches could accelerate vaccine development and manufacture in the future. For example, the Coalition for Epidemic Preparedness Innovations has an aspirational goal—"a moon-shot"—to make vaccines available in 100 days after determination of the pathogen's genetic sequence.

[64] Transcript from "Examining Emergent Biosolutions' Failure to Protect Public Health and Public Funds Hearing Before the Select Subcommittee On The Coronavirus Crisis of the Committee on Oversight and Reform House of Representatives One Hundred Seventeenth Congress First Session May 19, 2021."

Policy options that may help address challenges related to vaccine manufacturing

Policy option	Opportunities	Considerations
Assess vaccine manufacturing capacity and operational readiness *Policymakers could routinely assess U.S. manufacturing capacity and operational readiness.* For example manufacturing capabilities could be pressure tested to determine the nation's overall capability to manufacture current vaccines and meet pandemic surge demands.[a] This could help address the challenges identified related to meeting new demands without negatively impacting manufacturers' ability to produce current vaccines.	Determining U.S. vaccine manufacturing capacity and operational readiness and routinely pressure testing it can help identify gaps as well as key technologies and approaches to address them.	Vaccine manufacturing capacity requirements may change based on the specific infectious disease and vaccine platforms being pressure tested.
Improve preparedness *Policymakers could provide support and coordination for public-private partnerships to strategically develop manufacturing capacity to respond to surge requirements.* To maintain this capacity, partnerships could manufacture prototype vaccine candidates against high-priority pathogens.[b] For example, manufacturing, testing through phase 1-2 clinical trials, and stockpiling prototype vaccine candidates against prioritized classes of pathogens could decrease the amount of time needed to validate and scale up manufacturing processes if a pathogen from those classes does emerge.[c]	Manufacturing, testing and stockpiling vaccine candidates could be mobilized in an emergency and more rapidly mitigate future pandemics. By leveraging strategic partnerships, policymakers could take steps to increase the availability of vaccines to more quickly address threats to the U.S. population.	May require new resources or reallocation of resources from other efforts. There may be a risk that the vaccines manufactured, tested, and stockpiled against prioritized pathogen classes miss certain pandemic pathogens. The stockpiled vaccines would need to be regularly replenished prior to expiration.
This could help address the challenges identified related to the ability of the federal government to ensure that the manufacturing capacity to respond to pandemics is available and operational.		

Source: GAO. | GAO-22-104371.

[a]Operational readiness includes having available, well maintained equipment and facilities as well as enough trained personnel. Further, operational readiness includes maintaining "warm" manufacturing capabilities—for example, by operating at least one shift daily—so that equipment remains operational and personnel retain manufacturing competency.

[b]As described in section 2, if able to be developed and manufactured early in a pandemic, monoclonal antibody candidates may also provide some initial benefit.

[c]One expert estimated the cost to produce and test a vaccine through phase 2 clinical trials would be approximately $50 million, with one-third of that cost required for manufacturing the vaccine.

5. Economics of Vaccine Development and the Role of Incentives

Vaccines confer significant public health and economic benefits. However, economists we spoke with stated that the benefits that vaccines provide are not necessarily commensurate with the return on investment from developing or manufacturing them. Experts attribute the low rate of vaccine investment to market failures (i.e., market interactions that fall short of what would have been socially beneficial), challenging markets for some vaccines, high costs, and risks of development. Experts also stated that uncertainty as to whether a vaccine, once developed, would be recommended for universal use—for example, for all children as opposed to a subset of individuals with certain risk factors—is an additional risk and negatively affects incentives to develop them as it reduces the number of people recommended to be vaccinated.[65] Policymakers have a number of mechanisms to encourage investment in vaccine development. Some of these mechanisms have been used by HHS and the Department of Defense (DOD), including funding for clinical trials, and offering a financial incentive for the successful development of vaccines for COVID-19. However, it is unclear whether policymakers have systematically examined how various tools can be used to incentivize vaccine investment.[66]

As discussed earlier, vaccines have far-reaching, positive effects on public health. In addition to health benefits, such as reducing death and preventing infectious diseases and certain types of cancer, vaccines also produce economic and social benefits. For example, a July 2020 report found that vaccination enhances economic growth due to improved health as well as productivity gains from better physical and cognitive performance.[67]

Vaccines also produce social benefits including improving equity in healthcare, increased life expectancy, and strengthening healthcare resources (see Figure 7). The July 2020 report also found that when infrastructure is developed to administer vaccines, it provides a basis for the provision of other health and social care services, particularly improving maternal and infant mortality in developing regions. Although making projections about the economic and social benefit of vaccines is complex, a 2005 economic article reported that current childhood vaccinations against tetanus, polio, measles, mumps, rubella, hepatitis B, and others, when considered together, create significant economic and social benefits.[68]

---

[65] One expert stated that vaccine entrants who enter a market first will have a larger market share. A 2014 report from McKinsey & Company found that first-to-market entrants into drug markets had a 6 percent market share advantage over later entrants. See M. Cha and F. Yu, "*Pharma's First To Market Advantage*," McKinsey & Company, Sept. 2014.

[66] Several entities have reported on large profits earned by pharmaceutical companies for COVID-19 vaccines. Economists we spoke to stated that, from a benefit-to-cost perspective, it makes sense for policymakers to invest significant funds in vaccine development, manufacturing capacity, and supply chain development to respond to an active pandemic to meet immediate needs and reduce loss of life. However, investing in vaccine technologies and manufacturing capacity in preparation for future pandemics has the potential to reduce costs for vaccines because these capabilities will not have to be developed rapidly or all at once in response to a pandemic event. Similarly, having vaccine candidates under development for pathogens similar to a potential future pandemic pathogen may further reduce development costs as well as the overall price for vaccines. According to one economist we spoke to, investment undertaken at a more measured pace can be cheaper because it does not stretch scarce (and thus expensive) inputs. The economist noted that procuring vaccines under less urgency facilitates entry of multiple competitors and allows a competitive tender process to be organized that favors low prices over speed.

[67] C.M., Rodrigues and S.A., Plotkin, "Impact of Vaccines: Health, Economic and Social Perspectives", *Frontiers in Microbiology*, vol. 11, article 1526 (2020): 1-15.

[68] Current childhood vaccines against diphtheria, tetanus, pertussis, Hib, polio, measles, mumps, rubella, and hepatitis B, when considered together, were estimated to have a benefit cost ration of more than five to one for direct costs and seventeen to one for societal costs. T.A. Lieu, et al., "Overcoming Economic Barriers to the Optimal Use of Vaccines," *Health Affairs*, vol. 24, no. 3 (2005): 667.

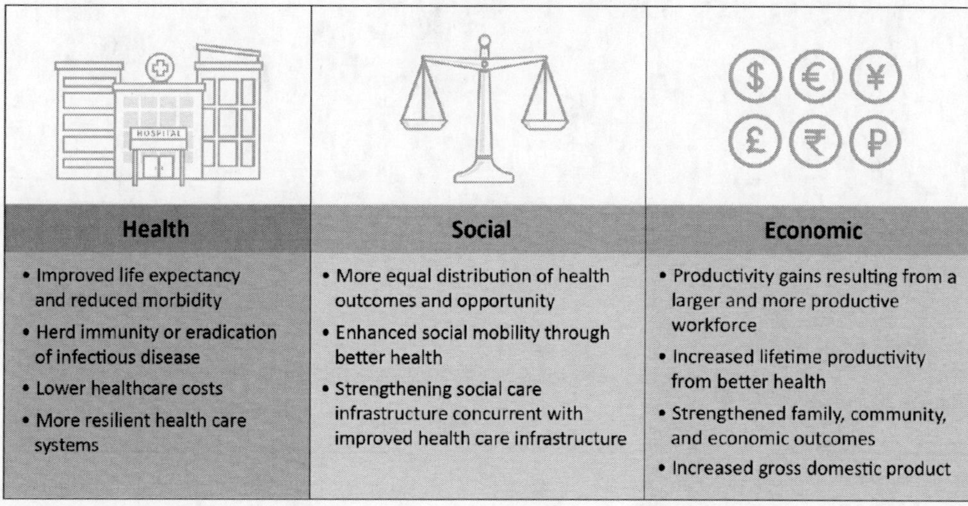

Source: GAO analysis and literature; Vectorfair.com/RealVector/dlyastokiv/stock.adobe.com. | GAO-22-104371.

Figure 7. Types of benefits vaccines provide.

5.1. Market Failures and Other Challenges Result in Fewer Vaccines

Market failures occur when interactions in the market lead to outcomes that fall short of what would have been socially beneficial. In the case of vaccines, market failures lead to vaccine developers producing fewer vaccines than what would have most benefited society, resulting in less protection from infectious diseases. Other challenges that contribute to low vaccine investment include markets that offer no or negative returns on investment, as well as the high cost and low probability of success in developing vaccines.

5.1.1. Positive Externalities

We focused on two specific market failures for vaccine development.[69] The first has to do with the nature of vaccines. Vaccines offer protection to those who are vaccinated as well as providing some level of protection to those who are not by reducing the spread of infectious disease (see Figure 8). In economics, this situation is known as a positive externality. Because this protection is inherent to all vaccines, developers are unable to price their products based on this additional benefit and, as a result, are not rewarded for preventing the spread of the disease. Consequently, developers tend to underinvest in vaccines, even though society would benefit from having more vaccines available.

[69] Other market failures may also explain underinvestment in vaccines. For example, vaccine research is a "public good" as the benefits of scientific and technological advances can extend to others, regardless of who is making the investment, without reducing anyone else's access to the advances. Researchers and developers cannot fully capture the financial benefits of this research and tend to invest less than what the social value of this knowledge is, leading to a situation where government action can improve upon market outcomes. Similarly, one economist we spoke to stated that there is a market failure associated with developers being limited in how much they can charge when a pandemic arises. In this situation, the price is not set by the market but by government purchases, and governments can limit prices, which means that the developers' expected revenue is low.

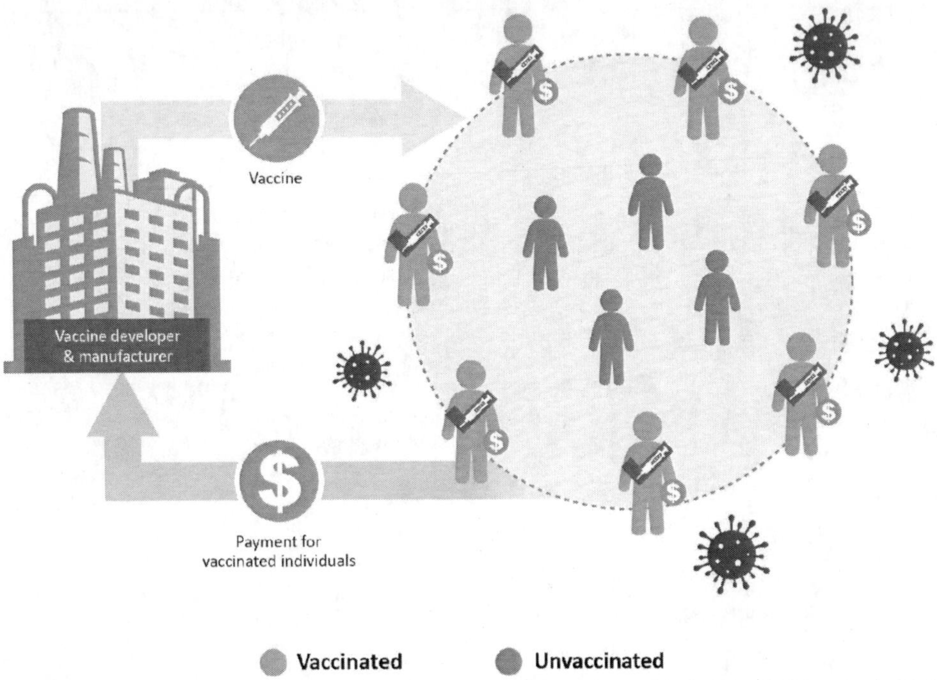

Source: GAO analysis and Maksim/martialred/Nizwa Design/dlyastokiv/stock.adobe.com. | GAO-22-104371.

Note: This figure is not intended to demonstrate vaccination levels commensurate with herd immunity. For more information on herd immunity, see GAO-20-646SP.

Figure 8. Vaccines provide some level of protection for individuals who are unvaccinated.

5.1.2. Imperfect Information

The second type of market failure is caused by the inability of developers to fully account for the disease risk in the price of the product because of imperfect information. Vaccine developers have little information on how likely a particular healthy person is to contract the disease or seek vaccination to avoid becoming sick. However, when an individual contracts the disease, the developer knows that the individual is likely to seek treatment.[70] Developers can use this information to charge much higher prices for therapeutics than vaccines. As a result, the return on investment from vaccines is commonly lower than that of therapeutics. With price incentives skewed away from vaccines and toward therapeutics, vaccines make up only about 1.5 percent of global pharmaceutical sales.[71]

In an example of a disease where workers employed in an industry may be at higher risk of being infected than workers not in that industry, workers in that industry who are at higher risk would be willing to pay a higher price for a vaccine. Workers not in that industry who are less likely to become infected would not be willing to pay as much. However, all workers could become infected and suffer adverse health consequences. If the vaccine's price was too high,

[70] The developer may have some information about the probability distribution of a particular infectious disease in the population. However, an individual's likelihood of contracting the disease depends on many other factors including the individual's behavior and the availability and use of preventive measures, which are unknown to vaccine developers. In the case of therapeutics, the developer can indirectly observe who has contracted the disease by observing who seeks treatment for it.

[71] T.A. Lieu, et al., "Overcoming Economic Barriers." 675.

only workers in the industry would choose to get vaccinated, leaving others unprotected. If a significant portion of the market—in this case, workers not in the industry—chose not to purchase the vaccine because of its price, then the developer would have less incentive to produce the vaccine.

5.1.3. Challenging Markets due to Uncertain Demand

Some markets offer little, no, or negative returns on investment, presenting challenges to vaccine developers. Such markets include vaccines that are developed for infectious diseases that occur only in developing countries, are considered low priority, or may result in future pandemics but are not currently an issue.[72] Experts told us that because of low returns or uncertainty in these markets, developers have little financial incentive to invest in such vaccines. Experts stated that infectious diseases that primarily affect developing countries which have little ability to pay for vaccines provide little incentive for investment. For example, a May 2020 study estimated that the rate of investment return on a portfolio of vaccines for nine infectious diseases identified by the Coalition for Epidemic Preparedness Innovations as high priority, many of which affect developing countries, was negative 61 percent, implying that the private sector is unlikely to address this need without public-sector intervention.[73] In these instances, international organizations, such as the Coalition for Epidemic Preparedness Innovations and philanthropic entities such as the Bill and Melinda Gates Foundation fund research in these infectious diseases.[74] (See textbox for an example of a challenging market).

Challenging Market for Group A *Streptococcus* Vaccine

Group A *Streptococcus* causes, among other things, strep throat, scarlet fever, and rheumatic fever. Currently, there is no vaccine, even though about 500,000 people worldwide die due to Group A *Streptococcus* infections annually, including between 1,100 and 1,600 deaths in the U.S. The pathogen is one of the top 10 causes of death from infectious diseases worldwide and is considered endemic in lower income areas of the globe. While NIAID supports research to develop a vaccine with several candidates in various phases of development, one expert told us that to produce a Group A *Streptococcus* vaccine at a price that could be purchased in lower income countries (less than $2 per dose), a business case analysis anticipated that total sales would be between $200 million and $300 million annually, which is not sufficient to incentivize developers to invest in such a vaccine.

Source: GAO analysis of information from literature and an expert meeting. | GAO-22-104371.

Further, infectious diseases that are considered lower priority can have limited market potential. For example, one expert told us that Epstein-Barr virus, which can cause mononucleosis rarely results in death, and therefore is considered a low priority for vaccine

[72] NIAID officials stated that it conducts research to develop vaccine candidates that is not subject to the same market challenges that private sector developer's face.

[73] The study estimated a rate of return for a portfolio of 141 trial vaccines to address infectious diseases from the Coalition for Epidemic Preparedness Innovations' Priority Pathogen List including: Chikungunya, MERS, SARS, Marburg, Rift Valley Fever, Lassa, Nipah, Crimean-Congo hemorrhagic Fever, and Zika virus. See J. Vu et al., "Financing Vaccines for Global Health Security," *National Bureau of Economic Research*, May 2020.

[74] The Bill and Melinda Gates Foundation is a philanthropic organization that funds global health efforts. A priority area for the Gates Foundation is to develop effective and affordable vaccines, medicines, and other health tools.

development.[75] Another expert stated that companies would be more encouraged to develop a vaccine for a larger or more defined population, such as children or people over the age of 65. For example, CDC recommends that all individuals 50 years or older should receive the vaccine for shingles.

Vaccines for pathogens that may cause future pandemics but are not currently a significant issue also face uncertain market demand. Because developers receive no return on their investment unless a pandemic occurs, there is little incentive to invest in these vaccines. Further, even if a pandemic event does occur, the demand for a vaccine may still be uncertain. If an outbreak quickly dissipates, the market for the vaccine may be limited because individuals may not seek a vaccine and governments may be unlikely to purchase it. For example, a May 2020 report found that the SARS and Zika epidemics ended before vaccine development was complete, and federal funding agencies reallocated funds that had been committed to vaccine development for these diseases, leaving manufacturers with financial losses and setting back other vaccine development programs.[76] The article also found that, even with successful development and licensure, commercial markets still may not sustain multiple vaccines for which relatively few doses may need to be manufactured. One expert said that the potentially low number of doses to be manufactured increases the uncertainty of the potential return on investment and therefore risk for vaccine developers, which creates an even lower incentive to develop a vaccine during any subsequent infectious disease outbreak and hinders preparation for future pandemics.

Another expert told us that vaccines placed on vaccine schedules—the lists of vaccines recommended for children and adults in the U.S.—and recommended for universal use generally have large markets and are often covered by insurance. However, the lack of assurance that a vaccine would be considered for inclusion on the vaccine schedule can also hinder investment. For example, experts told us that, following review by the CDC's Advisory Committee on Immunization Practices, a vaccine for meningitis B was not recommended for universal use.[77] This recommendation effectively reduced the number of people who would be receiving the vaccine and, therefore, the return on investment.[78]

---

[75] According to CDC, Epstein-Barr virus is one of the most common human viruses in the world. It spreads primarily through saliva. Epstein-Barr virus can cause infectious mononucleosis, also called mono, and other illnesses. Most people will get infected with Epstein-Barr virus in their lifetime and will not have any symptoms. Mono caused by Epstein-Barr virus is most common among teens and adults. Other infections sometimes go along with mononucleosis, which may need to be treated with antibiotics. NIH noted that its researchers have developed vaccine candidates for Epstein-Barr virus. For more information see https://www.cdc.gov/epstein-barr/index.html.

[76] See N. Lurie, et al., "Developing COVID-19 Vaccines at Pandemic Speed," *The New England Journal of Medicine*, vol. 382, no. 21 (2020): 1969.

[77] CDC's Advisory Committee on Immunization Practices is comprised of medical and public health experts who make recommendations on the use of vaccines in the civilian population of the U.S. Its recommendations serve as public health guidance for safe use of vaccines and other related products. If adopted by the CDC Director, CDC's Advisory Committee on Immunization Practices' recommendations are published as official HHS/CDC recommendations in the *Morbidity and Mortality Weekly Report*.

[78] According to CDC, in 2019, there were about 371 total cases of meningococcal disease reported. CDC recommends that adolescents between the ages of 16 and 23 consult with their clinician to determine whether they should receive the vaccine.

5.1.4. High Development Costs and Low Probability of Success

Two additional challenges further contribute to the low return on investment: high costs and low probability of success.[79]

- *High costs.* According to a 2018 study, vaccine development from discovery to licensure can cost billions of dollars and can take over 10 years to complete.[80]
- *Low probability of success.* The same study found that on average, vaccine candidates have a 94 percent chance of failure.

5.2. Mechanisms to Incentivize Vaccine Development

Several mechanisms can potentially be used to incentivize additional investment in vaccines. These mechanisms either subsidize some portion of the development process or provide rewards for successful development. Given the market failure associated with vaccines, it is unlikely private investments will sufficiently support the development of all socially beneficial vaccines. Policymakers could fill this gap by taking actions to incentivize investment in new vaccines to better address infectious disease; improve overall societal, health, and economic outcomes; and prepare for future pandemics. To do so, policymakers need a combination of tools to incentivize investment. HHS has leveraged some mechanisms to incentivize vaccine investment, most recently to respond to the COVID-19 pandemic.

5.2.1. Incentives for Vaccine Investment

We identified several mechanisms with the potential to incentivize vaccine investment. According to experts, policymakers need access to a wide range of mechanisms, because different mechanisms are better for some infectious disease scenarios than for others.

Policymaker interventions can be broadly classified into push and pull incentives (see Table 4). Push incentives subsidize the costs of developing a product or general research in vaccines by providing funding for grants to academic institutions, tax credits for R&D, and low or no cost manufacturing. Pull incentives increase revenue once a vaccine receives authorization or licensure. This can be done, for example, by guaranteeing to purchase a certain quantity or promising a cash prize for successful authorization or licensure. Other examples of pull incentives include patent extensions and priority review vouchers (which can be sold for revenue or used for faster review on a future drug or biologic application).

Experts we spoke to stated that different incentives work better for developing vaccines for some infectious diseases than for others. For example, push incentives such as grants, may be beneficial because they can encourage the use of a particular technology, such as certain vaccine platforms. However, grants do not necessarily result in the development of a vaccine. Tax incentives may be useful in incentivizing research into a particular area, but they do not work for developers without tax liability. Similarly, offering unused manufacturing capacity, public or private, for no or low cost to vaccine developers to produce vaccine candidates for

---

[79] One economist we spoke to stated that some factors impair how lucrative a market is, but they aren't market failures if they don't generate a wedge between a firm's commercial incentives and social benefits. Factors, such as high cost and low probability of success are not market failures, but they may serve to amplify them.

[80] D. Gouglas et al., "Estimating the Cost of Vaccine Development against Epidemic Infectious Diseases: a Cost Minimisation Study," *The Lancet Global Health*, vol. 6, no. 12 (2018): pp. e1386-e1396.

clinical trials can encourage developers to proceed with testing of candidates that they might not have been able to otherwise. This mechanism also has the benefit of keeping manufacturing capacity "warm" (i.e., available and ready to be used) and personnel at these facilities trained so they can quickly respond to potential pandemics. One expert told us that the cost to move a vaccine candidate through phase 2 clinical trials is about $50 million, with one third of that cost spent on manufacturing vaccines in support of the trials.

Table 4. Potential mechanisms to incentivize vaccine development

Mechanism	Definition	Opportunities	Challenges
Grants (push)	Financial assistance that may cover some or all of the costs associated with vaccine R&D	• Support basic research that cannot be incentivized with pull funding	• Do not guarantee development of a product
Tax incentives (push)	Reductions in tax liabilities to defray some of the costs of R&D	• Support basic research that cannot be incentivized with pull funding	• Do not guarantee development of a product • Can be very costly • Beneficial only if the developer has a tax liability
Advanced purchase commitments (pull)	Agreements to purchase vaccines in the future, after they are fully developed	• Product can be stockpiled for future use or used to vaccinate people immediately, or both • In many cases, paid only if a product is developed and receives emergency use authorization or licensure • Developers can be incentivized to select the most promising products	• Can be expensive, especially if several products are incentivized
Subsidizing manufacturing capacity (push)	Allowing excess manufacturing capacity to be used to manufacture vaccines for clinical trials at low or no cost	• Developers can be incentivized to take vaccines to clinical trials due to lower manufacturing costs • Excess capacity can be used to respond to future infectious disease outbreaks	• May be expensive to maintain facilities for manufacturing • May not ensure sufficient capacity to respond to all potential infectious diseases scenarios
Prizes (pull)	Reward for receiving authorization or licensure of a vaccine product	• Product can be stockpiled for future use, used to vaccinate people immediately, or both • In many cases, paid only if a product is developed and receives emergency use authorization or licensure	• Do not reduce the cost of R&D • Would have to be sufficiently large to induce investment
Patent extensions (pull)	An extension on a patent that exceeds the usual time limits	• Greater protection from competition and a longer period to benefit from higher prices may encourage greater innovation	• Patents can result in higher prices, making the vaccine too expensive for some patients or governments
Priority review voucher (pull)	Award for the development of drugs and biologics, including vaccines, for tropical diseases, rare pediatric diseases, and material threat medical countermeasures, which can be sold or redeemed for faster review of a future application.	• Potential for additional revenue could provide an incentive to develop vaccines for tropical diseases, rare pediatric diseases, and medical countermeasures	• The financial reward—that is, the amount of revenue earned from sale of a priority review voucher—could decline if more vouchers are awarded and available for sale

Source: GAO. | GAO-22-104371.

Pull incentives also have opportunities and challenges. Advanced market commitments are most beneficial when a vaccine will be administered to a large number of people, such as the entire population of a country. However, when a vaccine will be used by a smaller number of people, such as during a regional epidemic, the number of doses of the vaccine to be purchased may not be enough of an incentive. In these instances, a prize may be more appropriate. One benefit of pull incentives is that, in many cases, developers are only paid if a vaccine is eventually produced and is authorized for emergency use or licensed.

Pull funding is intended to supplement, not replace, push funding. For example, pull incentives may not incentivize sufficient at-risk manufacturing capacity for developers, leading to fewer vaccines than would have been beneficial from society's perspective. A combination of pull and push funding may be needed to assure sufficient vaccine supply can be manufactured. Additionally, a combination of push and pull incentives may allow for program costs to be lower than with pull incentives alone, while avoiding some of the inefficiency created by push incentives.

Experts we spoke to stated that the best mechanisms to incentivize vaccine investment would:

- Reward the development of new vaccines
- Keep prices low and thus allow vaccines to be accessible to as many people as possible
- Incentivize several pharmaceutical companies to produce vaccines by allowing benefits from incentives to be available to all pharmaceutical companies, not just some
- Be simple
- Be transparent to operate
- Develop a capacity that allows for better responses to endemic infectious diseases as well as prepare for potential future epidemics or pandemics

5.2.2. Federal Use of Vaccine Incentives

Some HHS programs have incentivized the development of vaccines. For example, the priority review voucher programs are intended to encourage development of drugs or biologics for tropical diseases, rare pediatric diseases, and material threat medical countermeasures.[81] If an application meets the criteria for one of the priority review voucher programs, FDA can award a voucher upon approval of the application.[82] These vouchers may be redeemed with submission of a future application, shortening FDA's targeted review time from the standard 10-month review to 6 months.[83] The vouchers may also be sold or transferred to another company, which may then choose to use it or similarly sell or transfer it.

---

[81] See 21 U.S.C. §§ 360n (tropical diseases), 360ff (rare pediatric diseases), and 360bbb-4a (material threat medical countermeasures). Material threat medical countermeasures are drugs and biologics used to prevent or treat harm from any chemical, biological, radiological, and nuclear agent identified as a material threat.

[82] From 2009 through 2019, FDA awarded 31 priority review vouchers to drug sponsors. Of those, available data indicate that 17 were subsequently sold to another drug sponsor, providing revenue to the sponsor selling the priority review voucher. See GAO, *Drug Development, FDA's Priority Review Voucher Programs*, GAO-20-251 (Washington, D.C.: Jan. 31. 2020).

[83] For new drugs that do not contain a new molecular entity, FDA's goal is to review and act on 90 percent of standard applications within 10 months and 90 percent of priority applications within 6 months of receipt. For original biologics and new drugs that contain a new molecular entity, FDA's goal is to review and act on 90 percent of standard applications within 10 months following a 60-day filing period (a total of 12 months from receipt). Priority review reduces this time to 6 months following the filing period (a total of 8 months from receipt).

A partnership between HHS and DOD was established in May 2020 to accelerate the development, manufacturing, and distribution of COVID-19 vaccines.[84] This was accomplished through the award of contracts and other transaction agreements to six vaccine companies for different types of activities, including clinical development and manufacturing activities or the purchase of COVID-19 vaccine doses. These awards were made, according to HHS and DOD officials, in anticipation that some of the vaccine candidates would subsequently receive authorization or licensure. By providing significant up-front funding to several of the companies, the government took on some financial risk, which enabled these companies to accelerate vaccine development and production.[85] As of October 2021, three COVID-19 vaccines that participated in the federal partnership were available in the U.S.

While HHS has used some mechanisms intended to incentivize development, it is not clear that it has examined how or under what circumstances different incentives can be most effective. In June 2021, BARDA officials told us that they were not aware of any HHS effort to examine market incentives for vaccines.

Further, experts we spoke with expressed concern that, if policymakers do not have the authority to implement appropriate incentives, they will be limited in their ability to help facilitate investment in new vaccines. If officials lack the authority to use different mechanisms, it may result in reduced preparation for future pandemics and weakened efforts to address infectious disease.

5.3. Policy Options That May Help Address Economic Challenges to Vaccine Development

We identified three policy options for policymakers that may help address economic challenges with incentivizing vaccine development. As mentioned previously, policymakers include Congress, federal agencies, state and local governments, academic and research institutions, and industry.

Policymakers could conduct a systematic assessment of the various mechanisms to incentivize vaccine development to determine which incentives could work best for infectious diseases identified as high priority, as discussed in section 2. Policymakers could also examine the authorities necessary to use these mechanisms and, to the extent that agencies lack such authority, take steps to obtain or provide it.

---

[84] This partnership was formerly known as Operation Warp Speed, but since May 2021 it is has been called the HHS-DOD COVID-19 Countermeasures Acceleration Group.

[85] See, *COVID-19: Efforts to Increase Vaccine Availability and Perspectives on Implementation,* GAO-21-443, (Washington, D.C.: Apr. 14. 2021).

Policy options that may help address economic challenges related to vaccine development

Policy option	Opportunities	Considerations
Evaluate factors that discourage vaccine investment *Policymakers could collaborate across sectors, such as government, academia and industry, to conduct a systematic evaluation of factors that discourage developers from investing in new vaccines.* This could help address the challenges we identified related to market failures, challenging markets, high costs, and low probability of success.	A clear understanding of the range of factors discouraging vaccine investment would provide the basis for effectively addressing those factors.	Collaboration between policymakers and other stakeholders to obtain all relevant viewpoints can be time-consuming and it may be hard to reach a consensus.
Evaluate mechanisms for increasing vaccine investment	Economic and societal costs from infectious diseases could be reduced.	Evidence on some mechanisms for incentivizing vaccine investment may not be available or sufficient to make determinations on the effectiveness of some mechanisms.
Policymakers could consider conducting a systematic evaluation of the effectiveness of different mechanisms to incentivize vaccine investment and determine what circumstances or time frames may make some mechanisms more or less useful. For example, policymakers could evaluate the effectiveness of mechanisms used to incentivize COVID-19 vaccine development. This could help identify when mechanisms to incentivize vaccine development is likely to be most successful.		
Evaluate authority *Policymakers could consider determining whether HHS, DOD, or other relevant agencies have the authority to use these mechanisms to incentivize vaccine development. For any identified gaps in authority, policymakers could consider seeking or providing such authority.* This could help address the challenges we identified related to incentivizing vaccine development.	Identifying and addressing any gaps in authority could allow policymakers to more effectively address the economic challenges to vaccine development.	Granting additional authority may not result in increased use of these mechanisms to address economic challenges. Even if incentives are used more widely, additional vaccines may not be produced due to technical and other challenges. Expanded use of incentives is likely to require more resources or a shifting of resources from other areas.

Source: GAO. | GAO-22-104371.

6. Agency and Expert Comments

We provided a draft of this chapter to DOD and HHS for review. DOD concurred without comment with the draft report provided by GAO. HHS provided technical comments on the draft report, which we incorporated as appropriate. Nine participants from our expert meeting also reviewed a draft of this chapter; we incorporated their technical comments as appropriate.

Karen L. Howard, PhD
Director,
Science, Technology Assessment, and Analytics

Appendix I: Objectives, Scope, and Methodology

Objectives

This chapter identifies and discusses:

1. technologies and approaches for vaccine research and development (R&D) and challenges that affect their use,
2. technologies and approaches for vaccine testing and challenges that affect their use,
3. technologies and approaches for vaccine manufacturing and challenges that affect their use, and
4. economic factors that affect vaccine investment and preparedness for future pandemics

Scope and Methodology

To address the first three of our objectives, we assessed available and developing technologies and approaches that vaccine developers could use for R&D, testing, and manufacturing of vaccines. For the fourth objective, we assessed available and potential mechanisms for incentivizing vaccine development. To do so, we reviewed scientific literature describing current and developing tools; interviewed experts from government, academia, the nonprofit sector, and the research industry; and collaborated with the National Academies of Sciences, Engineering, and Medicine to convene a 3-day expert meeting to discuss the objective topics.

Limitations to Scope

We focused our assessment on U.S. vaccine development. However, with pandemics posing a global threat, the policy options we identified include actions U.S. policymakers can take alongside international partners. The technologies and approaches to vaccine development, testing, and manufacturing discussed in this chaptert are not an exhaustive list of all possible methods. We selected technologies and approaches we identified as most promising from our review of the literature and from discussions with stakeholders. We do not discuss technologies and approaches related to how vaccines are distributed after they have been manufactured, as that was not within our scope. The list of mechanisms for incentivizing vaccine investment are also not exhaustive of all possible methods.

Literature Search

In the course of our work we conducted literature searches with ProQuest using search terms including "vaccine technology," "clinical trials," "vaccine manufacturing," and "vaccine economics," among a wide selection of keywords relevant to vaccine research and development. We conducted a broad search of materials published within the last 7 years, including scholarly articles and government reports. We used the results of our literature review to address our objectives as well as identify experts to interview and to participate in our expert meeting.

Interviews

We interviewed stakeholders and experts with a diverse set of perspectives on the science, administration, and economics of vaccine development.

To address technologies, and approaches for vaccine R&D, we discussed developments in vaccine platforms and ways researchers can identify and characterize pathogens and antigens. To address vaccine testing we discussed the design and purpose of preclinical testing, clinical trials, and ways vaccine testing could be conducted more efficiently and effectively. For manufacturing, we discussed emerging vaccine manufacturing technologies and infrastructure approaches to support greater flexibility, productivity, and capacity. To address the economic landscape of vaccine development, we discussed the market for vaccines as compared to other pharmaceutical products, the development costs and time requirements of vaccines relevant to other products, how these factors influence the choices made by pharmaceutical companies in deciding whether to develop vaccines, and government efforts to encourage vaccine development. For all relevant objectives, we spoke with stakeholders about key issues affecting the adoption of the technologies and approaches we identified.

Expert Meeting

To address all of our objectives, we held an expert meeting from January 25-28, 2021. This meeting was held in collaboration with the National Academies of Sciences, Engineering, and Medicine and was divided into six sessions, each moderated by two or three representatives from GAO.[86] The topics of each session were: (1) Technologies and Approaches for Research and Development, (2) Technologies and Approaches for Vaccine Manufacturing, (3) Technologies and Approaches for Preclinical Studies and Clinical Trials, (4) Pathogen Scenarios, (5) Economic Factors that Impact Vaccine Investment, (6) Lessons Learned and Next Steps.

Meeting participants were selected if they had expertise either broadly or specifically in at least one area related to our four objectives. We provided the National Academies of Sciences, Engineering, and Medicine with descriptions of the expertise needed by expert meeting participants. From this information, the National Academies provided an initial list of experts to potentially participate in the expert meeting. We reviewed the list and provided an additional list of experts based on our review of the literature. In addition to evaluating experts on the basis of their expertise, we evaluated them for any conflicts of interest. A conflict of interest was considered to be any current financial or other interest, such as an organizational position,

---

[86] This meeting of experts was planned and convened with the assistance of the National Academies of Sciences, Engineering, and Medicine to better ensure that a breadth of expertise was brought to bear in its preparation. However all final decisions regarding meeting substance and expert participation were made by GAO.

that might conflict with the service of an individual because it could (1) impair objectivity or (2) create an unfair competitive advantage for any person or organization. Of the 22 experts, some were affiliated with companies, government, or research-funding entities. We took these affiliations into consideration as potential conflicts of interest when conducting our analysis and preparing our report. We determined that these experts' relationships did not account for any inappropriate biases in our reporting. We did not suggest policy options that we have reason to believe will improperly promote or adversely affect any company. The comments of these experts generally represented the views of the experts themselves and not the agency, university, or company with which they were affiliated, and are not generalizable to the views of others in the field. Appendix V provides additional information on the meeting participants.

Policy Options

Based on our research, we developed a series of policy options. Policy options are not formal recommendations for federal agencies, or matters for congressional consideration, but they are intended to represent possible options policymakers can take to address a policy objective.[87] For each policy option we discussed potential opportunities and considerations. These are not listed in any particular order within each section, nor are they inclusive of all possible policy options.

Based on the goal of improving U.S. vaccine development capabilities, we decided on an objective designed to identify options that could help improve capabilities for developing vaccines more effectively and efficiently, including during emergencies. We limited policy options to those that fit the objective and fell within the report scope.

To develop the policy options, we compiled a list of possible options (19 in total) over the course of our work based on our review of the scientific and economic literature, interviews with experts, and our vaccine development expert meeting. We analyzed these options and removed ideas that were either redundant, not feasible to implement, or did not fit into the overall scope of our work. We then analyzed each policy option by identifying potential benefits and considerations of implementing them. The policy options and analyses were supported by documentary and testimonial evidence.

We conducted our work from June 2020 to November 2021 in accordance with all sections of GAO's Quality Assurance Framework that are relevant to technology assessments. The framework requires that we plan and perform the engagement to obtain sufficient and appropriate evidence to meet our stated objectives and to discuss any limitations to our work. We believe that the information and data obtained, and the analysis conducted, provide a reasonable basis for any findings and conclusions in this chapter.

Appendix II: Research and Development Technologies and Approaches

We identified four technologies and approaches that may improve vaccine research and development (R&D). This appendix provides three summaries of these technologies and approaches. Additionally, this appendix provides a summary of monoclonal antibodies, which are emerging as an important approach to preventing infectious disease.

---

[87] Policymakers is a broad term including, for example, Congress, federal agencies, state and local governments, academic and research institutions, and industry.

These summaries are based on documents we reviewed and interviews we conducted. Specifically, we reviewed scientific literature describing current and developing tools, interviewed experts from government, academia, the nonprofit sector, and industry, and collaborated with the National Academies of Sciences, Engineering, and Medicine to convene a 3-day expert meeting to discuss these technologies and approaches. Each summary includes information on what the technology or approach is, its maturity, and how it works.

Omics and Reverse Vaccinology

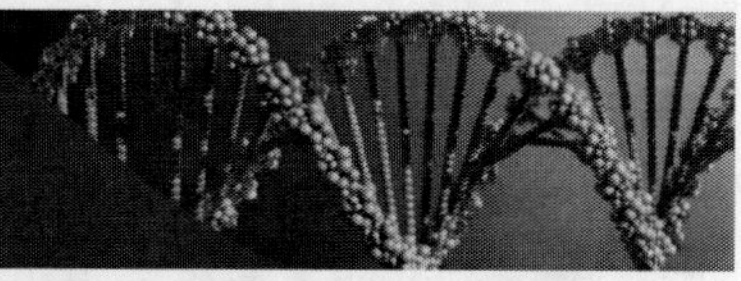

By integrating information from multiple fields of biology—collectively known as omics and including fields such as genomics and proteomics— researchers can better understand how pathogens cause illness and how different people respond to immunization. Reverse vaccinology applies omics approaches to identify potential vaccine candidates more effectively and shorten development time. In the future, such approaches could lead to a new generation of vaccines that are safer, generate a stronger immune response, and perhaps can even be personalized for vulnerable populations.

What is it?

Omics refers to the combined study of multiple areas of biology whose names end with "omics." The omics commonly used in vaccine development include genomics, transcriptomics, proteomics, and metabolomics (table 1).

Table 1: Some omic fields used in vaccine development

Field	Description
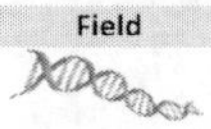 Genomics	Genomics is the study of the genome—the complete set of genetic instructions to create an organism. Studying the genome is the first step in reverse vaccinology and allows researchers to understand what information exists and, therefore, what could happen inside microbial organisms or human cells.
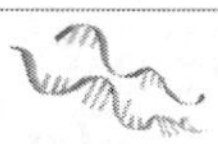 Transcriptomics	Transcriptomics is the study of RNA. RNA carries genetic instructions on what proteins should be made by the cells. Studying RNA allows researchers to understand what genetic information is being used and, therefore, what appears to be happening inside microbial organisms or human cells.
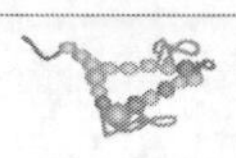 Proteomics	Proteomics is the study of the proteins made within a microbial organism or human cell. Proteins play leading roles in cellular structure, facilitating metabolic reactions, and responding to stimuli, among other things. Studying proteins allows researchers to more directly observe cellular processes.
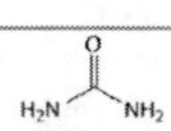 Metabolomics	Metabolomics is the study of small molecules, commonly known as metabolites, made within a microbial organism or human cell. Metabolites can be found in biological samples, such as saliva, blood, and urine. Studying metabolites allows researchers to understand what is or has happened within a microbial organism or human cell.

Source: GAO analysis and fizzgig/ logos2012/stock.adobe.com. | GAO-22-104371

Reverse vaccinology analyzes a pathogen's genome to identify the individual genes that are most likely to provide instructions for proteins that stimulate an immune response (antigens). This approach differs from traditional methods where the first step is to grow pathogens in a lab and characterize multiple antigens over many iterations.

How mature is it?

Individually, these omics fields are not new. However, recent advances in technology have allowed for integrated analyses that apply a combination of omics across large datasets, resulting in much faster development of vaccines, including those for COVID-19 (10 months to develop) and Ebola virus (5 years).

How does it work?

Within a cell, information generally flows from the genome (DNA) to proteins and metabolites via RNA. Researchers can use omics and reverse vaccinology to identify antigens faster and compare antigens to identify similarities across different types of pathogens. Using omics, researchers can also better understand human immune responses, including how specific populations would likely respond to a particular vaccine. Figure 1 shows how they were used for COVID-19.

Figure 1: Researchers used omics and reverse vaccinology to develop COVID-19 vaccines and prioritize vaccine recipients more quickly and effectively.

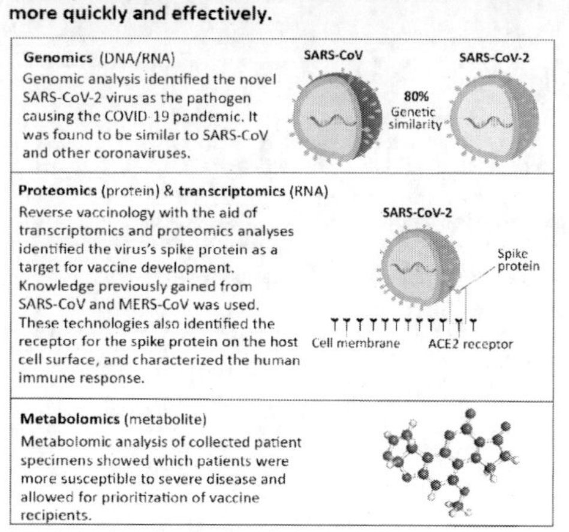

Source: GAO analysis and gamelover/fizzgig/stock.adobe.com. | GAO-22-104371

Source: Design Cells/stock.adobe.com (header). | GAO-22-104371

Next-Generation Vaccine Platforms

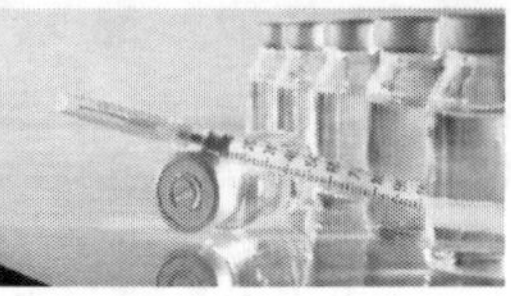

Next-generation platforms allow vaccines to be developed based on the pathogen's genetic information, instead of first growing the pathogen (e.g., a virus) in the lab. As a result, next-generation platforms are highly adaptable, and can potentially accelerate vaccine development.

What is it?

Next-generation platforms use an interchangeable system of components, allowing vaccines to be developed in a plug-and-play fashion. Next-generation platforms use a carrier to deliver genetic instructions for an antigen—the substance that stimulates an immune response—into the body. Platform based approaches can be scaled up more rapidly, potentially accelerating vaccine development, and can target multiple pathogens (table 1).

Table 1: Examples of next-generation vaccine platforms

Vaccine Platform	Description
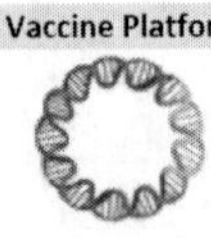 DNA	DNA vaccines use synthetic DNA coding for an antigen. The synthetic DNA is inserted into a DNA vector, which delivers it into the body. The body's cells then convert the DNA to mRNA which, in turn, is converted into the antigen.
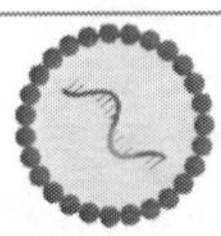 mRNA	Messenger RNA (mRNA) vaccines are encapsulated genetic instructions that allow the body's cells to directly produce the antigen and stimulate the immune system. Since mRNA is naturally unstable, it is first stabilized and then packaged in a carrier molecule. Lipid nanoparticles—tiny spherical capsules made of lipids—are the most frequently used carriers.
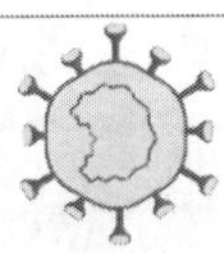 Viral vector	Viral vector vaccines use other viruses—genetically engineered to remove their disease-causing aspects—as the carrier to deliver the DNA code for an antigen into the body. Viral vector vaccines that reproduce themselves result in more antigen production and thus stimulate a stronger immune response.

Source: GAO analysis. | GAO-22-104371

How mature is it?

Next-generation vaccine platforms are a recent development. As of October 2021, the Food and Drug Administration (FDA) had licensed two next-generation viral vector platform vaccines for use in humans—one for dengue and one for Ebola, and had issued an emergency use authorization (EUA) for a viral vector COVID-19 vaccine. FDA had also issued EUAs for two mRNA vaccines for COVID-19, and one of these vaccines had also been licensed for certain individuals. FDA had not licensed any DNA vaccines for use in humans, but had licensed one vaccine for use in animals.

How does it work?

DNA vaccine platforms contain genetic instructions that induce the cell to make the antigen. The gene encoding the antigen is plugged into a DNA vector to make the vaccine. mRNA vaccine platforms contain synthesized mRNA encoding the vaccine antigen, which is then encapsulated in a lipid capsule to make the vaccine. Viral vector vaccine platforms contain copies of genes encoding the vaccine antigen. The gene is plugged into a viral vector to make the vaccine (fig. 1).

Figure 1: Vaccine platforms

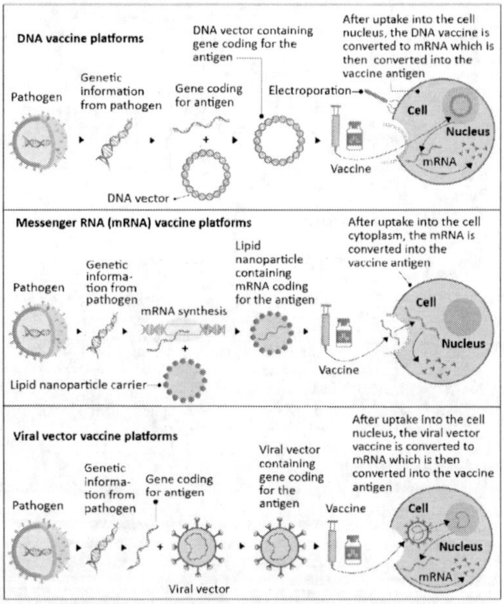

Source: GAO (analysis); Adaption of images depicting vaccine technologies with permission from Springer Nature: *Nature* ("The Race for Coronavirus Vaccines: A Graphical Guide,"Ewin Callaway) © 2020 and MariLee/fizzgig/Sir.Vector/stock.adobe.com. | GAO-22-104371

Source: Davizro Photography/stock.adobe.com (header). | GAO-22-104371

Nontraditional Methods of Vaccination

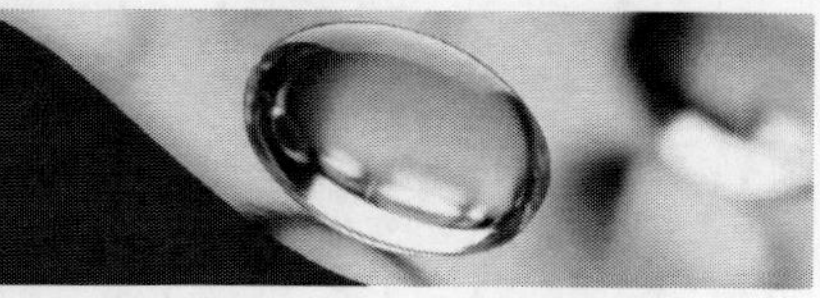

Most vaccines are currently administered by injection under the skin or into the muscle. However, injection can be associated with pain and cause anxiety for some individuals. Nontraditional ways of delivering vaccines such as via a nasal spray offer the potential for increased public uptake, better immune responses, and perhaps lower dosages.

What is it?

Three nontraditional approaches for administering vaccines may address challenges associated with traditional injections. *Dermal* vaccines are delivered by microscopic needle patches through the upper layer of the skin. *Nasal* vaccines are administered via either a mist or drops in the nasal cavity. *Oral* vaccines are delivered in the form of a pill or liquid (table 1).

All three approaches can eliminate the pain and anxiety that some people associate with traditional injections. Other potential benefits include decreasing the requirement for cold storage and reducing the need for trained personnel and injection supplies; these benefits may help increase vaccination rates. Nontraditional approaches can also potentially result in an improved immune response—the production of antibodies and activation of cells to fight a virus or some other microorganism that can cause disease.

Table 1: Potential opportunities and challenges of nontraditional vaccination methods

Nontraditional vaccination methods	Potential opportunities	Potential challenges
Dermal	• Pain free • Lower dosages • Easy to administer • Does not require cold storage	• Device development for simple, reliable, and reproducible delivery of vaccines.
Nasal	• Pain free • Cost effective • Easy to administer • Fewer supplies	• Vaccine may not remain in the nasal passage long enough for effective absorption.
Oral delivery	• Pain free • Cost effective • Easy to administer • Fewer supplies	• Must be formulated to protect against degradation in the stomach.

Source: GAO analysis. | GAO-22-104371

How mature is it?

The Food and Drug Administration (FDA) licensed the first oral vaccine in the 1960s for polio; only a few other oral vaccines have been licensed since then. More recently, dermal and nasal vaccines have been developed for seasonal influenza. Although many traditional (injected) vaccines have been successfully developed and administered over the last century, the number of vaccines available with nontraditional options of administering remains low. Researchers continue to focus on trying to develop nontraditional routes of vaccination.

How does it work?

Injected vaccines elicit a systemic immune response in the body's fluids, such as the blood. In contrast, vaccines administered via dermal, nasal, and oral routes produce an immune response in both the blood and in the mucous membranes—the protective lining in areas such as the mouth, nasal passages, and intestines. During this kind of immune response, the cells and antibodies in the mucous membranes block or destroy the invading microorganisms (also known as pathogens). The immune response is helpful in blocking the early stages of infection since most pathogens infect the body through the mucous membranes.

Dermal delivery uses patches covered with hundreds of microscopic needles made from sugar mixed with a vaccine, which dissolve into the skin after penetrating through its upper layer. For nasal delivery, cells in the nasal cavity encounter vaccines, stimulating an immune response in the respiratory tract that blocks a pathogen from entering the body. Oral vaccines are ideally absorbed in the intestines, which contain 70 to 80 percent of all antibody-producing cells in the body (fig. 1).

Figure 1: Nontraditional vaccination methods

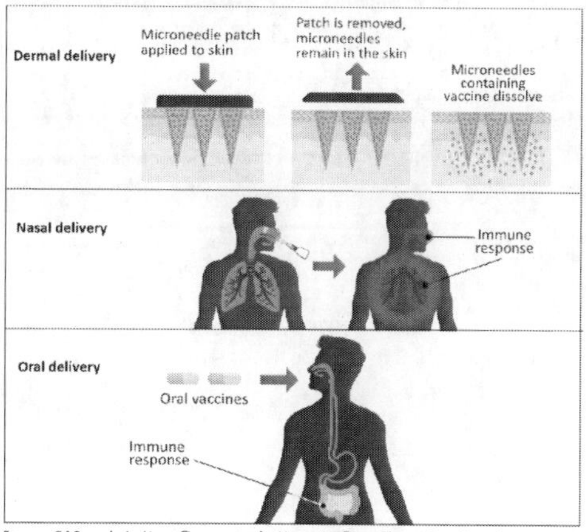

Source: GAO analysis, Harro© magazine by Harro Hoefliger, Bharat Biotech, and Melazerg/Pavlo Plakhotia/stock.adobe.com. | GAO-22-104371

Source: stevem/stock.adobe.com (header). | GAO-22-104371

Monoclonal antibodies

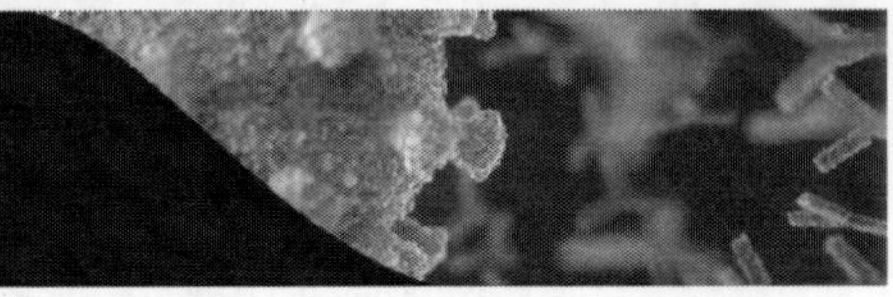

Monoclonal antibodies are not vaccines. They are laboratory-made proteins that mimic the human immune system's ability to fight off pathogens. These proteins can be developed quickly in response to potential pandemics and used to provide short-term protection against infectious diseases—either as a treatment or as a preventative before someone is infected. They can also be used to complement the human immune system to bolster the protective response in immunocompromised individuals, such as organ transplant recipients.

What is it?

Monoclonal antibodies are laboratory-produced versions of specific proteins that have been isolated from the antibodies naturally produced by the human immune system to respond to and neutralize invading pathogens. Monoclonal antibodies are emerging as an important approach to preventing infections. A recent study showed that monoclonal antibodies can be effective at preventing malaria, an infectious disease that currently lacks an effective vaccine. An August 2021 study reported that monoclonal antibodies reduced the risk of unvaccinated or immunocompromised people developing any COVID-19 symptoms by 77 percent.

Monoclonal antibodies are different from vaccines in that they do not stimulate long-term protection (table 1).

Table 1: Monoclonal antibodies and vaccines work differently to protect against disease.

	Monoclonal antibodies	Vaccines
What is it?	A protein that binds to a pathogen to mitigate effects of an infection	A modified pathogen or a part of a pathogen that triggers the immune system
How is it used?	To provide treatment or short-term protection to avoid infection	To stimulate the immune system to fight against a pathogen
How quickly does it work?	Immediately	Several weeks after all required doses are given
How long does the protection last?	Weeks to months	Years to lifetime (some vaccines require boosters)

Source: GAO analysis. | GAO-22-104371

How mature is it?

Since their introduction in 1975, monoclonal antibodies have been developed primarily for use as therapeutics against non-infectious diseases, such as cancer. Of more than 100 monoclonal antibodies licensed by the FDA, only seven are used to prevent or treat infectious diseases. The high cost is a limiting factor, as manufacturing is complex, expensive, and requires specialized personnel.

How does it work?

Monoclonal antibodies mimic the immune system by binding directly to antigens, the components of a pathogen that stimulate an immune response, preventing them from initiating the infection cycle. During the COVID-19 pandemic, monoclonal antibody products were developed as therapeutics to treat SARS-CoV-2 (the virus that causes COVID-19). As of October 2021, there were four authorized monoclonal antibody treatments for COVID-19. Clinical trial data have also shown that monoclonal antibodies may be effective for pre-exposure prevention of COVID-19, but they have not been authorized or licensed for this use (fig.1).

Figure 1: Monoclonal antibody targeting SARS-CoV-2, the virus that causes COVID-19

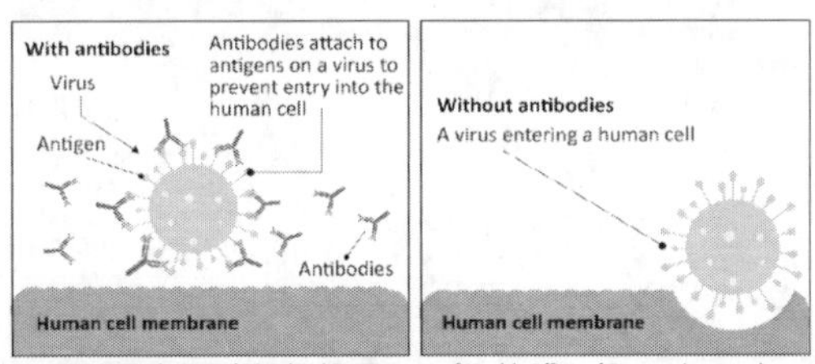

Source: GAO analysis, and Maryland Department of Health Office of Preparedness and Response, and lilerlok_xolms/stock.adobe.com. | GAO-22-104371

Most monoclonal antibodies have been administered intravenously, but some have been administered by intramuscular or subcutaneous injection. Monoclonal antibodies can target a specific pathogen or be combined into mixtures known as cocktails to target a broad range of variants of the same pathogen. A variant has one or more mutations that differentiate it from other variants of the same pathogen in circulation, and those mutations may protect the virus from being neutralized by an existing monoclonal antibody or vaccine.

Source: ktsdesign/stock.adobe.com (header). | GAO-22-104371

Appendix III: Testing Technologies and Approaches

We identified six technologies and approaches that may improve vaccine testing. This appendix provides five summaries of these technologies and approaches.

These summaries are based on documents we reviewed and interviews we conducted. Specifically, we reviewed scientific literature describing current and developing tools, interviewed experts from government, academia, the nonprofit sector, and industry, and collaborated with the National Academies of Sciences, Engineering, and Medicine to convene a 3-day expert meeting to discuss these technologies and approaches. Each summary includes information on what the technology or approach is, its maturity, and how it works.

Organ Chips

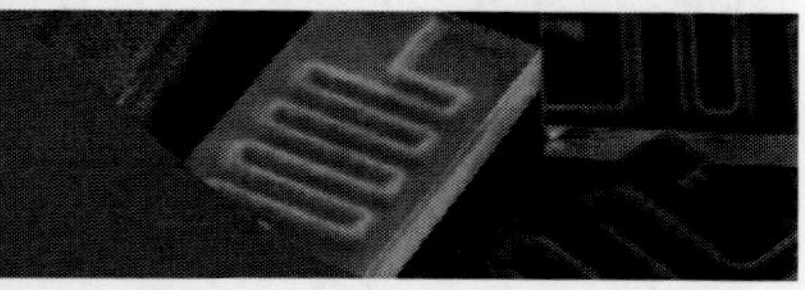

Organ chips are small experimental laboratory tools that contain human cells and mimic how organs and systems in the body work. When used individually, they allow researchers to study a particular part of an organ's function. When linked together, they can mimic the interconnectedness of multiple organs in the human body. Organ chips offer a potential alternative to traditional animal testing and could eventually expedite the development and testing of vaccines and drugs, among other things.

What is it?

Organ chips are designed to reproduce the functioning of human organs or tissues as realistic models. Inside these chips, which are about the size of a computer memory stick, are tiny channels lined with living human cells (fig. 1). Researchers control the external and internal environment around the cells to mimic certain conditions within the human body. For example, they can create movement to mimic breathing motions in the lungs and muscle contractions in the heart. This modeling allows researchers to replicate and study the structural and functional complexity of human organs.

Figure 1: Example of an organ chip

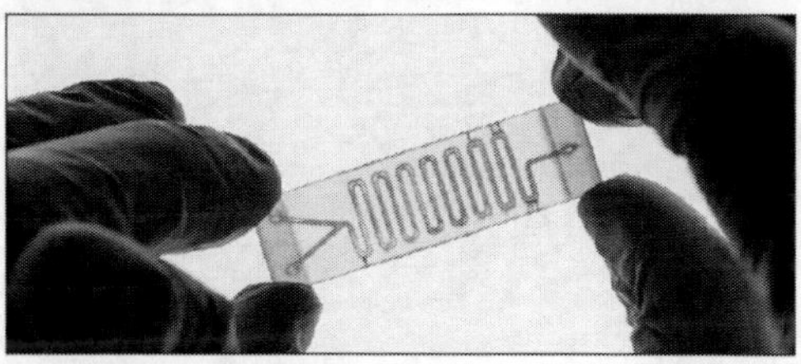

Source: luchschenF/stock.adobe.com. | GAO-22-104371

The interaction of multiple organs can be studied by linking two or more organ chips and also by incorporating multiple lines of cells from different organs onto one chip. Using these systems, researchers may be able to gain a deeper understanding of how a vaccine works or how a drug is absorbed, distributed, or metabolized by the body.

How mature is it?

Organ chip technology has been in development for over a decade. Recent advances allow for analyses using integrated multi-chip systems to study complex interactions among multiple organs and tissues, including liver, lungs, heart, intestines, bone marrow, kidneys, and lymph nodes. However, further advances in design may be needed to investigate some types of organ and cell functions. For example, more complex designs may be needed for chips containing multiple types of cells that differ from one another in the amount of time they need to grow and their responses to various stimuli.

How does it work?

Organ chips contain tiny channels that mimic the flow of substances like blood and air through tissues and organs, similar to what occurs in the human body. For example, a lung organ chip may have a main channel that is divided in half lengthwise to create a top and bottom. In the upper section, lung cells interact with air that flows through the channel. In the lower section, blood vessel cells interact with the flow of a liquid medium that imitates blood. Crucially, the divider between these sections is permeable, allowing the exchange of molecules between the different types of cells. Researchers can then study the effects of bacterial or viral infections by introducing the pathogen to the air flow channel. They can also test drugs by administering the drug into the blood in the lower channel (fig. 2).

Using organ chip technology in this way, researchers might be able to study how SARS-CoV-2 infects the lungs when a patient contracts COVID-19 without relying on animal studies, which may not reliably predict human responses.

Figure 2: A chip containing lung cells and blood vessel cells can be used to study the effects of pathogens or drugs in the human lungs.

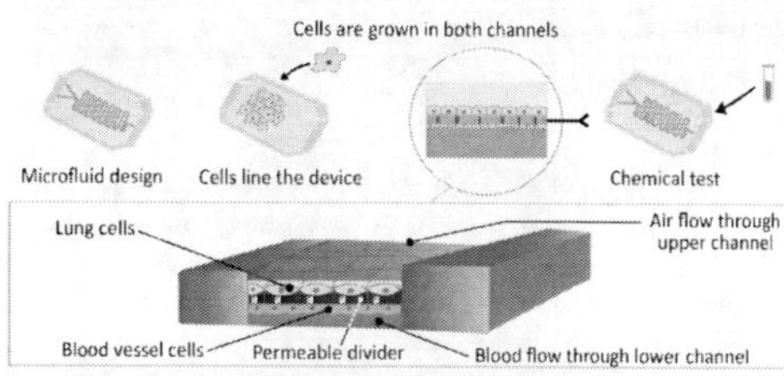

Source: GAO analysis, Wyss Institute at Harvard University, and J.E. Sosa-Hernández et al., "Organs-on-a-Chip Module: A Review from the Development and Applications Perspective," Micromachines, vol. 9, no. 10 (2018): 536. License: CC BY 4.0. https://creativecommons.org/licenses/by/4.0/legalcode. | GAO-22-104371

Similarly, different types of organ chips could be used to understand other pathogens or to study the effects of vaccines. For example, in one study, researchers administered a flu vaccine to lymph node chips to observe patient-specific antibody responses, which demonstrated the chip's potential as a preclinical tool to study human responses to vaccines.

Source: luchschenF/stock.adobe.com (header). | GAO-22-104371

Artificial Intelligence and Machine Learning

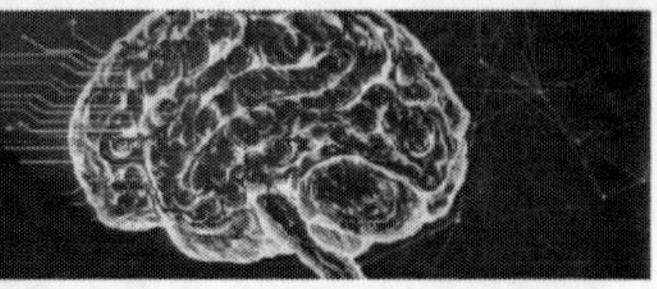

Artificial intelligence and machine learning (AI/ML) techniques use computer systems and algorithms to produce data-driven insights that allow vaccine developers to make discoveries during research and development (R&D) and clinical testing. Some of these insights may allow for more efficient clinical trials and generate predictions that could result in safer, more effective vaccines in less time.

What is it?

AI/ML is a set of advanced technologies that can perform complex tasks and analyze vast amounts of data to develop new insights, including for designing vaccines (table 1). Early AI technologies often used computer programs to make rules-based decisions. Later, the incorporation of mathematics and probability led to ML, which uses a variety of data analytics approaches to improve prediction.

Table 1: AI/ML techniques used in vaccine development

AI/ML techniques	Description
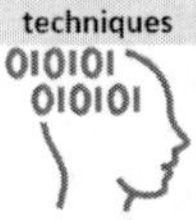 Artificial intelligence	Artificial Intelligence (AI) refers to the capacity of computers or other machines to exhibit or simulate intelligent behavior. AI-based approaches have been used in vaccine design to predict potential epitopes—the part of an antigen to which an antibody binds.
 Machine learning	Machine Learning (ML) is a family of statistical and mathematical modeling techniques that use data to train an algorithm or system to perform tasks. ML has been used to identify antigens from protein sequences.
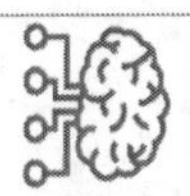 Deep learning	Deep Learning is a class of ML that processes input data to provide outputs that can be used to extract findings. Deep learning has been used to simulate coronavirus spike proteins and identify possible targets for vaccine design.

Source: GAO analysis of literature; kornkun/stock.adobe.com. | GAO-22-104371

How mature is it?

AI/ML techniques have advanced to the point where they are being used throughout vaccine development. However, the use of AI/ML in clinical trials is less mature due to limitations on access to patient data and other issues. Also, techniques like deep learning require large quantities of data which may not be available during a clinical trial.

How does it work?

In the early stages of vaccine development, researchers use AI/ML techniques to mine biological data to screen and identify antigens for potential use in vaccines. Deep learning methods can help researchers identify antibodies for their potential to bind to a given antigen, which may accelerate and improve the development of a new vaccine.

During clinical trials, researchers can use AI/ML to identify suitable participants, optimize design variables, and predict responses (fig. 1). For example, using data sources such as electronic health records (EHR) and genomics data, researchers may determine who is suitable based on trial criteria. They can then identify the optimal number of patients needed for the trial. Once data collection begins, researchers can analyze the data coming in, which may help identify subgroups likely to respond differently to various vaccines or dosages, among other things.

Figure 1: Artificial intelligence (AI) and machine learning (ML) can use various types of data to enhance vaccine development

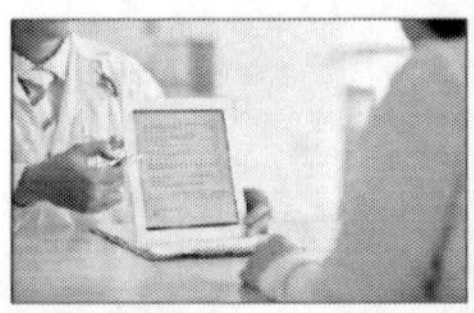

ML can use health record data to efficiently identify and select patients for trials.

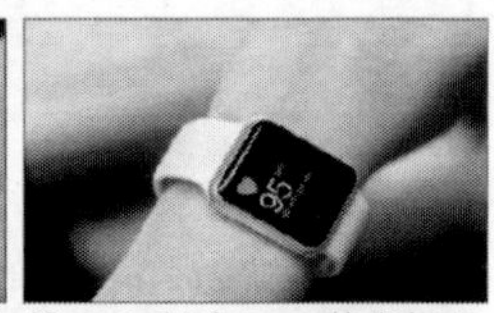

ML can use data from wearable devices to detect relevant events in real time.

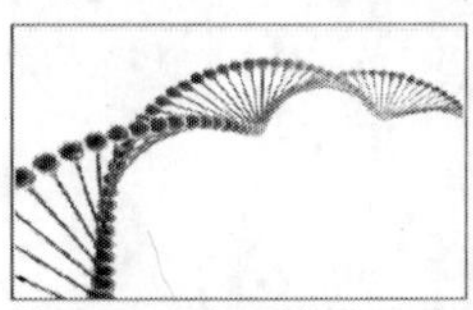

ML can use omics data to identify sets of genes that predict the ability of a vaccine to induce an immune response.

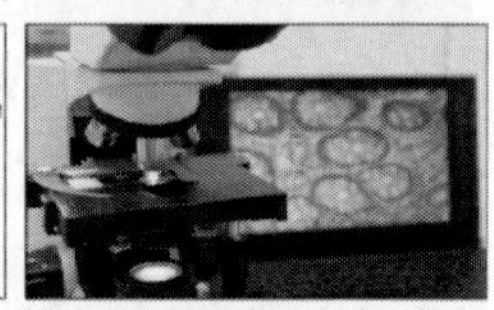

ML can use imaging data to analyze virus structures to more quickly design vaccines that will prevent infection.

Source: GAO analysis and Dragonimages/ballball14/arcyto/Jezper/stock.adobe.com. | GAO-22-104371

AI/ML techniques can also help vaccine developers predict the immune response a vaccine may induce. Using these techniques to analyze omics data from the blood of trial participants who have received the vaccine may allow researchers to predict whether someone will have a high or low antibody response and the likelihood of experiencing an adverse event. This approach has been used in vaccines developed against yellow fever, influenza, and malaria, and may improve the ability to estimate vaccine effectiveness.

Source: peshkov/stock.adobe.com (header). | GAO-22-104371

Electronic Health Records

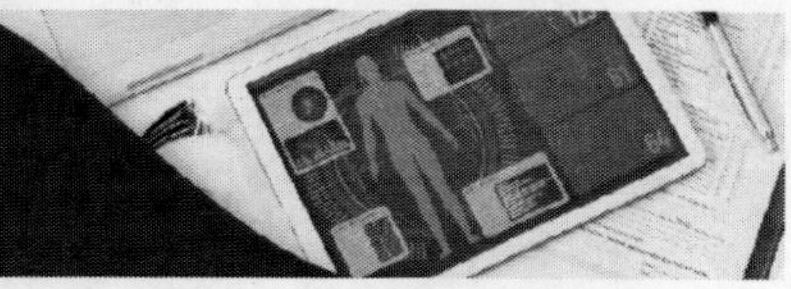

An electronic health record (EHR) is a digital record of a patient's medical information. EHRs could be used in clinical trials to streamline patient recruitment and data collection, and improve data accuracy. EHRs can facilitate post-trial follow-up of large numbers of patients, which can help researchers better understand how long a vaccine's immunity lasts. EHRs also provide a data source that can be used to generate real-world evidence included in prospective clinical investigations.

What is it?

EHRs store patients' health data, which include both structured data (e.g., diagnosis codes and lab results) and unstructured narrative data (e.g., clinical notes about symptoms and pathology reports). Because EHRs are used primarily in direct patient care, they are typically used and maintained by health care providers. EHR systems may also allow clinical researchers to access, combine, aggregate, and analyze many types of data for research purposes (table 1), including vaccine studies.

Table 1: Examples of data typically stored and not stored in electronic health records (EHR)

Examples of structured data stored in EHRs	Examples of narrative data stored in EHRs	Data unlikely to be stored in EHRs
• Date of birth	• Symptoms of illness	• Place of birth
• Sex	• Family history of illness	• Gender identity
• Vital signs	• Meaning of physical exam findings	• Survivorship care planning
• Most lab test results	• Some lab test results	• Living conditions
• Medications prescribed	• Pathology reports	• Psychological distress
• Diagnosis (coded)	• Diagnosis (descriptive)	• Patient-reported outcomes

Source: E. Kim et al., "The Evolving Use of Electronic Health Records (EHR) for Research," *Seminars in Radiation Oncology*, vol. 29, no. 4 (2019): pp.354-361. | GAO-22-104371

How mature is it?

EHRs have been widely adopted in clinical care, but are not in widespread use for clinical trials. Standardized data formats are being developed, and new Department of Health and Human Services rules are addressing interoperability issues. The rules should help address that some EHR systems are not interoperable with electronic data capture systems that manage clinical trial data. As a result, researchers have not always been able to easily transmit data from EHRs for analysis. Interoperable systems allow clinical care staff to enter data into patient records during the patient's visit and the patient's data—such as demographics, vital signs, and medications—automatically populate forms or other records.

How does it work?

EHRs could be used throughout the clinical trial process, subject to privacy protections. At the beginning, they can reduce the need for paper-based recruitment and manual entry of participant data. Researchers can search databases to identify people who meet the criteria to participate, then study coordinators can contact individuals to obtain consent to enroll them in the trial and use their EHR data. Participants could then be assigned to either an experimental group that receives the vaccine or a control group that receives a placebo. As the clinical trial proceeds, researchers can capture and analyze data from EHRs—potentially during a patient's visit to a clinic—which may provide access to many types of data for review that can supplement the data collected for clinical trials and facilitate post-trial follow-up to assess safety and effectiveness (fig. 1).

Figure 1: Streamlining the clinical trial process with electronic health records (EHR)

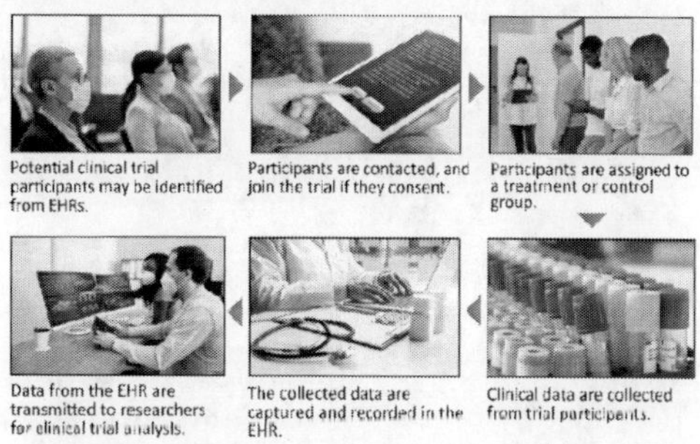

Potential clinical trial participants may be identified from EHRs.

Participants are contacted, and join the trial if they consent.

Participants are assigned to a treatment or control group.

Clinical data are collected from trial participants.

The collected data are captured and recorded in the EHR.

Data from the EHR are transmitted to researchers for clinical trial analysis.

Source: GAO analysis and luchschenF/Roman/Vinnstock/Popov/LightfieldStudios/Thitiphat/stock.adobe.com. | GAO-22-104371

EHRs are also used to monitor vaccine safety once a vaccine has been licensed and is given to patients. FDA's Biologics Effectiveness and Safety system monitors data in EHRs and other sources to detect adverse events and study specific safety questions for vaccines including for sub-populations such as individuals who are pregnant or have pre-existing conditions.

Source: metamorworks/stock.adobe.com (header). | GAO-22-104371

Standardized Assays and Common Control Groups

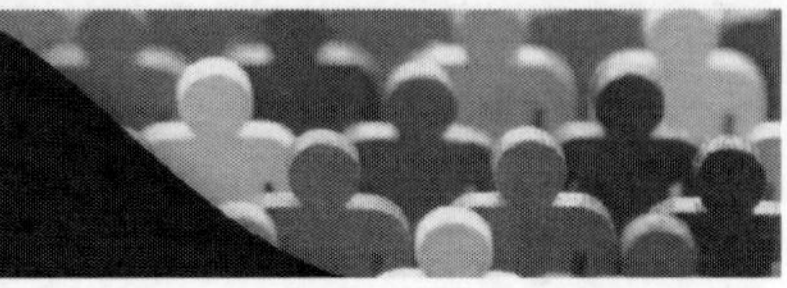

Using standardized assays and common control groups together can help vaccine developers better identify effective vaccine candidates. With this approach, multiple vaccine developers use the same assays (tests that measure a vaccine's immunogenicity, or ability to induce an immune response) to test multiple vaccine candidates and share a single control group during the clinical trials for those vaccines.

What is it?

Standardized assays are tests that vaccine developers may use in evaluating candidates, allowing them to measure immune responses the same way (table 1).

Table 1: Selected assays used in vaccine development

Purpose	Assay description
Humoral antibody response	Measurement of total or functional antibody levels in the blood
Cell-mediated immune response	Measurement of immune cell responses upon exposure to specific antigens

Source: GAO analysis and M. Dotzert, "Assay Development: Vaccines," *Lab Manager*, vol. 14, no. 5 (June 2019): pp.40-43. | GAO-22-104371

A common control group may be a single group of placebo-receiving clinical trial participants that is shared by multiple vaccine developers. Members of a common control group do not receive a vaccine. They generate clinical trial data that are compared to data from participants in other groups who may receive different vaccines or different versions or dosages (amounts) of the same vaccine. This approach eliminates the need for each developer to recruit its own control group, reducing the total number of participants needed. In addition, participants outside the control group have a greater chance of receiving a vaccine candidate than a placebo, which may increase clinical trial participation.

How mature is it?

Standardized assays have been used in vaccine trials, including phase 3 clinical trials of COVID-19 vaccines, according to The National Institutes of Health. Assays may require modifications during the vaccine development process, which is a challenge to standardization. However, some international organizations are collaborating to develop standardized assays for use against known pathogens in advance of potential future outbreaks to enable faster development of vaccines.

Common control group trials were first used over 20 years ago to accelerate the process of drug development. Since then, they have been used mostly in phase 2 and phase 3 clinical trials of different drugs and drug dosages. However, it may be difficult to use common control groups in clinical trials of multiple vaccine candidates in part due to logistical challenges of coordinating among multiple developers in a single trial.

How does it work?

To develop a standardized assay, researchers generally begin by obtaining blood samples from patients who have contracted a disease. This information helps vaccine developers understand how a patient's immune system responds to the pathogen and builds immunity. Developers can then find ways to measure immune responses, such as developing tests to detect pathogen-specific antibodies. They evaluate these assays for precision and may refine them based on performance criteria as vaccines are being developed. Researchers then write standard protocols defining the methodology to allow the assay to be used in the same way by other vaccine developers. This may involve preparing biological reference standards—rigorously evaluated samples used to determine whether an assay is functioning correctly—which can help ensure that data produced in different laboratories are comparable.

Once developers have completed all preclinical testing requirements and agreed to the common control group design, enrollment of participants begins. Each person is assigned randomly to either a group in which they receive one of the vaccine candidates or a common control group that receives a placebo (fig. 1).

Figure 1: Example of a possible trial design using standardized assays and common control groups

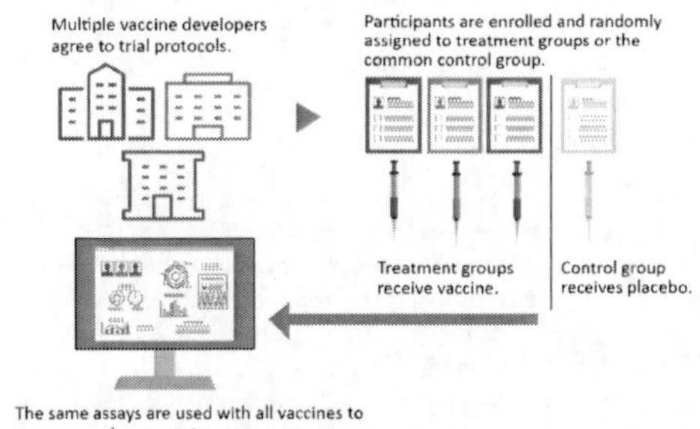

Source: GAO analysis and Kornkun/pp7/stock.adobe.com. | GAO-22-104371

Combining standardized assays with common control groups allows for apples-to-apples comparisons of the vaccine candidates. Investigating multiple vaccines at once could help identify the most effective vaccines against a disease and provide more rapid and reliable results.

Source: Jakub Krechowicz/stock.adobe.com (header). | GAO-22-104371

Virtual Clinical Trials and Wearable Devices

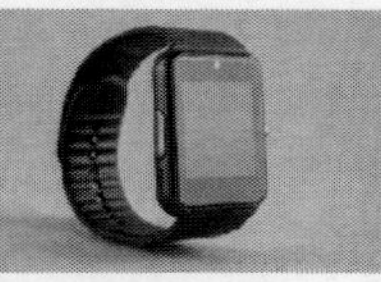

Virtual clinical trials, also referred to as decentralized trials, and wearable devices, also referred to as digital health technologies, work together to capture health data remotely, potentially eliminating the need to travel to a clinic or office to participate in a clinical trial. This approach makes it easier for more people to participate, thereby broadening the pool of potential candidates. Virtual clinical trials may also streamline data collection and reduce errors by eliminating the need for staff to collect and record data.

What is it?

Virtual clinical trials may use web-connected devices to extend the reach of clinical investigations to where participants live and work without compromising study design (table 1). Once clinical trial participants are connected electronically, they can submit their data via wearable devices as well as mobile phones and tablets. Researchers then use the data to assess outcomes and observe physical activity remotely. This approach has been used, for example, to test new medicines and assess the effect of behavioral interventions to treat depression.

Table 1: Comparison of traditional and virtual clinical trials

Clinical trial element	Traditional clinical trial	Virtual clinical trial
Study design	May use a randomized control trial design	May use a randomized control trial design
Health monitoring	On-site	Remote
Patient reported data	Submitted periodically during clinic visits	Submitted more frequently via devices

Source: GAO analysis. | GAO-22-104371

Wearable devices can look similar to commercially available fitness trackers and sometimes use clothing-embedded sensors to collect health data continuously as people go through their daily routines. Many wearable devices measure heart rate and blood pressure, allowing for monitoring of cardiac events. Wearables have also been developed to measure sleep and movement disorders, monitor glucose levels, and measure tremors experienced by patients with Parkinson's disease.

How mature is it?

The first virtual clinical trial began in 2011 but experienced technical challenges and was not completed. Since then, companies are increasingly leveraging digital capabilities to conduct virtual trials. These advances allowed some planned traditional trials to be conducted virtually during the COVID-19 pandemic. For example, researchers used some elements of virtual trials—such as remote screening to determine patients' risk status and remote reporting of symptoms and study data—in clinical trials to test vaccines against COVID-19.

How does it work?

While traditional clinical trials require a physical, centralized site where patients report for in-person visits, a virtual trial begins with online recruiting followed by informed consent and participant enrollment, also handled electronically. If a vaccine is designed to be self-administered (e.g., dermal, nasal, or oral delivery) and does not require special storage, it could potentially be sent to participants' homes in a fully virtual trial. However, vaccine trials would likely retain some features of traditional trials such as in-person vaccination. Study staff may also prompt participants via apps and text messaging for adherence to other study protocols (e.g., reporting symptoms) and conduct clinical evaluations via telemedicine. Participants can perform some clinical procedures such as using a finger stick device to obtain a drop of blood for analysis, results of which may be mailed back to researchers. When wearable devices are used, the data would be collected and transmitted to researchers via a smartphone app or web-based interface (fig. 1).

Figure 1: Possible data collection process for virtual trials

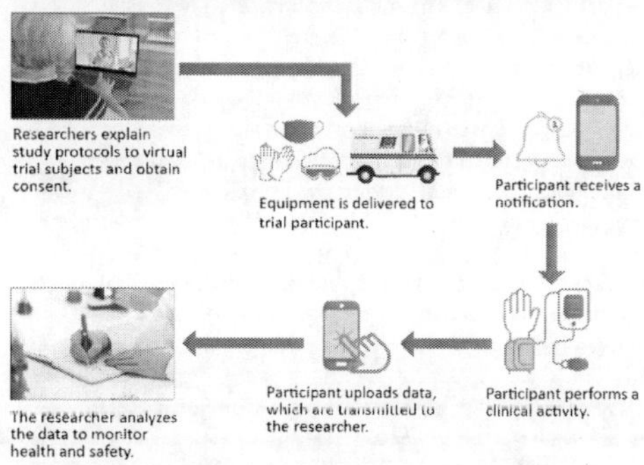

Source: GAO analysis and StudioRomantic/sla009/Agus/Sir.Vector/yurolaitsalbert/Backwoodsdesign/AAVAA/stock.adobe.com. | GAO-22-104371

Researchers might assess outcomes of virtual clinical trials by conducting interviews remotely and tracking participants' electronic health records (EHR). For example, researchers can connect telemedicine equipment such as blood glucose-monitoring devices via wireless data transmission to EHR systems. This allows clinical data to be sent directly to patient records, enabling real-time data collection of more data for faster clinical trials and more robust analysis.

Source: matthew_100/stock.adobe.com (header). | GAO-22-104371

Appendix IV: Manufacturing Technologies and Approaches

We identified five technologies and approaches, collectively known as bioprocess intensification that may improve vaccine manufacturing. This appendix provides a summary of these technologies and approaches.

This summary is based on documents we reviewed and interviews we conducted. Specifically, we reviewed scientific literature describing current and developing tools, interviewed experts from government, academia, the nonprofit sector, and the research industry, and collaborated with the National Academies of Sciences, Engineering, and Medicine to convene a 3-day expert meeting to discuss these technologies and approaches. Each summary includes information on what the technology or approach is, its maturity, and how it works.

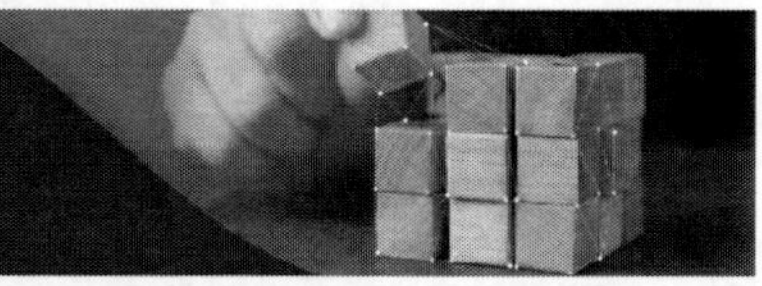

Bioprocess Intensification

Bioprocess intensification can improve vaccine manufacturing flexibility and productivity through flexible facilities, more productive equipment, and improved technologies. To improve flexibility, vaccine manufacturers can use modular bioprocessing systems, single-use systems, and cell-free synthesis that provide the ability to rapidly switch between vaccines, scale up production, or relocate production capacity. To improve vaccine manufacturing productivity, manufacturers can use process optimization technologies to, for example, improve the cells and growth ingredients used to produce vaccine antigens and automated, continuous processing systems that run with fewer interruptions.

What is it?

Bioprocess intensification combines flexible facilities, more productive equipment, and improved technologies to enhance vaccine manufacturing flexibility and productivity while reducing costs and time. Modular bioprocessing systems have flexible infrastructure components, similar to building blocks, that may replace the fixed rooms and areas dedicated to specific bioprocessing steps and provide the ability to rapidly switch between vaccines, scale up production, or relocate manufacturing capacity. Single-use systems are equipment and materials composed primarily of disposable, sealed, pre-sterilized plastic components designed to be used once. Continuous processing systems consist of automated equipment that seamlessly integrates all vaccine production and processing steps, including filling and packaging—also known as fill-finish. Process optimization includes, but is not limited to, improving the cells and cell growth ingredients used to produce vaccine antigens—the component of the vaccine that stimulates the immune systems. Cell-free synthesis uses biological molecules in place of living cells to make the vaccine antigens (fig.1).

Figure 1: The three parts of bioprocess intensification

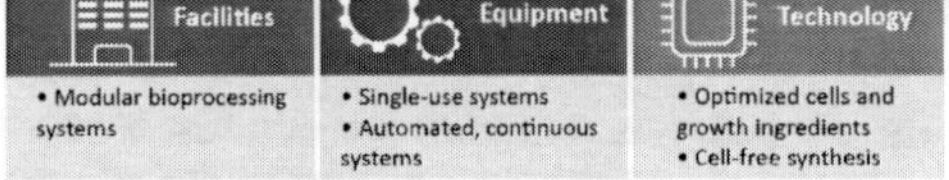

Source: GAO. | GAO-22-104371

How mature is it?

For decades, other industries, such as chemical manufacturing, have used flexible facilities, more productive equipment, and improved technologies similar to those used in bioprocess intensification. Over the past 20 to 30 years, these three categories have been used for pharmaceutical applications, including vaccine manufacturing. For example, single-use systems began to emerge in the early 1980s and continue to be adopted over traditional fixed systems. Further, in the last two decades, cell-free synthesis has surged to meet the increased production demand of inexpensive proteins and small molecules, most recently for generating the mRNA used in the COVID-19 mRNA vaccines.

How does it work?

Bioprocess intensification can be applied at different points in the vaccine manufacturing process. Modular bioprocessing systems work by breaking manufacturing components into smaller functional blocks, such as prefabricated rooms, which may be added into existing facilities to increase flexibility. These systems typically include single-use systems that replace fixed equipment and materials with disposable equipment and materials that are discarded after each use. This eliminates the need for cleaning and sterilization required for fixed equipment. Continuous processing systems integrate and automate all manufacturing steps with few or no interruptions, unlike traditional processes that stop after certain steps, such as cell growth. Process optimization uses approaches to improve the efficiency and productivity in each step of manufacturing. For example, improving cell growth characteristics and growth ingredients used in antigen production can greatly increase yields without adding capacity. Cell-free synthesis combines purified biological molecules in reactor vessels to synthesize antigens, which are then formulated into vaccines. This eliminates the need to grow large amounts of living cells to produce the antigen used in the vaccine (fig.2).

Figure 2: Bioprocess intensification

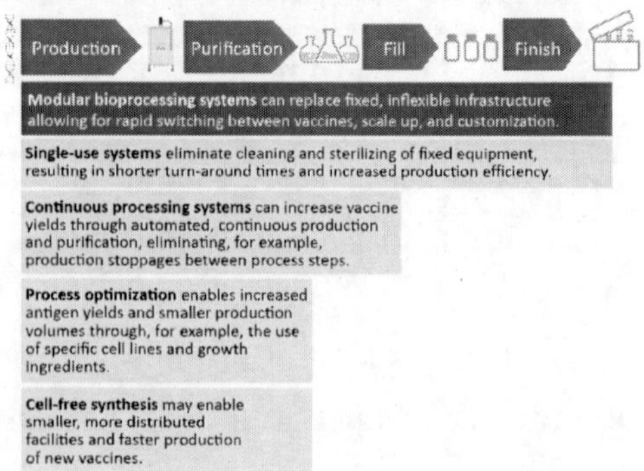

Source: GAO analysis of scientific literature and rashadashurov/tutti_frutti/StockBURIN /divstock/stock.adobe.com. | GAO-22-104371

Source: whyframeshot/stock.adobe.com (header). | GAO-22-104371

Appendix V: Expert Participation

We collaborated with the National Academies of Sciences, Engineering, and Medicine to convene a 3-day meeting of experts to inform our work on vaccine development; the meeting was held virtually on January 25-28, 2021. The experts who participated in this meeting are listed below. Many of these experts gave us additional assistance throughout our work, including ten experts who provided additional assistance during our study by sending material for our review or participating in interviews; and 9 experts who reviewed our draft report for accuracy and provided technical comments.

Phyllis Arthur, MBA
Vice President, Infectious Disease and Diagnostics Policy
Biotechnology Innovation Organization

Maria Elena Bottazzi, PhD
Associate Dean of the National School of Tropical Medicine and Professor of Pediatrics and Molecular Virology & Microbiology
Section Head, Pediatric Tropical Medicine Professor of Pediatrics and co-director, Texas Children's Hospital Center for Vaccine
Development
Baylor College of Medicine

James E. Crowe Jr., MD
Director of the Vanderbilt Science Center and Professor of Pediatrics & Pathology and Microbiology & Immunology and Ann Scott Carrell Chair
Vanderbilt University Medical Center

Patricia M. Danzon, PhD
Celia Moh Professor Emeritus
The Wharton School, University of Pennsylvania

Greg Frank, PhD
Senior Director of Infectious Disease Policy Biotechnology Innovation Organization

Dana Goldman, PhD
Distinguished Professor of Pharmacy, Public Policy & Economics and Leonard D. Schaeffer Chair and Interim Dean of the Sol Price School of Public Policy
University of Southern California

Jesse Goodman, MD, MPH
Director of the Center on Medical Product Access, Safety and Stewardship (COMPASS)
Professor of Medicine and Infectious Diseases
Georgetown University

Tina Hernandez-Boussard, PhD, MS, MPH
Associate Professor in Medicine (Biomedical Informatics), Biomedical Data Science, Surgery & Epidemiology and Population Health
Stanford University

Peter J. Hotez, MD, PhD
Dean of the National School of Tropical Medicine and Professor of Pediatrics and Molecular Virology & Microbiology
Texas Children's Hospital Endowed Chair in Tropical Pediatrics
Baylor College of Medicine

Beth Junker, PhD
Principal Consultant and Owner Bioprocess Advantage LLC

Ruth A. Karron, MD
Professor of International Health and Director, the Center for Immunization Research
Johns Hopkins University Founding Director
Johns Hopkins Vaccine Initiative

Jason Kelly, PhD
Co-founder and CEO Gingko Bioworks

Jerome Kim, MD
Director General
International Vaccine Institute

Michael Kremer, PhD
Gates Professor of Developing Societies Harvard University
Non-resident Fellow
Center for Global Development

Kelvin Lee, PhD
Gore Professor of Chemical and Biomolecular Engineering
University of Delaware

Tracy Lieu, MD, MPH
Director of the Division of Research Kaiser Permanente Northern California

Nicole Lurie, MD, MSPH
Director, CEPI-US and strategic advisor to the CEO, Coalition for Epidemic Preparedness Initiatives (CEPI)
Professor of Medicine
George Washington University Senior Lecturer
Harvard University

Jewel Mullen, MD, MPH, MPA
Associate Dean and Associate Professor University of Texas at Austin
Dell Medical School

Justin Sanchez, PhD
Life Sciences Research Fellow Battelle Memorial Institute
Christopher Snyder, PhD
Joel Z. and Susan Hyatt Professor Dartmouth College

Thomas Thomou, PhD
Senior Scientist/Engineer Gryphon Technologies

Eric Van Gieson, PhD
Program Manager
Biological Technologies Officer, DARPA

Chapter 2

Building Trust and Battling Barriers: The Urgent Need to Overcome Vaccine Hesitancy*

Committee on Oversight and Reform

Thursday, July 1, 2021

House of Representatives Committee on Oversight and Reform
Select Subcommittee on the Coronavirus Crisis
Washington, D.C.

The subcommittee met, pursuant to notice, at 9:08 a.m., in room 2154, Rayburn House Office Building, Hon. James E. Clyburn (chairman of the subcommittee) presiding.

Present: Representatives Clyburn, Waters, Maloney, Velazquez, Foster, Krishnamoorthi, Scalise, and Miller-Meeks.

Chairman CLYBURN. Good morning. The committee will come to order.

Without objection, the chair is authorized to declare a recess of the committee at any time.

I now recognize myself for an opening statement.

We're here this morning to discuss an issue of broad, bipartisan concern: the critical need to overcome vaccine hesitancy so that more Americans get vaccinated against this deadly virus.

I would like to thank Ranking Member Scalise for joining me in inviting witnesses to testify at today's hearing. This is not a partisan issue. The virus is equally dangerous for Democrats and Republicans, and the vaccines are equally safe and effective for Democrats and Republicans.

I would like to also thank today's witnesses for taking the time to testify about this critical issue.

The coronavirus vaccines authorized in the United States are proven to be safe and effective, and they have enabled our country to make significant progress in containing the virus and saving lives.

---

* This is an edited, reformatted and augmented version of Hearing before the Select Subcommittee on the Coronavirus Crisis of the Committee on Oversight and Reform, House of Representatives, Serial No. 117–34, dated July 1, 2021.

In: COVID-19 Vaccines
Editor: John Schroder
ISBN: 979-8-88697-150-7

We have a graph here that speaks for itself. As more and more Americans get vaccinated, fewer and fewer are dying from the coronavirus.

Yet too many Americans remain unprotected against this deadly disease because they are hesitant to receive coronavirus vaccines. This vaccine hesitancy is allowing the virus to continue to spread in areas with large unvaccinated populations and increasing the risk that vaccine-resistant variants will emerge.

Polls show that up to one in five American adults say they are strongly opposed to getting a coronavirus vaccine. Vaccination rates are particularly low in the South and rural West. In both regions, less than 40 percent of the total population of multiple states is fully vaccinated. In my home state of South Carolina, for example, only 39 percent of the total population is fully vaccinated.

Most concerning, we are still losing hundreds of Americans to the coronavirus every day. Nearly all of the more than 8,500 Americans who died from COVID–19 last month were unvaccinated. I want to repeat that: Nearly all of the more than 8,500 Americans who died from COVID–19 last month were unvaccinated. If more Americans got their shots, we could reduce coronavirus deaths to nearly zero.

At this critical juncture, we must not lose sight of the work that remains to fully stop the spread of the virus in the United States. We must undertake dedicated efforts to overcome vaccine hesitancy and redouble our outreach and education so that we can find a way to convince those who are reluctant of the importance of getting vaccinated.

We must overcome access barriers and address informational needs, particularly in communities of color, so that we can make it easier for everyone to get vaccinated. We must identify innovative ways to increase vaccine uptake.

The Biden administration has made tremendous progress in making coronavirus vaccines available to all eligible Americans. They are continuing to work to enhance vaccine access for all communities and to promote confidence in the vaccines. Their unprecedented efforts have helped to vaccinate more than 179 million Americans in record time. But more work is needed to prevent backsliding on this hard-fought progress.

I look forward to hearing from our witnesses about the strategies that are effective to overcome vaccine hesitancy and increase vaccine uptake and about how we can better inform the American public and encourage those who may be hesitant to feel confident in getting these shots.

Once again, thank the members and guests for being here today. And I now yield to the ranking member for an opening statement.

Mr. SCALISE. Well, thank you, Mr. Chairman. Appreciate you holding this hearing.

Thank our witnesses for coming today.

As Americans move into the Fourth of July weekend, Independence Day takes on special meaning this year. Thanks in large part to the vaccines, this is the first holiday weekend where virtually all of America is back open, free. Families and friends will celebrate together. Grandmothers will visit and hug their grandkids. Crowds will gather again for fireworks.

Every one of us on this subcommittee can tell the American people there is total bipartisan agreement on this subcommittee: The vaccine ended this pandemic.

So how did we get to the point where America created the fastest vaccine in human history, manufactured, produced, and distributed enough vaccine to give a shot to every American who wants one? The story really begins 30 years ago, when the United States Trade Representative began negotiating international trade agreements in earnest. On a bipartisan basis, for three decades, USTR made protection of U.S. intellectual property a cornerstone of those agreements.

About 25 years ago, Congress decided to make a major push on biomedical research. The Republican-controlled Congress worked with President Bill Clinton to double the size of the National Institutes of Health. During the administration of George W. Bush, Congress made yet another major investment in NIH, with strong bipartisan support.

And then came former Energy and Commerce Committee Chairman Fred Upton, working with Diana DeGette across party lines. Their leadership brought us the 21st Century Cures Act. That was one of the most proud moments I worked as majority whip, on a piece of legislation that was bipartisan, working with then-President Obama. We doubled yet again our commitment to the NIH. And, just as importantly, we established in that bill the Emergency Use Authorization process, which these COVID–19 vaccines were ultimately approved based on. These are provisions, Emergency Use Authorization especially, that helped save millions of lives.

Operation Warp Speed, of course, then built on those decades of work. America created the fastest vaccine in human history. But all Americans should be assured and confident, the vaccines were not rushed. They were built off a platform decades in the making, with the best minds in public health and private sector coming together to create world-class innovations and breakthroughs in a step-by-step fashion.

If you want to get vaccinated, it is safe, effective, free, and available.

Today, nearly 154 million Americans are fully vaccinated. That's about 47 percent of the population. At least 180 million people, or 55 percent of the population, have received at least one dose. And remember, we're not vaccinating children under 12 years old. Many Americans, thousands and thousands of Americans, who contracted COVID–19 also have the antibodies. We're approaching that elusive goal now of effective herd immunity.

Every American, again, who wants to get vaccinated can now get vaccinated.

Scientists have made it clear that we don't need to achieve 100 percent vaccination for effective herd immunity. So, let's give folks who are hesitant the reassurance that they're not going to be forced by the Federal Government to do something against their will. It's ultimately every American's decision. But we want it to be an informed decision.

First, the vaccine works. Pfizer and Moderna's Phase III clinical studies found that their two-dose regimens were 95 and 94 percent effective, respectively, at blocking COVID–19, while Johnson & Johnson's one-shot vaccine was found to be 66 percent effective in its studies.

All three, however, have been found to be extremely effective in preventing people from getting severely sick from COVID. So, even if someone does get sick from the vaccine, the severeness of that sickness is dramatically reduced.

Since vaccinations began, emergency room visits related to the virus have declined 77 percent among older adults. As we saw, the highest percentage of COVID deaths in those early months were from seniors in nursing homes, especially, and the more vulnerable populations—diabetes, hypertension.

While some breakthrough infections were reported—that is, infections that occurred after vaccination—those illnesses tended to be milder than infections among unvaccinated people. As we know, no vaccine is 100 percent effective. A very small percentage of vaccinated individuals will get sick, but that is not evidence that the vaccination does not work.

Second, the vaccination is safe. Over 324 million doses of COVID–19 vaccine have been given in the United States from December 14, 2020, through June 28 of this year. COVID–19 vaccines were evaluated in terms of thousands of participants in clinical trials. The vaccines met the Food and Drug Administration's rigorous scientific standards for safety, effectiveness, and manufacturing quality that is needed to support Emergency Use Authorization that I talked about earlier.

Many people experience side effects after receiving the vaccine. We've seen reports of fatigue, fever, soreness. These last for a short period of time. A very small percentage of individuals experience an allergic reaction.

The bottom line is, for the overwhelming majority of Americans, the benefits of getting vaccinated clearly outweigh the small risks. COVID is a dangerous virus that has killed 600,000 Americans, but the risk of death from COVID drops dramatically for vaccinated individuals.

Let's all work together to get the facts out to the people of this country, particularly populations that have concerns or hesitancy. Let's present the evidence but also reassure individuals that this decision is their decision. I believe that this is the strategy that will ultimately maximize the number of Americans who choose to take the vaccine.

And as I'm closing, Mr. Chairman, I also would be remiss if I didn't point out the fact that this committee does need to hold a hearing on the origins COVID–19. As we've pointed out many times for over a year, this is a virus that killed over 600,000 people in America, 4 million worldwide. More and more evidence is growing in the scientific community that this virus originated in the lab in Wuhan, not naturally occurring from bat to animal to human. And, in fact, earlier this week, the Republicans on the committee, after over a year of calling for this hearing, held our own hearing. We brought in scientific experts. Every one of those scientific experts, Mr. Chairman, reported during their testimony that this vaccine, based on the genetic sequencing that we now see, started in the Wuhan lab. The evidence is overwhelming.

If China would've been honest with us in those early months— and I'm going back to September, at least, of 2019, well before the first cases were reported, where now we do know anecdotally that people with flu-like symptoms, both in the lab and near the lab, were starting to experience those symptoms. If China would've been honest back then, instead of waiting until March 2020, hundreds of thousands of American lives could've been saved and millions of lives globally could have been saved if they were forthright with us.

We still have many questions to ask based on the testimony we heard. In many cases, the people who can give those answers were invited and refused to come forward. Mr. Chairman, with your subpoena authority, you could compel them to come forward.

So, I will reiterate once again, for the ability for us to prevent something like this from happening again, the sooner, the better, we need to have a hearing on the origin of COVID–19 before the full committee.

I'll be happy to get you a copy of the transcript. In fact, C-SPAN carried the hearing that we held, so we can get you all of that information. A lot of important scientific information was presented. There is more scientific information that needs to come forward from people who refused to come forward.

So, I would urge that we have that hearing, again, and, with that, I yield the balance of my time.

Chairman CLYBURN. I thank the gentleman for his opening statement, and I look forward—I would like to get a copy of that, and you and I might be able to discuss that sometime in the not-too- distant future.

As all of us have just heard, there is a vote on. And we are going to work together here to make sure that everybody gets a chance to cast their vote and to return. Mr. Foster has cast his vote, and he's coming here. He'll be taking my place while I go vote. And we have several other members who need to go vote as well.

But before we do that—— Mr. SCALISE.

[Inaudible] have someone chair during your absence.

Chairman CLYBURN. I'm sure you would, but I think I'd better keep this gavel on this side of the aisle. Thank you so much, though. Thanks for the offer.

I'm going to introduce the witnesses so that we won't hold them up. And then I think Mr. Foster will preside while the three of us go cast our votes so that we won't miss that, OK?

Let me now introduce our witnesses.

Joshua Garza is a coronavirus survivor from Sugar Land, Texas. After turning down an opportunity to receive a vaccine, Mr. Garza contracted a severe coronavirus infection that rapidly destroyed his lungs. Mr. Garza was placed on life support and then suffered complete lung failure, requiring an emergency double lung transplant. After a miraculous recovery, Mr. Garza has shared his story publicly. He hopes to save lives by inspiring others to learn from his mistake and get vaccinated.

Dr. Georges Benjamin serves as the executive director of the American Public Health Association, the Nation's oldest and largest organization of public health professionals. He previously served as the secretary of health for the state of Maryland. He is a board-certified internal medicine—in internal medicine, a master of the American College of Physicians, a fellow of the National Academy of Public Administration, a fellow emeritus of the American College of Emergency Physicians, and a member of the National Academy of Medicine.

Welcome back, Dr. Benjamin.

Dr. Katy Milkman—and, Katy, I hope I'm pronouncing that correctly—is a professor of behavioral economics at the Wharton School of the University of Pennsylvania. Professor Milkman is an award-winning scholar who has applied her research to assist states and vaccine providers create incentives to increase vaccinations.

Dr. Jerome Adams served as our Nation's 20th Surgeon General. He also served on the White House Coronavirus Task Force during the previous administration. Prior to becoming United States Surgeon General, Dr. Adams served as health commissioner of the state of Indiana and as a vice admiral in the United States Public Health Service's Commissioned Corps.

Welcome, Dr. Adams.

Sophia Bush is an actress, activist, and entrepreneur. She has starred on the drama series "One Tree Hill" and "Chicago PD," along with numerous films. Ms. Bush's activism includes supporting the empowerment of women and girls, fundraising for those affected by the Deepwater Horizon oil spill, and serving as founder and board member of I Am a Voter, a nonpartisan movement to increase voter participation. Most recently, Ms. Bush has used her platform to educate others about the importance of vaccinations.

Will the witnesses please rise and raise your right hands?

Do you swear or affirm that the testimony you're about to give is the truth, the whole truth, and nothing but the truth, so help you God?

You may be seated.

Let the record show that the witnesses answered in the affirmative.

Without objection, your written statements will be made part of the record.

Mr. Garza, you are now recognized for your opening statement.

Statement of Joshua Garza, Coronavirus Survivor

Mr. GARZA. Good morning to everybody. My name is Joshua Garza. I'm 43 years old, residing in a suburb of Houston, Texas. Due to my initial hesitancy regarding the COVID vaccine, I passed on a chance to obtain the vaccine in early January. Due to underlying health issues that I was aware of and treating, I was eligible for the early dose. As a result of not following through with the vaccination, I ended up contracting the virus in late January and endured a four-month stay in the hospital, resulting in a double lung transplant to save my life.

When approached about the vaccine in early January, I felt that I was adhering to all the protocols. I wore the mask when out, made sure to be socially distanced, continued washing of hands, et cetera. At the time, I strongly felt that I was doing everything I needed to protect myself and my family. It's a decision that I have to live with for the rest of my life.

On January 28, I started to feel ill with the usual symptoms of the coronavirus. As my condition worsened, my wife and I decided to get tested on January 30. Results were sent to us the next day. My wife was negative, but I was given the dreaded results of being tested positive.

My condition worsened in the following days to a point where I no longer had enough strength to walk. My oxygen levels started to drop as a result of the virus attacking my lungs. I tried to walk to the front of the house and ended up falling due to oxygen levels being so low. My wife called an ambulance to take me to the hospital immediately. I was first admitted into a hospital on February 2.

The first hospital I was at ran the usual tests, but my condition continued to get worse. After receiving results from the testing, doctors were able to determine that my lungs were hit the hardest and deteriorating at a rapid rate.

After a two-week stay and countless tests, we received the news we did not want to hear. The doctors had done everything they could have done, and my condition was too far gone to fix. This hospital had given up on me, and I was not ready to give up.

I reached out to my family and explained the situation and said my final goodbyes, as I did not know what was to come or how long I had to live. The toughest call I had to make was to my 12-year- old son and let him know the situation.

After the call, I decided that I was not ready to give up. My wife and I decided, in order to continue fighting, I would have to transfer to a different hospital. This was February 13.

On February 14, I was able to secure a bed at Houston Methodist Hospital Medical Center. After being transferred to the Methodist—after being transferred, the Methodist staff started testing immediately. The doctors had the same conclusion, that my lungs were being destroyed by the coronavirus, but they had options for treatment not offered at the previous hospital.

I was moved to the ICU floor and was placed on an ECMO system to help my lungs function during this time. The ECMO system prolonged my life enough to get evaluated for a lung transplant. After evaluation, it was determined that I was a candidate for transplant. I was on the ECMO system for almost five weeks before being approved for the transplant list.

Once placed on the list, I waited three weeks in order to find a match. Successful transplant surgery was done on April 13. After surgery, I had to start the rehab process within the Methodist network and was released from the hospital on May 27.

Here is a photo of me on the ECMO system.

While in the hospital, I was faced with many uncertainties that are not controllable due to the situation. You have time in the hospital to reflect on life decisions and the outcome of each.

The amount of pain I endured during this ordeal is something I never want to replicate. If I could change my decision back in early January to go forward with the vaccination, I would.

We live in a country where we're free to make your own decisions. With respect to the coronavirus vaccine, I would ask my fellow Americans who are on the fence to think of not only yourself but also your family and community to avoid the pain and suffering many families have gone through, as many have lost loved ones due to COVID–19.

I have a second chance at life, and I intend to share my story as much as I can to help someone save their life.

Thank you.

Mr. FOSTER. [Presiding.] Thank you, Mr. Garza.

Dr. Benjamin, you are now recognized for your opening statement.

Statement of Georges Benjamin, MD., Executive Director, American Public Health Association

Dr. BENJAMIN. Thank you, Mr. Chairman and members of the subcommittee. I want to thank you for the opportunity to address you today.

You know, the SARS-COVID–2, the virus that causes COVID–19, has infected over 33 million individuals and taken over 600,000 lives. I just remind us that it would've been much worse had we not really implemented many of the important public health measures—masking, handwashing, social distancing, closing selected venues.

But the best tool we have in public health is vaccination. It's good that we have a safe and effective vaccine, but, you know, having a shot and getting those shots in the arms are really two different things.

And we've done a lot of things to really get to this point. You know, people have had—over 323 million doses have been delivered. We've really made substantial progress as a Nation. But it clearly isn't enough. As Chairman Clyburn pointed out, it does save lives.

But I want to focus my remarks on just the fact that I think we need a new strategy. And that is one that builds on the successful national strategy that we've certainly had but one that is grounded in communities. And I'm talking about one that's using old-fashioned, grassroots, shoe-leather public health.

And what often happens is that we get close to these benchmarks that we've set for ourselves and then we get complacent, and we don't finish the job. And we need to make sure that, in this case, we finish the job. And we really need to double-down particularly on the vulnerable populations—communities of color, communities that, quite frankly, have not taken the virus as seriously as others. So, we're really recommending a four-step approach that has been endorsed that we believe is community-driven. And this framework has, really, four components.

The first one is using data to identify those communities where there is a lower-than-expected level of vaccination.

Second, exploring which challenges those communities have to coverage—meaning, where are people not confident enough to get the vaccine and why? Because it's turned out that there are lots of reasons, there's a whole spectrum of reasons why people are not willing to get vaccinated, from simply haven't gotten around to it, to not having all the questions that they need to have answered answered and, therefore, they're not that confident.

And then engaging local community-based stakeholders to help design those solutions; and really monitoring what we do; and then, in a cycling manner, doing these things all over again until we get an adequate number of people vaccinated.

Over the last month, there has been a national effort to do this kind of strategy, and I'm pleased to report that we're beginning to see success in that strategy. But we need to double—redouble those efforts if we're going to be successful.

I think we should anticipate that, over the next part of this year, we're going to have intermittent outbreaks, and we're probably going to have those outbreaks over the next several years. The wayto kind of conceive that is, it'll be like these measles outbreaks that we have. We have a well-vaccinated population for measles, but we have a population where people are not adequately vaccinated, and people get infected.

This is a very, very severe disease, and we need to take it very seriously.

I also want to point out, because this disease is raging in many parts of the world and we, quite frankly, have not done enough as a planet to get that part of the world vaccinated, we are going to have entry of new variants for some time to come.

I know people are very worried about the Delta variant, and I am too, but just let me say, there is very likely to be a variant that develops in any of our communities where we're under vaccinated. And so, we need to be concerned about any of these new variants that occur and watch them very, very carefully. And I know the CDC has revved up its surveillance of these, but we just can't let our guard down.

So, I thank you for this, and I look forward to the opportunity to testify today, and I look forward to working with Congress and the administration and, quite frankly, our community in making sure we address this.

And let me just say one final thing to Mr. Garza.

Mr. Garza, I'm very glad, as a physician, that you're better and want to thank you very much for your advocacy.

Mr. FOSTER. Thank you, Dr. Benjamin.

Dr. Milkman, you're now recognized for your opening statement.

Statement of Katy Milkman, PhD., Professor of Operations, Information, and Decisions at the Wharton School; Professor, Division of Health Policy at the Perelman School of Medicine, University of Pennsylvania

Ms. MILKMAN. Thank you, Mr. Chairman and distinguished members of the committee, for inviting me.

I'll focus my remarks today on how behavioral science suggests we can encourage COVID vaccination by changing the cost-benefit calculus.

First, we should be making vaccination radically convenient to reduce its hidden costs. People are busy, forgetful, and generally far more dissuaded by "hassle" factors than we appreciate.

One recommendation is to prearrange vaccination appointments for unvaccinated Americans. Research shows that prescheduling people for flu shots, while making rescheduling easy, leads to a 36- percent increase in vaccination over simply telling people how to schedule an appointment.

If we can't give every unvaccinated American an appointment to get a vaccine, we can still repeatedly remind them of how to schedule one and convey that a vaccine has been reserved for them, as opposed to just made available, which evidence suggests will also help.

In two studies that included over 700,000 Americans and tested dozens of different text-reminder messages encouraging flu vaccination, my collaborators and I found that reminding people a vaccine was reserved or waiting for them boosted vaccine take-up in pharmacies and doctors' offices by 7 to 10 percent.

These types of reminders were proven to increase COVID vaccinations too, and they likely work because having a healthcare provider remind you to claim a vaccine that's set aside for you communicates the vaccination's recommended, suggests it will be easy, and because we strongly dislike giving up things that have been allocated to us.

I also want to discuss financial rewards. For someone who isn't rushing to get a vaccine, maybe because they're young and don't fear infection or because they're concerned about the indirect costs of vaccination, like lost income, incentives increase the immediate benefits of getting inoculated. Thirty-four percent of unvaccinated Americans surveyed this spring reported they'd be more likely to get a vaccine if they were paid $100 to do so.

A caveat, though, is that a recent study of unvaccinated Medicaid patients found cash payments only actually compelled more vaccination among people who already intended to get their shot but just hadn't gotten around to it.

Another caveat to cash payments is that research suggests paying people a small amount to get their vaccine could unintentionally convey that there's a health risk associated with vaccination, even though greater risks accrue to those who decline a vaccine. If you have to pay me to do something, I may incorrectly infer you're paying to offset a risk you're imposing on me.

In one study, people said they'd be more likely to get vaccinated if paid $100, but a payment of $20 would actually reduce their interest in getting a vaccine, probably because of the incorrect inferences low payments produce about risk.

Lottery payments for vaccination may help dodge this issue, as we infer different motives for guaranteeing a reward versus offering up a chance at a jackpot. Moreover, lottery incentives are generally cost-effective, in part because we tend to overestimate the chances of low-probability events. For instance, we act as if a chance that's one in a million of an event is more like one-in-a– 10,000 chance. So, when we're entered in a lottery, we overestimate our chances of winning.

And data from the benefits of Ohio's Vax-a-Million lottery are very promising. The week after that lottery was announced, Ohio's 16-and-up vaccination rate jumped 28 percent. And estimates suggest that lottery caused an extra 50,000 to 80,000 Ohio residents to get vaccinated in just the two weeks post-launch, implying a cost of about $85 per dose.

In Philadelphia, my collaborators and I recently designed a vaccination sweepstakes that uses what's called a regret lottery. We're drawing names from a Philadelphia residential data base but requiring those we contact to prove they were previously vaccinated to accept their winnings. Since all residents are entered in the lottery, some unvaccinated Philadelphians will be notified that they would've won a cash prize if only they'd gotten their vaccine, which is the regret component.

Past research shows that, because people imagine the regret they'd feel if they got that call and couldn't cash in, regret lotteries can be even more motivating than standard lotteries.

Our lottery's grand prize is also just $50,000, because we doubt a million-dollar jackpot is necessary. And half of the winners in each drawing will come from a preannounced ZIP Code with a particularly low vaccination rate to target incentives more efficiently.

It's too early to know the program's impact, but we hope it could be a model for motivating local vaccination.

And, finally, I want to discuss non-monetary incentives.

One survey found that offering Americans the opportunity to stop wearing masks after vaccination was highly motivating.

Giving only vaccinated Americans access to certain opportunities will also matter. Over 500 U.S. colleges and universities are requiring students to be vaccinated to return in the fall, and many employers are setting similar mandates.

Mandates are understandably controversial, but a recent review showed that workplace policies like vaccine mandates increased flu vaccination coverage by an average of 25 percent, whereas surveyed incentive programs only boosted vaccination rates by 9 percent. This means encouraging mandates that allow for medical and religious exemptions could increase vaccination rates immensely.

I'll close now but note that I've only provided testimony on evidence-based ways to change the costs and benefits associated with vaccination. There are many other ways to encourage vaccination and reduce health disparities, and I look forward to perhaps discussing some later in this session.

Thank you very much.

Mr. FOSTER. Thank you, Dr. Milkman.

Dr. Adams, you are now recognized for your opening statement.

Statement of Jerome Adams, MD., Mph, Former Surgeon General of the United States (2017 2021)

Dr. ADAMS. Well, thank you for the opportunity to testify at this incredibly important and timely hearing.

The increasing spread of the Delta variant makes this conversation all the more urgent, but the COVID–19 pandemic is just the latest example of how our efforts to address overall vaccine hesitancy must improve.

And I want to applaud your use of the phrase "vaccine hesitancy," because I never say "anti-vax." There is a small, albeit vocal, contingent who are what I call "vaccine-resistant," but most vaccine-hesitant people simply have questions or barriers that, when addressed with compassion, can be overcome. Or, as I often say, the more people know we care, the more they care what we know.

Herd immunity is about having enough people with antibodies by vaccination and/or prior infection to stop disease spread. So, in other words, we could achieve sufficient protection to contain COVID outbreaks with less than 70 to 80 percent of all people in the U.S. vaccinated. That's good news, because we also have to quite simply acknowledge we may never achieve 70-percent nation- wide vaccination rates.

What we need to focus on, in my opinion, is defining micro-herds and striving to achieve overall containment through vaccination within those smaller groups, because that's really where outbreaks start. Your herd could be your church, your workplace, your child's sports team, the neighbors you gather with, and especially your family. The more these smaller herds achieve 70-percent-plus vaccination rates within their groups, the less likely the virus and variants will find quarter to spread within the larger population. And moving on to populations and interventions, the most important lesson you should take from this hearing is that we absolutely must change our strategy from broad mass-vaccination campaigns to more focused education and engagement of smaller groups and individuals.

We're well past the days of vaccine eagerness, where you could simply set up at the local sports stadium or fairgrounds and expect people to drive miles and wait for hours for a vaccine.

My conversations with community nonprofit public health and healthcare groups and organizations have revealed a number of strategies to combat vaccine hesitancy, which I'd invite the select committee to consider. They're grouped into three main "mis"es that I think we need to focus on: misinformation, mistrust, and a misperception that access is no longer an issue.

I'd refer you to my written testimony for more details and 10 key recommendations I've gleaned from my engagement with these groups, and which address these "mis"es. But at a very high level, they are:

One, make the conversation about more than just COVID.

Two, recognize and address continuing access issues as a matter of health equity.

Three, we've got to get more shots in doctors' offices.

Four, encourage and fund efforts to better understand hesitancy at the ground level and empower people with factual information.

Five, work with states to award micro grants to community groups who are doing the work on the ground.

Six, through the Department of Labor and Small Business Administration, fund an effort to have businesses and employers understand the benefits of encouraging and offering vaccinations.

Seven, through the Department of Education, support school- based vaccination clinics for COVID and all other vaccines students have fallen behind on, because guess what: Our kids are at as much and possibly more risk from other vaccine-preventable diseases as they are from COVID right now.

Emphasize—No. 8—the non-health benefits of vaccination. Focusing on the social positives of the vaccine to a constituency that in many cases fears the social harms of COVID more than the potential health harms is more likely to motivate behavior change.

Nine, work with vaccine manufacturers and the FDA to gather the data necessary to move toward full approval of vaccines. I really, really hope the committee hears me when I'm saying this. This is something that people on the ground level are continually saying. It took five months to go from Phase III trials to EUA. It's taken already longer than that to go from EUA to full licensure of these vaccines, and the American public wants to know why.

And, number 10, stop talking about vaccine hesitancy in political terms, for goodness' sake, and find different and credible spokespersons for different groups. I've never heard a single person say, "I'm not getting vaccinated because I'm a Republican." I've heard plenty of people say, "I won't get vaccinated because I don't trustthe government," "I don't trust the healthcare system." And when we focus on this mistrust, versus focusing on political ideology, we win people over.

In summary, vaccine hesitancy did not manifest itself out of nowhere, especially in communities where trust of the medical establishment is tenuous at best. Our country needs to fundamentally change how it values and invests in caring, quality, and expert public health services and communication.

Because vaccine hesitancy, quite frankly, isn't the root problem. It's just the latest symptom, the latest example of our collective failures to engage, educate, enable, and empower all citizens to be their healthiest selves.

So, thank you for the opportunity to testify today, and I look forward to taking your questions.

Mr. FOSTER. Thank you, Dr. Adams.

Ms. Bush, you are now recognized for your opening statement.

Statement of Sophia Bush, Actress, Activist, Entrepreneur

Ms. BUSH. Thank you, Mr. Chairman, Ranking Member Scalise, and honorable members of the committee, for the opportunity to testify before you today.

My name is Sophia Bush, and I am a storyteller. As an actress, an activist, an entrepreneur, and the host of the "Work in Progress" podcast, I have committed myself to learning about people and communities so that I might highlight the change-makers working to unite and propel us all toward a better future.

In being afforded the opportunity to tell people's stories, I have found both my personal purpose and the passion for what lies ahead for us as a Nation. And I feel incredibly privileged to have this opportunity to carry their voices into the chamber with me today.

In early 2020, like so many of my fellow citizens, my workplace shut down, and shortly thereafter I was locked down at home.

I was terrified of COVID. As a child with severe asthma, I suffered bouts of pneumonia that further weakened my respiratory system, and, as an adult, what might present as a seasonal cold for my coworkers has quickly turned into bouts of bronchitis that have sent me to the hospital for emergency breathing treatments. Even with the unearned privilege of my less at-risk group, one with better racial outcomes, and with my financial ability to access quality healthcare, I wondered if I would be one of the young Americans to suffer severe complications or carry a deadly virus home to my family.

I was inspired by the urgency with which the global health community mobilized to sequence the virus, develop a vaccine, all thanks to decades of prior research on coronaviruses. Researchers around the world collaborated like never before in response to the greatest public health threat of our lifetime.

So, I jumped at my chance to get the vaccine the moment I was able to, to protect myself and my parents, my coworkers' and friends' families.

I jumped at the opportunity to take my best friend to get her mRNA vaccine. She was five months pregnant at the time and has a clotting disorder, and that made her cautious about receiving a vaccine. But being acutely aware of what contracting COVID could mean for her and her baby, she, too, jumped at the chance to protect them both once experts confirmed the vaccine's safety for pregnant women.

I drove us home with tears in my eyes that day. To be honest, I also cried the day my parents received their second mRNA vaccine, because, for me, vaccines represent love.

My grandfather was a United States Navy man—I have his tags on the desk with me today—and he used to tell stories about polio. My mother, too, remembers the relief when her family stood in line for that vaccine.

Vaccines are acts of love made possible by innovation. And I believe that, in innovation, we have historically seen the best of America. That is where we are exceptional. From skyscrapers to airplanes, eventually landing on the Moon, we are innovators. And the COVID vaccine, in my opinion, is our generation's shot at a Moon landing. This is a step for humankind made possible by science.

Two of the largest groups of unvaccinated people exist in communities you've mentioned: communities of color and rural populations. There have been concerted disinformation and misinformation campaigns to discourage communities, including these, from vaccinating themselves against COVID–19.

We cannot allow people dubbed a threat to this Nation by our own intelligence agencies, no matter if they are anonymous internet marauders or members of our own governing body, to peddle disinformation that keeps us from protecting ourselves and others. Those are harmful stories.

And medicine is not partisan. Science is not partisan. Public health must be supported to the best of our Nation's ability, all of us, by nonpartisan political will.

It is on us to remind our loved ones that this pandemic is not over. New variants, as you mentioned, including the more transmissible Delta variant, are circulating at an alarming rate.

And even before the proliferation of these variants, experts were anticipating a fourth wave in areas with low vaccination rates. We were warned just this week that we could see dense outbreaks in rural areas because not enough of those communities are vaccinated.

And on the subject of community inequity, as the chairman mentioned, Black and Brown communities have suffered unspeakable losses through this pandemic. And it should come as no surprise to us that some people of color who felt abandoned by our government in 2020 may have hesitated to believe that the government would protect them now against COVID–19.

We must collectively come to terms with our historical—with our history of medical trauma and the abuse on Black and Brown Americans. And we must provide culturally competent, evidence- based messaging that is community-specific if we want to prevent more devastation this fall.

We need to spread the word about where people can find more information about the vaccines. My dear friend and science communication lead for the COVID Tracking Project, Jessica Malaty Rivera, likes to say that science isn't finished until it's been communicated with empathy. So, we must work to make sure that our policies and the stories we tell about them, the ways in which we communicate the science, are trustworthy, transparent, and inclusive.

Public health must be our number-one priority, because, by nature, public health requires us to work on behalf of the public. Our doctors and researchers do, and each of us can do the same by standing up for our communities and getting vaccinated to stop the spread.

My fellow millennials watching and the innovative Gen-Z'ers out there, we are looking to you. You can reclaim your academic institutions and your precious milestones in person by getting vaccinated to protect yourselves and your loved ones so that you can write the stories of your futures. I genuinely believe that, together, we can do this.

Thank you for your time.

Mr. FOSTER. Thank you, Ms. Bush.

And thanks to all of our witnesses for your testimony.

Each member will now have five minutes for questions, and so the chair will now recognize himself for five minutes.

And, first, I have to say, you know, as a scientist, I often daydream that we can simply—when there's an issue that has to be communicated to the public, you can just say, here are the statistics, here are the numbers, here's the cost-benefit analysis, and then every one of my constituents will analyze that, apply the statistics to themselves, and say, OK, decision's clear, when do I get vaccinated, for example.

But it's not like that. You know, this job is to get an often-irrational primate to behave rationally. And so, very often, you have to inject sort of an equal and opposite irrationality into that primate with the sort of passion that you described in your testimony. It's important. Or the—what Dr. Adams mentioned about regret and even worrying about future regret. And so, I think—and it all rings true to you as a human being, even once you appreciate the statistics perfectly.

You know, I hosted a telephone townhall last week where we had doctors, public health experts, and we took questions from people about their concerns. And I understand—well, first off, we have to start with the science, and we have to get the science clear, that there is a definite net benefit. And we have to be honest with the public that the risks are not zero, but the benefits are so much more probable, that you must—you must analyze that yourself, and you must really, I think, take that rational approach to your life and your family's. But we need more than that. You know, we need the sort of passion that we saw in the testimoneys here.

You know, there—well, just in terms of the statistics, you know, I think all of us struggle to find, what are the right statistics to simply explain this to people? And the one that I've found as effective as any is that, if you looked at the 180,000 Americans who lost their lives from COVID–19 in May alone, less than 1 percent of those had been reported as being fully vaccinated.

That means 99 percent of those who died in May had vaccines available, by and large, and chose not to get vaccinated and paid the ultimate price. Not to mention their families, not to mention those who simply became sick and are going to, you know, live with, potentially, a life of long COVID. That's something that's hard to measure, hard to quantify, but it's going to be real, the reality for probably millions and millions of Americans.

So, it's time to get the shot here. You know, vaccines are a public health issue, and, as everyone has mentioned, they are not and should not be a partisan issue.

Just this morning, my colleague on this committee, Dr. Miller- Meeks, and I published a joint op-ed in USA Today urging all Americans to get vaccinated.

And, without objection, I'd like to ask unanimous consent that that op-ed be entered in the official—yes, I presume you're not going to be objecting to our op-ed?

Mrs. MILLER-MEEKS. No.

Mr. FOSTER. All right. Great. Yes, it's always nice to stack the committee when there's an answer you want to get.

Mr. FOSTER. Now, Dr. Benjamin, in your written testimony, you referenced a national poll that found that certain words and approaches make people feel safer in getting the vaccine. Could you say a little bit about that?

You know, one of the big irrationalities of human beings is that, you know, labeling or a few words just twist our opinions beyond all rationality. Can you say a little bit about the words that work?

Dr. BENJAMIN. Yes. Thank you for that.

Yes, one of the challenges we have is that words matter. And, you know, we try to make sure that you don't stigmatize people, as the Surgeon General pointed out, that you—what I do is, I ask people what their concerns are and then ask them to—then I try to address those specific concerns. I try not to make an assumption that I know what their concerns are.

And then using words that they're comfortable with. You know, the fact that the vaccine was developed over many years is important as part of that communication. Using words when you talk about who described—who developed the vaccine. Make sure that they understand it was people—scientists, researchers, people in their community, so they don't think these are some abstract people somewhere that went into a back room and made this, you know, "mad scientist" type of image of how the vaccine got developed, that it was very thoughtful people.

Pointing out, for example, that there are—particularly for the African-American community, very, very important—that African Americans were part of both the development of the vaccine—in fact, leaders in the development of the vaccine, that African Americans were involved in the studies themselves and, in fact, there was a Herculean effort, because we're not really very good at getting diversity in these studies, but, in this case, there was good diversity in these studies.

So, doing things like that to make sure that people understand what actually happened. And so, it's not just the message, but it's also the messengers——

Mr. FOSTER. Yes.

Dr. BENJAMIN [continuing] which is very important. Mr. FOSTER. Thank you.

And I believe my time has expired, and I will now recognize Representative Miller-Meeks for five minutes for her questions.

Mrs. MILLER-MEEKS. Thank you, Mr. Chair, Representative Foster.

First, I'd like to thank the chairman and the ranking member for holding this important nonpartisan hearing today.

And I would like to thank our witnesses for their testimony, even those that are virtually—or also those that are virtually.

I have been to every county in my district, all 24 counties in southeast Iowa, to administer the COVID–19 vaccines. I also attended a function on getting young people to run for office and administered vaccines there when a pharmacist brought the vaccine. I've also penned an op-ed on this topic with my colleague, Representative Foster, as he indicated, which was published today in USA Today on this exact topic. And I've done multiple interviews and sent letters encouraging the American people to get vaccinated.

I cannot emphasize how important I think it is to get vaccinated so that we can all return to normal.

To date, three vaccines are approved under the Food and Drug Administration Emergency Use Authorization process.

And, Dr. Adams, you mentioned something which is near and dear to my heart and for which I and other members of the Doctors Caucus—I'm an M.D. and a former state director of the Iowa Department of Public Health—sent to the FDA talking about this exact issue.

Can you explain how the Emergency Use Authorization is different from the full biologics license application approval?

Dr. ADAMS. Well, thank you very much for that question.

And it is important for people to understand that, during the EUA process, we are—or the FDA is evaluating to determine whether or not the risk is less than the benefit of an intervention. It hasn't gone through the full licensure process. And so, it is a bar that is especially important in the midst of a pandemic, because people are dying each and every day from COVID–19, but it is certainly not full licensure.

Now, that said, I want to hit a point that Representative Scalise mentioned earlier. Three-hundred-plus-million people vaccinated so far in this country—or doses delivered in this country. This vaccine has, again, been administered to more people and we have more safety data on it at this point than we've had for any other vaccine in history—in history—at this point of administering it to people. So, I, as a doctor, feel it's safe. I got vaccinated. My 15-and 16-year-olds have been vaccinated. But, that said, I continue to hear from the public that the lack of an update on licensure is something that's hanging over their heads. And that's why it's important that the committee address this.

Mrs. MILLER-MEEKS. So, you would agree with me and other members of the Doctors Caucus when we have asked the FDA to look at real-world evidence of the millions of vaccines administered both in the United States and globally, that that should be enough study data information to give full authorization for these vaccines?

Dr. ADAMS. Well, absolutely. Dr. Fauci and I worked closely, and Dr. Collins from the National Institutes of Health, with these organizations throughout the process to get to EUA, and we looked at data within the United States and outside of the United States. And when you go beyond the United States, you're well over 300 million doses that have been administered. We have even more safety data.

I just personally, as a physician and as someone who was inside this process, really, myself, don't understand why we haven't had more of an update yet.

Mrs. MILLER-MEEKS. Thank you for that. And, Dr. Adams, I want to say also that I remember meeting you at an ASTO) meeting here, and so it's a pleasure to see you again.

I'd also like to say that you mentioned herd immunity. And, in April, in this committee, I asked Dr. Fauci and Dr. Walensky both for herd immunity and the typical average of herd immunity, which you have said is around 70 percent.

Granted, we don't know what it is for this virus. But I think it's important—and I'm in an agricultural state. We know what herd immunity is. And the goal is to get as many people vaccinated as possible, and especially in the risk groups.

But you also mentioned about side effects. And there are so many questions I would love to ask, but I'm going to direct this next question to Ms. Bush.

And, Ms. Bush, your testimony was very compelling, because you mentioned the anxiety that you had, given your health risk. But we also know that, for children, there are tremendous mental health effects associated with not being in a normal school environment, coupled with stunted social and emotional growth of children 12 and over, and it far outweighs the potential effects of a vaccine.

So, what would you say to young people and to parents of children between 12 and 18 as far as getting the vaccine?

Ms. BUSH. Well, I think, again, you know, to the doctor's points, this is about how we protect our communities. I might have been less at risk than my parents, who are older and both immunocompromised, but I still got vaccinated for them and, admittedly, was terrified of this.

And I think the notion that households like some of our friends, who have some children over 12 and some children under 12, could be better protected if kids 12 to 18 were vaccinated, the likelihood that as we reach closer and closer to herd immunity, we will have less incidents of infection is incredibly important.

And it's our responsibility, in my opinion, to get vaccinated for ourselves, our loved ones, and also for those who can't, for immunocompromised people, immunocompromised children. This is a community action that we can take.

And, hopefully, the sooner we reach that herd immunity, the sooner we cross that threshold, all of these kids will be able to get back to the in-person learning that they need for their mental health and also for their cognitive development.

Mrs. MILLER-MEEKS. Thank you so much.

And, Mr. Chair, I know that my time has expired, but I just wanted to say that I thank the witnesses for talking about ending the mask mandate. We asked about this in April, given the data we had, and it should've been ended earlier so that people could see there was another benefit to getting vaccinated other than the lottery system, which I found tremendously interesting.

Thank you, Mr. Chair. I yield my time.

Chairman CLYBURN. [Presiding.] Thank you very, very much.

The chair has now returned via remotely. But thank all of you for your questions.

I do have questions that I would like to raise. As I mentioned earlier, I represent a largely rural district, and I am deeply concerned about vaccination rates in our rural communities. Although the CDC has warned that rural Americans may be at higher risk of severe illness and death from the coronavirus, rural communities are falling behind on vaccinations, and we are seeing cases rise in rural communities with large unvaccinated populations.

Over the next two weeks, I will be having five townhall meetings. Three of them will be in rural communities. And we will have the vaccine available at all of those meetings.

And I would just like to ask Mr. Garza: What would you have me tell my constituents who may not be sure that they want to get vaccinated?

Mr. GARZA. Yes, sir. I think the most important thing to explain is, the side that probably doesn't get shown very much is the side of somebody who went through it, like myself.

You know, you're in the hospital. There are so many uncertainties that you don't know about. And I think you have to explain the—there are just so many—it's hard to explain, being that I was there, and I experienced it, and a lot of people haven't experienced it yet. Maybe these people haven't—they don't know of people that have gone through it. Maybe they don't know of somebody who lost a loved one. You know, I knew of people who contracted the virus and, you know, they were fine within a week or two, and they were back to normal. And I felt like that was the norm.

I got hit very hard, so I went through the experience. You know, you sit in a hospital, you see on a daily basis—you see the people die on a daily basis. I think that needs to be, you know, brought to light. I think it—you know, it's nothing we really want to talk about, you know, all the time, but it's the truth.

And there's ways to protect it, and that's by taking the vaccination and going forward with it. And, you know, I would say, just share the stories as much as you can, because it's something that needs to be out there and for people to know that there is a consequence to not getting the vaccination, and it could happen to you and your family or your community. And that's something that we don't want to do, we don't want to see that happen, you know, but it's happening.

And I think people are on the fence either way, so I would share the stories as much as you can and explain, you know, the situation that—what could happen versus what they see.

Chairman CLYBURN. Well, thank you for that.

And I want to say to our staffs and our technical people here today that I would love very much to get your story. I was not here for your testimony; I'm going to listen to it. And I'm going to ask the staff to see whether or not we can make your testimony and your case available to more people in rural communities.

I can see us getting your story out to various community groups, at least throughout my district, and rural churches so that morepeople will know a little bit more about the dangers of not adhering to the science when it comes to this coronavirus.

So, I want to thank you so much for being here with us today. And, Dr. Benjamin, I want to thank you once again. You may have said strategies before I came back. Is there anything you would add to what Mr. Garza has said to us about getting the word out to rural communities?

Dr. BENJAMIN. Yes, sir. I think that one of the things you want to do is, particularly as you do in your townhalls, you know, you want to prep the community. That means going, you know—as you know, just like an election cycle, getting people going out door-to- door, making sure people are well-educated about the townhall, the opportunity to be vaccinated there, and trying to get some of their questions answered, having not only probably your health department there but also maybe some other community messengers.

And you know the folks we're talking about. You know, I've been to your events, as you know. We've known each other for a long time. And the kind of community outreach workers that you've had for some of the educational sessions that you've done at the university that go door-to-door, bang on doors, getting those folks out to talk to folks so that, when Mrs. Jones comes in, you know, she knows the community messenger that is trying to encourage her to get vaccinated so that it's not someone that doesn't know her or him.

And so, I just think that we need to put our arms around the community and just, as they say, show them the love when they come into those events.

Making sure that they have adequate transportation, providing rides to both your townhall and if the vaccination is at a different site, getting their vaccination there and back.

Recognizing that, yes, people do sometimes not feel well for either their first shot, quite often that second one, but they'll be fine afterwards.

And making sure that they can get off work and working with the local employers to give them time off. And, of course, I'm an advocate for paid time off when they do that.

Chairman CLYBURN. Well, thank you so much for your testimony.

Thank you, Mr. Garza.

The chair now recognizes Ms. Waters, Chairlady Waters, for five minutes.

Ms. WATERS. Thank you very much, Chairman Clyburn.

And I'd like to thank our witnesses for being here today to talk about a subject that's bothering so many of us. We are so concerned about our communities and the hesitancy that is displayed daily. We know all the stories about why people are hesitant, why they are suspicious. We know the distrust because of the way we've been treated in the medical community with experiments and et cetera.

We know all of that.

And we are talking to people and warning them ad nauseam. We're saying, you may die if you're infected and you have not been vaccinated.

So, we've done all of that. So now I'm really looking at incentives. I'm looking at what incentives work and how we can involve maybe the private sector in supporting us with incentives to get particularly young people out.

Now, either of you have any knowledge or experience that you can share with us about whether or not incentives work and whether or not it is ethical to do incentives?

First, Dr. Adams, what do you think?

Dr. ADAMS. Well, thank you so much. And, actually, I would direct the question to Dr. Milkman, because she wrote the book on this. She is the expert on this.

Ms. WATERS. Oh, she did?

Dr. ADAMS. Yes, she did. And she is the expert on the panel on incentives.

But what I would say to you very quickly is, you need to have the right incentive for the right audience. And a blanket incentive isn't going to work for every population, because it's not going to address the concerns the particular populations have. So African Americans may respond to different incentives than Hispanics and Latinos, than rural communities.

But, again, I'll throw it to the expert who is here, Dr. Milkman. Ms. MILKMAN. Sure. No, the evidence that incentives work is building. We have decades of evidence that they work for changing health behaviors in other contexts. Of course, we only have a little bit of evidence to date on how well they're working for COVID–19 vaccinations.

But, as I mentioned earlier, the Ohio Vax-a-Million data is already looking very promising. There was a 28-percent increase in vaccinations in the week following the announcement of that, and we believe that, in the two weeks following, there were an extra 50,000 to 80,000 vaccinations given.

Now, you asked a question about particular communities and do they work differently in different communities, and I wish we knew more about that. One thing that we're pioneering in Philadelphia, where I co-designed the Philadelphia Vax sweepstakes, is a kind of lottery incentive that's actually focused on communities where there are low vaccination rates.

So, we are running a citywide sweepstakes, but we are giving half of the prizes in each round, in each drawing, to a particular ZIP Code that's under vaccinated. And I think we should be doing more to target those under vaccinated communities.

A nice thing about lottery incentives is that they draw tremendous media attention. We think that's part of why they're so effective. People get very excited. There's vivid stories, which is important. We just talked about the importance of stories. You have vivid stories now of winners, happy stories that people like to hear about.

And so, I strongly encourage more communities to think about doing localized incentive programs.

Ms. WATERS. Well, thank you. This——

Dr. ADAMS. And, ma'am, work sites. Incentives at work sites are key, working with businesses. People spend more of their waking hours at work than what they do at home.

Ms. WATERS. Uh-huh.

Dr. ADAMS. And the people are going back to work.

Active is a company, an electronics manufacturer, that's working with Texas on the border to vaccinate people on both sides.

Again, it's important that—and I encourage the committee and I put in my written testimony that you all should work with businesses, the Department of Labor, and SBA to encourage and empower work sites to offer incentives and onsite vaccinations.

Ms. WATERS. Now, you may be the wrong experts to ask about this, but, of course, I was at the BET Awards this past weekend, and I was looking at Lil Baby and Rapsody and these rappers and how thrilled young people were with them, the young people that they have around the stages screaming.

What about that? Entertainment, athletes, rappers, do you think they could be helpful, you know, in helping us to get certain groups of people out?

What do you think, Dr. Benjamin?

Dr. BENJAMIN. Absolutely. The right messenger is very important.

And I can tell you what we've learned, you know, from our tobacco work, our anti-tobacco work, is that peer-to-peer education is very important, so getting young people to talk to other young people and getting them well-educated.

You know, just up the road here in Maryland, my colleagues at the University of Maryland have barbers that are talking to folks in the community. You know, lots of stuff gets talked about in the barber shop while you're in that chair.

And we did it through a—you know, when I was here in D.C. as a health officer, we used lay barbers and others to educate the community about a range of health threats. And we believe this would be effective.

A dean at the University of—in New Orleans at Tulane also has a barber program, a community program. It turns out it works.

Ms. WATERS. Well, thank you so very much. Like I said, I know we've all been preaching and talking, so we've got to be creative. We've got to come up with some new ways by which to do it.

Thank you very much for being here today. Thank you all.

Chairman CLYBURN. Thank you very much, Chairlady Waters.

The next—do we have anyone present on the Republican side for the next question?

Ms. Velazquez, you are now recognized for five minutes.

Ms. VELAZQUEZ. Thank you, Mr. Chairman, for holding this important hearing, important to the communities that I represent, communities of color and underserved communities.

And I want to thank all the witnesses for being here.

So, recently, I introduced the Building COVID–19 Vaccine Confidence Act of 2021, which directs the CDC to fund grants to local health departments and nonprofit organizations to conduct outreach to combat vaccine hesitancy, especially in communities of color.

Dr. Benjamin, what are the top three recommendations to create a successful, culturally competent, multichannel, targeted vaccine campaign?

Dr. BENJAMIN. So, I think the first thing is to make sure that you engage the community as part of your design. It is important that we not go in and think that we know what the community needs or what the community thinks. I think that's the first thing. Second, make sure that the—you know, that we make it convenient for people to get their vaccine. And that's extremely important.

And that——

Ms. VELAZQUEZ. So that means opening up vaccine sites where they are.

Dr. BENJAMIN. It means the sites where they are, it means getting them rides, but also, again, asking them what they need.

Ms. VELAZQUEZ. Sure.

Dr. BENJAMIN. When we were trying to do lots of education around infant mortality, it turns out that pregnant women wanted to—needed a place that was safe that they could simply do their laundry. We would've never thought about that. But, you know, just creating a welcoming environment for people to do things that they want to do.

And I think the third thing, of course, is that, if you're going to use incentives, that those incentives are focused. Now, I would like to argue that the most important incentive is that you don't get real sick and die. But people are not good at thinking about risk, but they do respond to targeted incentives that they find valuable.

Ms. VELAZQUEZ. Right.

Dr. BENJAMIN. And it doesn't have to be a lot of—— Ms. VELAZQUEZ. Thank you.

And, Dr. Benjamin, reports suggest that there may be a need for a booster shot. A New York Times article from May raised public skepticism over the COVID–19 vaccine's efficacy, and, just a few days ago, The New York Times indicated the vaccine could lead to years of protection.

So how do we educate the public on the facts and address these concerns?

Dr. BENJAMIN. Yes. One of the challenges is that we're doing science in real-time. In the old days, we would all go into a back room, we'd spend several years exchanging newspapers and articles, and debate amongst ourselves, and then we'd come out and tell the public what we thought our consensus was. That's now occurring in the public, and so the public is hearing the scientific debate.

I think it's important that, as we communicate that stuff, that we tell people that, first of all, we don't know if we need boosters yet. We might. There may be certain populations that need boosters and not others. It may be that if you got a particular vaccine from a different platform, you know, mRNA versus the adenovirus ones, et cetera, with different efficacies. It may be that if we mix and match these vaccines you get better coverage and maybe the booster may be different.

The answer is, we don't know. We need to tell the public we don't know—tell them everything we know but tell them also what we don't know. And then, as we know more, we should do that.

By the way, I know that they're working on creating boosters, but we're not there yet.

Let me say one final thing, is that, you know, the variants are going to drive that booster discussion probably more than anything else.

Ms. VELAZQUEZ. Right. Yes.

Dr. BENJAMIN. The story that we saw in the paper the other day, I think they were talking about assuming that the strain that we are protected from stays stagnant. If we get something that is much more virulent and escapes the vaccine, then we will clearly need a booster down the line.

Ms. VELAZQUEZ. Thank you.

And, Dr. Milkman, a recent poll found that more than half of unvaccinated Americans preferred to get a vaccine from the doctor's office instead of a pharmacy or a vaccinationsite.

So, what can be done to reach vaccine-hesitant individuals who may not have a local doctor, such as individuals experiencing homelessness or undocumented individuals?

Ms. MILKMAN. Yes. That's a fantastic question. And I think one of the things I'm most encouraged by is the fact that there are opportunities to do, sort of, door-to-door—and that can also be, you know, going to shelters and so on—outreach and have physicians who are willing to travel and have those conversations in that setting. Even if it's not your physician, knowing that it is a doctor you're talking to and having that conversation face-to-face can be very important.

And so, I think we need to be looking to tactics along those lines, rather than expecting people to come into pharmacies and request vaccines. The more we can go to the community and bring the information and expertise to them, the better.

Ms. VELAZQUEZ. Thank you, Mr. Chairman. I yield back.

Chairman CLYBURN. Thank you very much for yielding back.

Now, I am told that Mrs. Maloney is on her way. I don't know if she's in the hearing room yet. Is she?

She is not.

I will ask the witnesses to bear with us as we observe a five- minute recess. We will recess for five minutes to give members time to get back from this vote.

[Recess.]

Chairman CLYBURN. Let me thank the witnesses for their indulgence.

And I understand that Mrs. Maloney has returned and let me now recognize Chairlady Carolyn Maloney for five minutes.

Mrs. MALONEY. Thank you, Mr. Chairman. Thank you for your leadership.

I am very concerned about the lagging vaccinations and the rates of the vaccinations in younger Americans. According to the CDC, just half of Americans between the ages of 18 and 39 have received one or more doses of the vaccine, compared to more than 85 percent of Americans age 65 and older.

Ms. Bush, I really admire that you have been so outspoken on this issue. What message do you have for young Americans who have yet to get vaccinated?

Ms. BUSH. Thank you very much, Representative.

I think it's incredibly important for us to acknowledge the facts and then also acknowledge how we feel about them.

We are seeing that overall COVID cases are dropping, but only among the vaccinated. And the rates of infection, hospitalization, and death among the unvaccinated remain unchanged since January of this year. And we know that more and more young people have contracted COVID, and we know that it is not just adults. COVID–19 is among the top 10 pediatric killers currently.

So, this does matter for all of us; this does matter for young people. And I understand that there is an air of invincibility at times, especially because in the initial stages of the outbreak of the pandemic we thought that this was something that mostly affected older Americans. That's simply not true.

And especially for young people, who have so much of their lives ahead of them, who have dreams that they're building on and academic careers to pursue, so much of that is magic, frankly, because it happens in person, because of who we meet, who we fall in love with, where we wind up working, and I don't want young people to lose those opportunities.

And Representative Waters asked how entertainers and rappers and activists and athletes can play a part. What I would encourage any young person watching to think about today is how many of us you know through a screen or through a sport who you've seen get vaccinated, and our bodies are literally our jobs.

When I watched Megan Rapinoe and Sue Bird not only go get vaccinated in Seattle but volunteer at a vaccine site, I knew that that would be meaningful to young people, to see icons, professional athletes, whose bodies are their business, whose bodies have to run like gladiators, go out and get a vaccine to protect themselves and also their families.

And so, my hope is that, if you're a little less interested in politics than most of us in this room, that perhaps the people who you look up to, the athletes and the entertainers, et cetera, who you know don't really have anything to do generally with what's happening in these rooms, believe in medical science, believe in the innovation, understand that, as we look at a global number of over— 3 billion?—of over 3 billion vaccines that have been administered, we're doing great.

This will save lives, and, in particular, it will allow young people to get back to the futures that they're pursuing.

Dr. ADAMS. Congresswoman Maloney, if I may jump in really quickly. This is Dr. Adams.

One of the points I made in my written testimony was that the Department of Education should support school-based vaccination clinics. And that will especially help with our sports teams.

When you look at Jon Rahm—when you look at Chris Paul, who missed an NBA playoff game; Jon Rahm, who lost millions of dollars because he had to drop out of a golf tournament; when you look at the NC State baseball team, there are numerous examples of people whose lives were harmed by the social consequences of not getting vaccinated as opposed to the health consequences.

And young people, in many cases, aren't going to be scared into getting the vaccine by the health harms, but we need to help them understand how getting vaccinated will help them get their lives back to normal. When they go back to school, some of them in just a few weeks, they won't have to quarantine if they're exposed to someone. They won't have to wear masks, in most cases, if they've been vaccinated. It's important to show the benefits that actually matter to that group of people.

Mrs. MALONEY. Reclaiming my time, as I only have a very limited amount of time, I wanted to ask a question about my home state of New York.

In my home state of New York, we've offered 50 full-ride scholarships to any New York state public college or university to people under the age of 18 who get vaccinated. We also offered lottery scratch-off tickets with a grand prize of $5 million to those 18 and older and free baseball tickets, among other incentives.

Dr. Milkman, what strategies should we be using to increase vaccination rates among younger Americans and anyone else?

Dr. Milkman?

Ms. MILKMAN. Thank you for the question, Congresswoman.

I think it's wonderful what New York is doing. I think, actually, it's fantastic to see these kinds of incentives that, in particular, appeal to young people.

I think, in addition to college scholarships, we could think about, are there ways that we can particularly target young people? And Congresswoman Waters earlier mentioned celebrities. There are lots of things that we could offer in lotteries besides just scholarships that might be even more exciting to young Americans.

And I think there's an opportunity to try to get artists engaged, you know, free concert tickets or an opportunity to meet your favorite musician for lunch. Those are the kinds of things that we could consider also putting on offer in lotteries as prizes that might particularly appeal to young people. And having the kinds of events that were mentioned in Seattle, where sports icons come out and you could go meet them and get your vaccine.

So, I think the more we can engage with artists and entertainers and get them involved, the better we'll do.

Mrs. MALONEY. Thank you.

My time has expired. Thank you.

Chairman CLYBURN. Thank you, Mrs. Maloney.

I don't know that Congressman Krishnamoorthi has returned. I understand he may be on the way, but I don't want to hold our witnesses any longer than we need to. So, if the ranking member is not here for his closing statement, I'm going to proceed to my closing statement. And I will interrupt myself if Mr. Krishnamoorthi were to return.

So, before we close, I would like to enter into the record 21 letters the select subcommittee has received in recent days from organizations representing healthcare providers and advocates. I won't read off the names of all 21 organizations, but each of these groups has written to emphasize the critical importance of overcoming vaccine hesitancy so that we can increase vaccinations across the country and contain this deadly virus.

I'm going to ask unanimous consent that these letters be entered into the official hearing record. And unless there are objections, I'm going to order that they be in.

Without objection, so ordered.

Chairman CLYBURN. In closing, I want to thank Mr. Garza, Dr. Benjamin, Dr. Milkman, Dr. Adams, and Ms. Bush for testifying before the select subcommittee today. We appreciate your personal stories, your expertise, and your leadership.

I would also like to thank the ranking member for his participation in this effort.

We need to inform all Americans of the truth: Coronavirus vaccines are safe and effective.

To overcome hesitancy around the country, we must meet the skeptical where they are. We must enlist community organizations and trusted community messengers to inform the groups they represent.

We must also continue working to break down barriers in vulnerable communities, including technology, transportation, and language disparities, to reach those who want the vaccine but are unable to get it.

We must also recognize that there are many unvaccinated Americans on the fence, not opposed to getting vaccinated but not eager enough to have done so already. We can learn from those states who have come up with smart ways, such as lotteries, free giveaways, sweepstakes, and other incentives, to increase uptake among those who need extra encouragement.

The American public is still at risk. The more that the coronavirus continues to circulate, both in the United States and globally, the greater the risk that deadlier, more contagious, and vaccine-resistant variants could emerge. To lower this risk and to end the pandemic once and for all, it is crucial to get as many people vaccinated as quickly as possible.

We need to continue developing and implementing innovative solutions to encourage everyone to receive their vaccinations. I look forward to working with all of you on this panel, with my colleagues on both sides of the aisle, and with the Biden administration to do so.

But before I close this hearing, I wish to recognize Representative Krishnamoorthi for five minutes.

Mr. KRISHNAMOORTHI. Thank you, Chair Clyburn. Can you hear me?

Chairman CLYBURN. Yes.

Mr. KRISHNAMOORTHI. I wanted to just ask the panel a couple questions. And I'm sorry I'm running back and forth with votes and press conferences and so forth.

But the question is this, which is: Can any of the panelists speak to—and I apologize if you covered this before, but can any of the panelists speak to what has been effective in encouraging people who are hesitant about taking the vaccine to do so now?

And the more specific that you can be in terms of any examples of what has worked, I would be most grateful.

Ms. MILKMAN. I'd be happy to take this one for a moment and then turn it over to others.

Some of the key things that we've seen that do work are lotteries. Lotteries are working. There was a 28-percent increase in vaccination among those 16 and up in Ohio after the announcement of the Ohio Vax-a-Million and an estimated 50,000 to 80,000 additional doses delivered in the two weeks after that lottery was announced.

We know that people also respond to large incentives, payments on an order of magnitude of $100, though there is some risk that small incentives can actually backfire by signaling, "We have topay you; it must be risky to take this vaccine," which is inaccurate, but an inference people make. So large incentives work.

And people are also very motivated by reductions in restrictions, like not having to wear masks anymore. That means a lot to a lot of people.

Another thing that works very well are mandates, even though they're unpopular for good reason. However, we know that when there is a mandate it's highly effective. And 500 colleges and universities are mandating that people be vaccinated when they come back to campus in the fall. That's going to make a huge difference. And larger numbers would help, especially given that we know there are low vaccination rates among the young. And so that's another strategy we could think about encouraging.

And employers can also impose mandates. And I think we should be looking at whether or not there are ways to encourage more employers to do that, given the huge impact it has and the externalities of vaccination on your community.

Mr. KRISHNAMOORTHI. Are there any particular messages, especially with young people, that seem to work better than others in getting them to get vaccinated, obviously aside from saying that you have to do it, from a mandatory vaccination standpoint?

Ms. MILKMAN. It's important to hear from people who they trust and who they respect and admire. There was a discussion about, you know, musicians, athletes, the kinds of people we look up to. Young people respond more to that than to hearing from a politician.

Everyone responds well to hearing from a trusted medical source. So, if young people have a doctor, they're used to having conversations with, having those in-depth conversations can be really powerful, as well as just seeing role models.

But social norms spread, meaning I see my friends doing something and that makes me much more attracted to doing it. So, the more we can also convey to young people how many other young people are making the choice to get vaccinated, make that really visible on social media, that's going to help as well, because it will propel more and more. There's a snowball effect when we see someone else who looks like us doing the thing that we are contemplating doing.

Mr. KRISHNAMOORTHI. Would something as simple as having people who have been vaccinated get online and basically share that they were vaccinated, would that make a difference?

Ms. MILKMAN. It should. We know that it makes a difference in other contexts. When young people see on Facebook a number of their friends have voted, for instance, it increases their likelihood of voting. And the closer the social connection, the bigger the impact.

So, the more visible we can make it when young people vote and the more, we can ask them to tell their friends, communicate to their friends, send a message to their friends, the better.

Mr. KRISHNAMOORTHI. And has there been something that has not been done in that vein that should be done? I would imagine that there's a lot of social media campaigns that involve what I just referred to, but perhaps I'm wrong about that. But can you think of other things that need to be done on social media that haven't been done that would be effective?

Ms. MILKMAN. Well, one thing that I advocate for—and this applies to all populations, but young people in particular—is, I've been advocating for radical convenience, so whatever we can do to make it feel like the lightest possible lift to get this vaccine. Like, you wake up, you roll out of bed, and, boom, it's done.

So, college campuses bringing it to your dorm room, right? Your friend shows up and escorts you to the vaccine center, and you already have an appointment, everything's set up for you. I think that would help a lot with this population, and I don't think we've done enough of that.

Mr. KRISHNAMOORTHI. Thank you so much. I yield back.

Chairman CLYBURN. Thank you very much for your questions. And thanks, once again, to the panelists who are here today.

Without objection, all members will have five legislative days within which to submit additional written questions for the witnesses to the chair, which will be forwarded to the witnesses for their response.

Chairman CLYBURN. This hearing is now adjourned. [Whereupon, at 10:35 a.m., the subcommittee was adjourned.]

Chapter 3

Building Vaccine Confidence: Our Shot at Curbing the Pandemic in Chicago and Beyond*

Committee on Oversight and Reform

Wednesday, November 10, 2021
House of Representatives Committee on Oversight and Reform
Select Subcommittee on the Coronavirus Crisis
Washington, D.C.

The subcommittee met, pursuant to notice, at 1:08 p.m., in Conference Room C, Malcolm X College, 1900 W. Jackson Blvd., Chicago, IL, and via Zoom. The Hon. Raja Krishnamoorthi presiding.

Present: Representatives Krishnamoorthi and Foster.

Mr. KRISHNAMOORTHI. The subcommittee will come to order.

The title of today's hearing is "Building Vaccine Confidence: Our Shot at Curbing the Pandemic in Chicago and Beyond."

Without objection, the presiding member is authorized to declare a recess of the committee at any time.

I now recognize myself for an opening statement.

I would, first of all, like to thank Congressman Foster, my fellow subcommittee member, for joining me today, and all of today's witnesses for taking the time to testify about the critical issue of building vaccine confidence.

I would also like to thank Chairman Clyburn of the Select Subcommittee on the Coronavirus Crisis for his strong leadership and for lending us the resources for this important hearing today.

President Biden, Governor Pritzker, and Mayor Lightfoot have successfully vaccinated millions of Americans, over 222 million in total, including 8.3 million here in Illinois and 1.6 million in Chicago. That is over 75 percent of all Americans, Illinoisans, and Chicagoans over the age of 12 who have received at least one dose of vaccine.

---

* This is an edited, reformatted and augmented version of Hearing before the Select Subcommittee on the Coronavirus Crisis of the Committee on Oversight and Reform, House of Representatives, Serial No. 117–51, dated November 10, 2021.

In: COVID-19 Vaccines
Editor: John Schroder
ISBN: 979-8-88697-150-7

In just five months, the vaccine prevented 140,000 deaths across the country.

We know that the vaccine is effective. We know that it is safe. And we also know that widespread vaccination is the way to end this pandemic. So, why aren't more people getting vaccinated?

After all, without the vaccine, people are six times more likely to get coronavirus, and 11 times more likely to die from it. And vaccinations offer better protection against the coronavirus than immunity from a prior infection. Unvaccinated people who had recovered from a prior COVID infection are five times more likely to get COVID again than those who are vaccinated who had a prior infection.

With the vaccine, families can confidently gather for the holidays. Kids can see their grandparents. Children can spend more time in school and less time quarantining.

The Federal Government has provided millions of dollars in aid to end this scourge. The American Rescue Plan provided $350 billion across the country, including about $275 million here in Illinois. Chicago's vaccination efforts were fueled by almost $100 million in Federal funding.

Yet, many Americans remain unvaccinated. Nationwide, more than 20 percent of all adults and children over the age of 12 have not yet received even one dose of vaccine. Illinois has done better than the rest, and Chicago the same. Yet among adults and children over the age of 12, 23 percent have not started a vaccine series here in Illinois.

We now have an unprecedented opportunity to increase vaccine uptake here in Chicago and across the country. Just last week, Federal regulators approved the vaccine for children ages 5 to 11. I should say that my own five-year-old got vaccinated last week, and she got a poke present in return.

We owe it to our children to get shots in their arms quickly and equitably. They will spend more time learning, and, importantly, they will be able to get back to playing sports and socializing. They will have access to reduced-price nutritional meals, we well as other important social services.

President Biden, Governor Pritzker, and Mayor Lightfoot are all working hard to get shots to our kids. They are ensuring that vaccines are readily available at locations parents know and trust, like doctor's offices, children's hospitals, and schools.

Chicago is closing its public schools this Friday so parents can get their children vaccinated, and they are offering a small monetary award for children who get vaccinated.

As we vaccinate young children, we must continue to address vaccine hesitancy in historically underserved communities. We must continue the hyperlocal outreach that is working in Chicago. That means sending trusted messengers into their communities, and it means overall building vaccine confidence.

We are going to hear from many people today about how well this approach works.

We are going to hear from Mayor Lightfoot, who spearheaded the Protect Chicago 77 program, a community engagement program working to ensure 77 percent of Chicagoans 12 and older, across all 77 Chicago communities, have started their vaccinations by year's end.

Chicago is getting close; it is at 75 percent, and climbing. To help get to 77 percent, every Chicagoan can talk to friends and loved ones about the vaccine. Businesses can require vaccinations for their staff and patrons.

And we don't want to just hear from government leaders. We will be hearing from people who are out in their communities, doing the hard work of on-the-ground outreach.

Ms. Martha Martinez, the supervisor at an outreach program at a public library in Elgin, will tell you about how she and her team talk to community members every day. Dr. Omar Khan is both a medical doctor and a Muslim-American community leader. He will tell us how he has tailored his work to those in his community. Mr. Don Abram works for the Interfaith Youth Core, which funds local groups that are working to increase vaccine uptake.

They all agree on one thing: hyperlocal, on-the-ground outreach works. And the empirical evidence supports this approach.

Financial incentives are great, and they do a great job of ensuring a large number of people get vaccinated when they become eligible. But they don't work for everyone.

Employer vaccine requirements can also help fill the gaps. At United Airlines, implementing vaccine requirements increased the vaccination rate to 99 percent. Chicago and Illinois have both implemented vaccine requirements for public employees, keeping children and others in the care of public workers safe. And we are looking forward to hearing what Dr. Ezike has to say about this, as well.

Among the vaccine hesitant, many more want time to wait and see if the vaccine works. And many just want to talk to someone who can answer their questions. By funding and empowering hyperlocal outreach on-the-ground efforts, Chicago and Illinois are helping residents get the answers they need from the people they trust. And that is going to be an ongoing theme, I think, of today's hearing, which is finding trusted messengers to do that hyperlocal, on-the-ground outreach.

With hard work in the weeks ahead, we will keep children in schools and let families come together for Thanksgiving and the Christmas and winter holidays. I look forward to hearing from our witnesses how to meet those goals by building vaccine confidence in Chicago and beyond.

Now I would like to recognize Congressman Foster for his statement.

Mr. FOSTER. Thank you to the committee and to my friend, Congressman Krishnamoorthi, for convening this hearing, and to both panels of witnesses for their participation. I would also like to thank several organizations in attendance that have been critical to the COVID vaccination efforts in my district: the Will-Grundy Medical Clinic; VNA Health Care; and Advocate Aurora Health.

As one of two Ph.D. scientists in Congress, I always look to the research and data when making decisions, and the decision to get vaccinated is one place where the data could not be more clear: all three of the FDA-approved vaccines are extremely safe and extremely effective.

We run into two classes of arguments in the discussion over vaccinations. One is a scientific one based on pure self-interest, and a second one less scientific. It is based on your duty to your family and your community, and ultimately your country and all humanity because of the danger that one person being infected presents to eventually all of humanity.

So how do we know that they are safe and effective? First, the vaccines were tested on primates, for whom they were over 90 percent effective and had no serious side effects. Then we moved on to three different phases of human trials.

Across each of these three phases, the first of these phases, between 30,000 and 50,000 people received each vaccine, and each person was monitored closely for any adverse reactions or COVID infections. Again, the vaccines proved to be up to 95 percent effective at preventing COVID infections, and even better at preventing hospitalizations and deaths. The side effects observed were rare and usually minor.

So, if you want more evidence, then even after the vaccines were approved and deployed at massive scales, the FDA and pharmaceutical companies continued to closely monitor people's reactions, keeping close records of any serious side effects or infections that have occurred. To date, 431 million shots have been administered in the U.S. If these shots were dangerous, we would know it by now. And if they didn't work, we would also know that.

But, in fact, this extensive data has shown the opposite. Although it is still possible for someone who is vaccinated to catch COVID–19 or to pass it on, unvaccinated people are six times more likely to get the disease and, depending on the study, 11 to 20 times more likely to die from it than a vaccinated person. Many of our hospitals are overwhelmed with COVID patients right now, and more than 95 percent of those patients are unvaccinated.

And as far as safety, after tracking millions of vaccination outcomes, the only common side effect is a sore arm and perhaps a day of flu symptoms. This certainly isn't fun, but neither is spending a month on a ventilator.

But everyone on the two panels before us today already agrees with these conclusions. So, what we are here to do today is to figure out how to effectively communicate these data and statistics and ultimately get shots in arms.

Our local health departments and their partner organizations in the southwest suburbs have been working around the clock to get our neighbors vaccinated. We have seen the Will County and DuPage County Health Departments, among many others, run highly successful vaccination campaigns for our communities of color. I am incredibly grateful for their dedication, and I look forward to hearing what further support we can give them to get us across the finish line.

Thank you, and I yield back.

Mr. KRISHNAMOORTHI. Thank you, Congressman Foster.

Now I would like to begin by introducing our first two panelists.

Chicago Mayor Lori Lightfoot has led an impressive campaign to vaccinate Chicagoans quickly and equitably.

Mayor, thank you for everything you have done and everything that you are doing to build vaccine confidence in Chicago.

Our second witness is Dr. Ngozi Ezike, Director of the Illinois Department of Public Health, who has been a constant advocate and a steady voice for our state's public health and for children's health.

Director, thank you for all that you are doing for our residents in Illinois.

I will begin by swearing in the witnesses.

If you would please rise and raise your right hand? [Witnesses sworn.]

Mr. KRISHNAMOORTHI. Thank you.

Let the record show that the witnesses answered in the affirmative.

Thank you and please be seated.

Without objection, your written statements will be made part of the record.

With that, Mayor Lightfoot, you are now recognized to provide your testimony.

Statement of Lori E. Lightfoot, Mayor, City of Chicago

Ms. LIGHTFOOT. Thank you, Congressman Krishnamoorthi and Congressman Foster, and members of the Select Subcommittee on the Coronavirus Crisis, for holding today's hearing. I applaud your work and the unwavering support that you have shown municipalities across Illinois.

Though this journey is far from over, it is an honor to appear before you today to share the work that we have accomplished thus far and our plans for the future, which would not have been possible without cooperation from the government at all levels. So, I want to again thank the members of this body for the resources that have been provided to municipalities like Chicago. I also want to thank our State partners represented today by Dr. Ezike, who has been very instrumental in making sure that we are focused and coordinated in our efforts with the State.

From the moment COVID–19 hit Chicago, we were determined to listen to public health experts on the science and address its effects equitably and include our residents in the progress that we are making toward mitigating COVID–19. Thanks to this, we saw extremely strong rates of residents cooperating with public health orders and developed an equally strong community-led, hyperlocal response. We have been able to build vaccine confidence in our city because we started early on working with local leaders across disciplines to build a robust, city-wide response.

This started with the recognition that although all of Chicago was impacted by COVID–19, our Black and brown communities really bore the brunt.

For example, in April 2020, despite making up only 29 percent of Chicagoans, Black residents accounted for 75 percent of COVID- related deaths. That was seven times the rate of any other demographic.

To address this glaring and unacceptable disparity, my team, alongside community partners, created the Racial Equity Rapid Response Team, or RERRT, which forged partnerships with trusted community messengers across disciplines and utilized trusted locations to provide residents with information, testing, and eventually vaccine.

While this started with a focus on deaths in Black Chicago, we soon widened our aperture and worked to build the same kind of trusting relationships across Latinx Chicago.

To bolster this data-driven, hyperlocal approach, we launched initiatives like Protect Chicago Plus, in which we sought to vaccinate multiple generations within the same household simultaneously by going deep into these communities that were showing sustained rates of high-case infections. Here again, we used a network that we had built for testing and education to make progress in our hardest-hit zip codes.

We also then created Protect Chicago at Home, which mobilized our paramedics and vaccinators to provide in-home vaccinations for homebound or disabled residents and has been available to all residents free of charge since June of this year.

To date, more than 15,000 people have been served through this Protect Chicago at Home program. It is very, very popular.

And as of the last four weeks, 54.6 percent of the participants in this program were Black, and 18 percent were Latinx.

We also created a 600-strong work force of contact tracers, and we specifically targeted the underemployed with an earn-as-you- learn approach. Not only have they been doing contact tracing, but they have also been deployed to be vaccine Ambassadors in their communities.

Recently, as you mentioned, we launched Protect Chicago 77, which engages individuals in every single one of our 77 communities to ensure that at least 77 percent of residents aged 12 and over have received at least one dose of COVID–19 vaccine by the end of the year. These efforts have helped to save countless lives, including Marie Ann Jesus, parents of Portage Park resident Cessi. Cessi and her parents were desperate for a vaccine appointment when they met Brianna, who volunteered to connect them with vaccine appointments for residents after losing her grandfather to COVID–19. Twenty-four hours later, Cessi secured an appointment to protect her parents. Cessi's story and the story of countless others were made possible for the many volunteers, community leaders, and organizations who continue to pull their time, talents, and resources together to protect our most vulnerable communities and have allowed Chicago to retain its reputation as having the most equitable vaccine distribution strategy in the country.

I want to emphasize a couple of data points in my closing seconds. Ninety-nine percent of fully vaccinated Chicagoans have not tested positive for COVID–19, whereas 99.9 percent have not been hospitalized, and 99.9 percent have not died due to COVID. These numbers are pretty remarkable, but the flipside is the case for folks who remain unvaccinated.

My time is up, but I appreciate the opportunity to speak with you here today. Thank you.

Mr. KRISHNAMOORTHI. Thank you, Mayor.

Now I would like to recognize Director Ezike for your testimony.

Statement of Ngozi Ezike, MD, Director, Illinois Department of Public Health

Dr. EZIKE. Congressman Krishnamoorthi and Congressman Foster, thank you so much for inviting me to be here today to speak about our vaccination efforts to protect all of Illinois from COVID–19. And thank you for your leadership at the Federal level to promote these life-saving efforts to keep our country safe.

As of November 9, 2021, more than 16 million vaccines have been administered in Illinois, leading to about 62 percent of the population with at least one dose. And more importantly, 57 percent of the total population is fully vaccinated against COVID–19.

By age, the share of Illinoisans who are fully vaccinated is about 84 percent for individuals over the age of 65; 66 percent for adults aged 18 to 64; and 54 percent for youth age 12 to 17. Following the authorization of vaccine for children age 5 to 11, just on October 29, younger children have started to get vaccinated. As of November 7, over 15,000 doses have been administered to children age 5 to 11, including your own.

Mr. KRISHNAMOORTHI. Thank you.

Dr. EZIKE. We are currently averaging more than 53,000 doses administered per day Statewide, and the seven-day rolling average of doses administered in Illinois is more than twice as high as our most recent lull, at roughly 19,000 doses per day, back in mid-September. There is no doubt that the local health departments, health care providers, retail pharmacy partners, employers, and so many other partners across Illinois have worked tirelessly together to implement a very successful Statewide vaccination effort, and we are celebrating this achievement thus far, but still understanding that there is a lot more work to do.

We know that there is a wide variance in vaccination rates across the State, so the numbers can sometimes hide the details. For example, about 95 percent of seniors in Kendall County are fully vaccinated, and that compares to 34 percent of seniors being vaccinated in Alexander County. For youths age 12 to 17, 70 percent are fully vaccinated in DuPage County, while two percent are fully vaccinated in Harden County.

Racial differences have also persisted, including for young children just beginning to be vaccinated. Among those 15,000 doses administered through November 7, [inaudible] percent were administered to white children, and only 12 percent to Hispanic children, and three percent to Black children.

As we prepare to accelerate the next wave of vaccinations for children age 5 to 11, now is a good time to take stock of exactly what we have learned about strategies to increase those vaccination rates for all.

There was a time when there was incredibly high demand for the COVID vaccine before they were approved and as those first doses were rolled out in December 2020. But since April 2021, when the rate of vaccination actually began to slow in Illinois, the population of individuals left to be vaccinated is increasingly composed of people hesitant to the COVID–19 vaccine, in addition to the minority of Illinoisans who could be described as anti-vaccine or opposed to any form of vaccination.

In Illinois, those that are most likely to report vaccine hesitancy have primarily been younger people, people of color, and rural residents. Importantly, we also know that vaccine hesitancy and refusal can serve to reinforce social identity, in this case often tied to political or partisan and religious identities polarized through the pandemic. Research also reveals some of the reasons vaccine-hesitant people share for not receiving the vaccine include concerns with the speed of vaccine development, lower trust in the experts, and fears about the safety and effectiveness of the vaccine.

Our continuing vaccination efforts will rely in part on acknowledging and understanding vaccine hesitancy to best target remaining vaccine-eligible individuals. Every day we are vaccinating individuals who are likely to have expressed some hesitancy, otherwise they would have already been vaccinated since all adults were eligible in April.

These individuals are hesitant adopters, people who are both vaccinated and yet report some degree of hesitancy. In the current phase of the pandemic, addressing vaccine hesitancy should focus on creating more hesitant adopters by implementing interventions that are tailored to the specific concerns of specific populations. This has been our approach in Illinois to date, where we have spent a total of $225 million on the vaccination effort.

There is need for urgent action. The highest rates of COVID–19 vaccine hesitancy are found in the demographic groups that have already been the most severely affected by the pandemic. In Chicago, in Cook, for example, COVID–19 vaccine hesitancy for children was nearly three times higher among Black parents compared to white parents, while Black Chicagoans comprise a disproportionately greater number of COVID–19 deaths compared to other groups.

Attitudinal hesitancy may not be the only issue, however. Communities with lower rates of COVID–19 vaccination are also those with structural inequities and access to health care resources. For example, retail pharmacies have been a major source of both testing and vaccination, but research has persistently found that Black and Hispanic neighborhoods have fewer options for pharmacies and have to drive longer distances to the closest COVID–19 vaccination. All that we have learned to date will inform how we implement our ongoing efforts for the 5-to 11-year-olds. We are working to reach school-age children. We are going to use our pediatricians, our family doctors, our community health centers, all these places where parents can receive trusted information about the vaccine to reduce hesitancy.

To date, approximately 2,200 providers in Illinois have registered to administer the vaccine, and we plan to continue registering the additional providers, especially targeting communities where vaccination rates have lagged.

Federal support could significantly aid Illinois in our efforts to facilitate vaccination among hesitant individuals. The Federal Government should help mitigate and counter misinformation in the ongoing info pandemic that parallels the pandemic. This info pandemic fuels hesitancy and public confusion through the rapid and widespread dissemination of inaccurate messages. Knowing what is being spread and catching it early could allow IDPH and our many partners to respond swiftly to misinformation with simple, consistent, accurate counter-messaging. Unfortunately, current Federal funding is often restrictive and lacks the ability to rapidly re-allocate those funds to address the emerging needs and crisis situations as they arise.

Reorganizing public health funding is one way the Federal Government can help us implement the kinds of interventions necessary to refute misinformation and continue vaccinating hesitant individuals and populations.

Thank you so much for the opportunity to share Illinois' experience, and I am very happy to answer questions.

Mr. KRISHNAMOORTHI. Thank you so much.

I should have told you about the timer before, but there is a five- minute timer here, and we will try to abide by the time.

I would like to recognize myself for five minutes of questions. Mayor Lightfoot, I understand that Chicago has taken a data-driven approach to its vaccination program, and I am fascinated by this at-home vaccination strategy.

Can you explain some of the lessons Chicago has learned and how it has changed its approach based on what it has learned?

Ms. LIGHTFOOT. Well, I think one of the biggest things that we have learned is that there is not a one-size-fits-all approach, particularly when you are dealing with vulnerable communities. We have really spent a significant amount of time building partnerships, joining tables that have already been built, and really then using the data and sharing that data with local-based advocacy groups and stakeholders to craft really neighborhood-specific interventions.

One of the ones that really came out of that discussion was our at-home program. We started that using Johnson & Johnson to go into homes of our seniors. But we have seen such an embrace of it across particularly Black Chicago on the South Side, where we have seen lower rates of vaccine uptake, that we have literally been going door to door with vaccine Ambassadors and then signing up whole households for the at-home service. It has really been quite tremendous with us.

But what I would say is, again, one of the things that has been most important in our vaccine distribution program is the work that we did prior to the time that the vaccine hit by building those relationships with trusted community partners and messengers, and then using that infrastructure to push out vaccines, and then constantly being engaged with them to understand what the levels of hesitancy are.

I think Dr. Ezike got it just right. Based on polling that I have seen, both nationally and certainly here locally, there is a small percentage that are anti-vax, that are never going to reach it. The vast majority of people that remain unvaccinated are still vaccine hesitant. So, when we sent out those Ambassadors into neighborhoods, going door to door, we see the ability to really address people's concerns, make sure that we are informing them of the facts because, as you know, there is still a persistent drumbeat of misinformation out there about the vaccine, about the efficacy of it, the ingredients of it, what was used and so forth. When we are able to have those kind of one-on-one conversations, we are able to break through at remarkable rates.

Mr. KRISHNAMOORTHI. Thank you.

Dr. Ezike, rural areas, it seems like this is a really tough-to crack. Can you tell us what is working in rural areas, and can you give any specific examples?

Dr. EZIKE. You know, we have tried the door-to-door method that had worked in some areas, and we had a lot of pushback and resistance on that. So, what we have done, we have continued to do outreach, we have continued to partner with churches in the area, trying to find local people of faith who are willing to share the message, allow education to be spread, host events. But we have also had to make sure that we give other options, and so we have been very diligent about educating about monoclonal antibodies. We know that at the end of the day we need to save lives, and if we have people who are still on the fence, still hesitant, or absolutely not going to get a vaccine, part of the approach has to make sure that they do understand how they might take another option if they were, in fact, to get infected, although we continue to promote an ounce of prevention is worth a pound of cure.

We have also tried to make sure that there is access——

Mr. KRISHNAMOORTHI. Excuse me. If I could jump in, are there any trusted organizations in the rural areas, or trusted messengers, that seem to be more effective than others?

Dr. EZIKE. So, we think that using physicians from the local area, people who are recognized by people in that area. We have a strong rural health department at IDPH, and working with those physicians who are in the community, helping to have the town halls where people can ask the specific questions that are maybe holding them back. And when they see a physician or a nurse practitioner, another clinician that is known to them that is from the local community, sometimes that correct messenger is the person whose message will be received.

Mr. KRISHNAMOORTHI. Now, Mayor Lightfoot, what do you think? Who do you find to be—if there is a group or a class of people who are the most trusted messengers that you have found, who are they?

Ms. LIGHTFOOT. I think it is those local health care providers, first and foremost. But what we have also been able to deploy is people themselves who are vaccine hesitant, who then can tell the story to others about what it was that really got them to decide, no, the vaccine is something that I need for myself and for my family. Those are very powerful messengers.

Mr. KRISHNAMOORTHI. Excellent. Thank you.

Now I would like to recognize Congressman Foster for your questions.

Mr. FOSTER. Thank you.

You know, as a scientist, I am really proud of the work that researchers have done to develop and test vaccines to provide protection against this virus. In the early days of the pandemic, Congresswoman Donna Shalala, the former head of HHS, and I led a bipartisan letter urging maximum resources to be put into all vaccine manufacturers that had any chance of making a workable vaccine. This effort was eventually rebranded as Operation Warp Speed, and the Coronavirus Oversight Committee that we are convening here, we have been very active in overseeing that production effort and also making sure that when the first doses were available they were equitably distributed, which was not naturally going to happen.

So, I am very grateful for the work of the Federal, State, and local officials, as well as the health care providers and other community members who helped get the first millions of shots in arms in record time. And now with 423 million doses of coronavirus vaccines administered in the U.S. to date, we have seen that the vaccines are very safe and effective. The data show that the vaccines are literally lifesavers and that serious side effects are rare, and yet far too many Americans are still placing their lives and the lives of others at risk because of vaccine hesitancy.

So, Dr. Ezike, as a physician, what are the first arguments that you find most effective when you recommend that people get vaccinated or boosted as soon as they are eligible?

Dr. EZIKE. I continue to share the information about how layered approaches are important and how prevention is always our first line. I think I try to use the examples of vaccine-preventable illnesses that we don't see. I have been a physician for over 20 years. I have not treated one case of measles. But my tennis captain, her brother is deaf from the results of measles. So, in that short time, we can see what the vaccine has done.

The example of polio, I don't have children jumping double-dutch jump rope with braces on their legs from polio. The only reason that we don't have polio is because of the vaccine.

So, just reminding and level-setting about what vaccines are.

I know a big pushback that comes back is when we talk about Tuskegee in the African American community. We talk a lot about, oh, the Tuskegee experiment where public health officials did not do right by people of color. So, even understanding that example, acknowledging that something was done very wrong during that time, but remembering that in Tuskegee, in that instance, we had a situation where treatment was withheld. There were available antibiotics that were withheld from people who needed it. And in this case, we have that available treatment that we don't want to withhold from people of color or anyone else.

Mr. FOSTER. You are right, that will just compound the inequity that has been longstanding in our health care system.

Actually, you did a good job of answering my next question.

Mayor Lightfoot, are there other aspects of your city's approach that have helped convince Chicagoans that vaccines are safe and effective that you have not had a chance to mention yet?

Ms. LIGHTFOOT. Yes. I think, look, at the very beginning it was just getting out the basic information about the various clinical trials, the results of the effectiveness. That really helped to allay a lot of concerns initially. But right now where we are, there is really not a one-size-fits-all approach. You have got to simply start the conversation by listening and really getting an understanding of what the particular person's hesitancy is. It is that simple, but that complicated.

And we have all the data that you want. For example, in our city, if you are a person of color 50 years or older, you have a 50 times higher likelihood of death if you are unvaccinated. When you start talking to people one-on-one about those kinds of shocking statistics, that catches their attention.

But what we also try to do is draw out the misinformation that they have taken in so that we can disabuse them with the facts. But it really requires a lot of patience, a lot of listening, to go directly, and that is a lot of what the vaccine Ambassadors, the work that they are doing on a regular basis, and that is why I am proud of that program and why I think it has been wildly successful in bringing communities into care.

The other thing that we are really avoiding doing is shaming people in communities for not being vaccinated. So, we are trying to reinforce the Protect Chicago 77 with positive messaging. Any time a community makes measureable progress, we highlight that on various social media platforms, and I think that positive reinforcement is also helping considerably.

Mr. FOSTER. Thank you.

I have five seconds left, so I think I will yield back.

Mr. KRISHNAMOORTHI. OK. Thank you, Congressman. We are going to do one more round of questions.

So, Mayor, as you were talking, one thing that dawned on me is that when you have almost 80 percent of Chicago residents now having received their first shot, that has to touch almost every family in the city, at least that is what I am assuming.

Now, let me ask you this. This may be a loaded question, but do you find that family members are good Ambassadors to other family members? Because I hear the anecdotes both ways.

Ms. LIGHTFOOT. It really does go both ways. But if we can reach someone in that family, and then get them to be the Ambassador with their own family, to talk to mom, dad, grandma, other siblings, it does make a huge world of difference. That is why I think in part our initial push, Protect Chicago Plus, was so successful. We really concentrated on getting someone, particularly within an intergenerational household, who would be the messenger on the vaccine, who would bring the reluctant family members to a vaccinationsite. That is what I think made it very successful.

For example, the Belmont Cragin neighborhood, through most of 2020, before there was a vaccine, was a neighborhood where we saw exploding case rates, percent positivities in the high teens, or even higher in some instances. That community now is one of the most vaccinated in our city because of the hard work that was done through Protect Chicago Plus, working with trusted stakeholders, and we held a lot of vaccination opportunities all over, in schools, in houses of worship. You name it, we were there working with our partners in various pharmacies, with various doctors that were from that neighborhood. That neighborhood has had a remarkable recovery because of the hard work that was done prior to the time that we got vaccine, and then pushing it out and highlighting those local stakeholders who said, yes, I got the vaccine, and here is the reason why.

Mr. KRISHNAMOORTHI. Got it. Thank you.

Dr. Ezike, what can the Federal Government do to assist in increasing the vaccination rate? You mentioned something about disinformation or misinformation and social media. I would be curious about what are your observations there and what are you doing or what needs to be done by others to control that issue?

Dr. EZIKE. I think the infodemic, if you will, is a very powerful tool that is working negatively against the COVID response efforts, and I know most public health departments and other health partners don't really have the resources or the expertise to be able to monitor what the trends are in social media. So, by the time we are actually aware of some of these ideas that have just permeated and bathed the people, it is a very uphill battle to get on top of that because that news spreads so quickly.

So, if there was a way that the Federal Government could assist with monitoring the information that is out there so that we can jump and seize hold of some of these mistruths and disinformation earlier on, before it has had such a chance to percolate throughout society, we could probably avert many people from hearing the wrong news, or at least having the counter-message be ready.

Mr. KRISHNAMOORTHI. Getting in front of it. Dr. EZIKE. Exactly.

Mr. KRISHNAMOORTHI. Mayor, what do you think about the challenge with regard to youth? I see it has risen, the percentage has gone above 50 percent, and Dr. Ezike said this about Illinois as a whole. What strategies seem to be working with our youth? I am talking about 12 to 18 for right now.

Ms. LIGHTFOOT. Well, first of all, we have to get the parents. In that age cohort, you have to get the parents on board. Fundamentally, that is what it is really about. You have to make sure that young people are connected up with a pediatrician, because that is going to be the most likely place that you are going to see. And then for the older end of the teenage years into the early 20's, we have done a number of different things. We have popular influencers who are going directly to those young people talking about the vaccine. We have done D.J. radio takeovers where there is messaging through the whole program on popular radio sites in a variety of languages all talking about the safety of the vaccine. Of course, we have to get those people vaccinated first, but we have had a lot of success with that.

We have done a lot of digital assets deployed on social media platforms and elsewhere to really reach young people with the kind of messaging and imagery that is going to make a difference for them.

So, we have really been focused on that cohort, I would say initially 18 to 39, and now more recently 12 to 18, and we are doing the same thing, frankly, that marketers are doing, what works, how do you reach them, and that is where we are going.

Mr. KRISHNAMOORTHI. Thank you.

Congressman Foster?

Mr. FOSTER. Thank you. Back to the pure science for a moment.

Viruses constantly change through mutation, and new variants of a virus can spread more easily or make viruses resistant to treatments or other vaccines. One of the strongest arguments for getting yourself vaccinated is to reduce the number of chances the virus has to incubate a new variant, a new and dangerous variant of itself. The most prominent of these is currently the Delta variant, which is thought to be twice as contagious as the original virus. In fact, studies have shown that people infected with the Delta variant carry about 1,000 times more copies of the virus in their respiratory tract than those infected with the original strain.

Dr. Ezike, how has your department responded to the challenges from the onset of the Delta variant?

Dr. EZIKE. So, we obviously had a heads-up because we saw the information coming from around the world, and so we knew that this virus will find its way, this variant will find its way to us. So, we continued the messaging. Masking became another important tool on top of the vaccination, and just trying to spread through our community Ambassadors as well the information that this was a different virus. I kept using the line you are talking about COVID–19; we are dealing with COVID–21 right now. So, you have to understand that this virus has changed. It has newer properties, and they are not properties that work in our favor, and that is why we had to go back to the masking for all, and that is why we had to double our efforts for vaccination, understanding that this vaccine, we are fortunate that it also still offered protection even against this new variant and that the sooner we got as many people vaccinated—and, of course, we know this is a global issue in terms of vaccination—the sooner we would be able to slow the continued mutation and development of new variants.

Mr. FOSTER. So it may, in fact, be Aaron Rodgers who is that one-in-a-billion person who incubates through his selfish decisions, incubates a new variant that could put billions of people at risk.

Ms. LIGHTFOOT. I would be happy to talk about Aaron Rodgers all day long.

[Laughter.]

Mr. FOSTER. Really? OK. [Laughter.]

Mr. FOSTER. That is a little bit outside—let's leave Chicago for a moment here.

Illinois has worked hard to increase the vaccine uptake, and to do so equitably. Earlier this year Illinois Governor Pritzker launched a $10 million campaign to tackle vaccine hesitancy and spread awareness about coronavirus vaccines, and although more than 77 percent of Illinoisans over the age of 12 have now received at least one dose of the vaccine, vaccination rates are lagging behind in some parts of the state, and particularly the rural areas. This is not unique to Illinois. We are seeing it across the country. A recent study found that close to 40 percent of rural respondents nationwide were not vaccinated or eager to get vaccinated, compared to almost a quarter of suburban residents and a little over 20 percent of urban residents.

Dr. Ezike, how will the low vaccination rates in rural areas make your job difficult throughout the state?

Dr. EZIKE. Well, we have already seen the effects of the low vaccination as we have come off of this Delta surge. The area that was hit the hardest was the region that was the least vaccinated. We got to the extent in southern Illinois where there are literally no more ICU beds—not for COVID patients but for any patient. We were interfacing with our Federal VA partners, begging for beds that we could transfer patients to. We were asking hospital partners in other parts of the state to please allow us to transport patients.

So, we have already seen the effects of the low vaccination rates. In fact, when we looked at where we had limited ICU capacity, it matched in order—1, 2, 3—in terms of lowest vaccinated regions were the areas that had the lowest amount of beds and the highest rates, case rates of COVID.

Mr. FOSTER. This is a tragedy. Are there any states you are aware of that have been more successful at getting their rural populations vaccinated, any success stories at all, or is this just a problem with where rural areas get their information from?

Dr. EZIKE. It has been a very consistent problem, unfortunately. When I talk with my colleagues around the country that have similar rural populations, part of it is the demographic, some of it is politics. We know that everything is political, but it has also become, unfortunately, partisan, and that has made some people make a decision against the vaccine.

Even as people have seen family members become ill themselves, seen the head of their nursing department die, we have not seen people around them say, oh, I guess I need to get the vaccine. So, we continue to work with our partners. We hope that every day more and more people will make the choice, especially as we are talking about third doses for people. Those who haven't gotten their first are way behind, and it is still not too late to get started on the effort.

Mr. FOSTER. Thank you.

It appears my time has expired. I will yield back.

Mr. KRISHNAMOORTHI. Well, thank you so much, Mayor Lightfoot and Director Ezike. Thank you for your testimony.

Panel 1 is now concluded and you are both—I was told here to use the word "released."

[Laughter.]

Mr. KRISHNAMOORTHI. I will just say free to depart. So, thank you so much again for your wonderful testimony. Thank you.

Ms. LIGHTFOOT. Thank you.

Dr. EZIKE. Thank you.

Mr. FOSTER. Thank you very much for everything you do every day.

Dr. EZIKE. Thank you, sir.

Ms. LIGHTFOOT. Thank you.

Mr. KRISHNAMOORTHI. I now invite the witnesses on our second panel to approach the witness table.

[Pause.]

Mr. KRISHNAMOORTHI. OK. We are joined today by five witnesses for our second panel.

Dr. Helene Gayle is the President and CEO of The Chicago Community Trust.

Dr. Omar Khan serves as the Co-Chair of the Muslim Community Center's Health and Awareness Committee.

Ms. Martha Martinez is the Supervisor of the Pandemic Health Navigator Program at the Gail Borden Public Library District in Elgin.

Mr. Don Abram is a Program Coordinator at Interfaith Youth Core.

And Mr. Ben O'Donnell is an Ironman athlete and coronavirus survivor.

Thank you all for being with us today. I will begin by swearing in the witnesses.

If you could please rise and raise your right hand? [Witnesses sworn.]

Mr. KRISHNAMOORTHI. Let the record show that the witnesses all answered in the affirmative.

You may be seated.

Thank you again for joining us.

I should mention that the microphones are sensitive, but please speak directly into them.

Without objection, your written statements will be made part of the record today.

With that, Dr. Gayle, you are now recognized to provide your testimony, and you have five minutes.

Statement of Helene D. Gayle, MD, President and CEO, the Chicago Community Trust

Dr. GAYLE. Great. Thank you so much. I would really like to thank you and Representative Foster, as well as Representative Clyburn and the other members of the subcommittee, for holding this field hearing.

This year the Chicago Community Trust partnered with the Rockefeller Foundation and local partners to develop the Chicagoland Vaccine Partnership, so I am going to focus most of my comments around this partnership. This work is coordinated with the work that you heard from our public sector, and in that vein I want to say how grateful we are to have public-sector leaders like the ones that you heard from who have done so much to protect the health and well-being of our most vulnerable residents and communities. They have had to make some tough choices in order to keep us all safe and healthy, and to make sure that equity was at the center of this response.

However, still, although vaccines are widely available and effective, many Chicagoans, as you heard, particularly Black and Latinx residents, remain unvaccinated. That is why we launched the Chicagoland Vaccine Partnership, which is a collaboration of more than 170 organizations dedicated to building a healthy and resilient Chicagoland.

The Partnership recently made over a million dollars in grants to community-based organizations who could get the people that they work with every day vaccinated. These grants supported a diverse range of organizations that are deeply rooted in their communities, organizations like food pantries, churches, youth boxing programs, and violence prevention organizations, organizations that are not often thought about as part of the public health response. The program has developed things like speakers bureaus and an ambassador program to help develop the knowledge base among trusted messengers. We have hosted convenings with public health departments and community leaders to answer community members' questions. We have begun a program to help community members gain access to public health careers. And now, with the vaccines that we have talked about being available for those who are 5 to 11 years old, we have declared November a month of action to educate families about vaccines and promote vaccinations for all.

Despite these efforts, we know that disparities in vaccine rates persist. To better understand why, we worked with the research group Mathematica to conduct a survey to talk to people in our communities and hear what they had to say about the COVID vaccine. Data from the first wave of this survey have had some revealing insights.

First, most vaccinated responders listed doctors, health care providers, scientists, and the CDC as the most trusted source of information about the COVID vaccine, and most of these who were vaccinated were motivated to get vaccinated to prevent death and serious illness within themselves, but also to protect their households and family members.

But for unvaccinated respondents, lack of trust stood out as the largest issue. While nearly everyone knew where to go to get a vaccine and how to schedule an appointment, most of the unvaccinated recipients wanted more time to wait and see if the vaccine worked, and many believed it was developed too quickly. They also worried about getting sick or experiencing side effects, and only about a quarter agreed that the vaccine was safe or effective.

The unvaccinated did not trust vaccine information from sources like the CDC, scientists, religious leaders, news media, or government officials. Only seven percent reported trusting Federal Government officials. Only four percent reported trusting state and local officials.

In communities of color, and for Black Americans in particular, we understand why there is that hesitancy, and Dr. Ezike referred to generations of discrimination in medical research and practices that have caused harm and distrust. So, we understand why some of this longstanding hesitancy and distrust exists. We also know that there are language and technical barriers to accessing vaccines in Black and brown communities.

It is clear that we need more than brochures, public service announcements, and financial incentives. But equally important, we know that we need trusted messengers, one-to-one conversations, and persistence in education and empowering hard-to-reach and skeptical populations. We need to ensure that issues like childcare and paid leave are addressed so that people can get the vaccine and deal with any potential side effects. And we have to develop easy-to-understand messages that describe how the vaccine testing and production process was safely compressed into a shorter timeframe while still validating and supporting people who do want and need more time.

There is no silver bullet for building trust and overcoming the obstacles that are faced in communities with lower vaccine rates. We need to meet people where they are and build solutions that meet their needs. We believe this vaccine partnership can serve as a model to be scaled and replicated more broadly and be an important bridge to building trust in communities beyond this crisis.

At the Chicago Community Trust, we have made closing the racial and ethnic wealth gap our highest priority. We cannot have a thriving economy on the household, community, or regional level if we don't do all we can within our reach to prevent further harm from the COVID–19 pandemic. Ensuring the equitable uptake of the COVID–19 vaccine is key to achieving it. It is both the prudent public health response and a critical first step toward a just and inclusive economic recovery.

Thank you.

Mr. KRISHNAMOORTHI. Thank you, Dr. Gayle.

Now I would like to recognize Dr. Khan for your five minutes of testimony.

Statement of Omar Khan, MD, Co-Chair, Muslim Community Center's Center's Health and Awareness Committee

Dr. KHAN. Thank you. I would like to thank Representative Krishnamoorthi and Representative Foster, again, for your time and inviting us here to speak with you all and share in our experiences on the ground at a hyperlocal level, as Representative Krishnamoorthi had mentioned.

COVID has been an international devastation, and many local communities have had to step up to disseminate complex information and provide accurate and up-to-date statistics from reliable and credible resources. It has been a challenge for many, including our own communities at the Muslim Community Center and The Douglas Center. I am the Co-Chair of the Health and Awareness Committee at the Muslim Community Center, or also referred to as MCC, which has locations in the northern Chicago suburbs, as well as a location in the city of Chicago. These locations include mosques, schools, and, at the core, community centers.

I am also the Director of Health and Wellness, Administration, and Development at The Douglas Center, which is located in Skokie, Illinois. The Douglas Center provides community day services for adults with intellectual and developmental disabilities. Both organizations play key roles in many people's lives, and both organizations had to unfortunately close their doors to their patrons at some point during COVID.

Challenges have been faced within numerous communities in regards to comprehension of information, sources of information, and hesitancy. Many have expressed concern of side effects, long-term effects, and the speed in which vaccines were developed. Unique challenges that we have identified within the two organizations that I work with are language barriers, cultural sensitivities, faithbased concerns, and with the special needs population sensory challenges when it comes to face masks, adhering to hygiene guidelines, and comorbidities and chronic illnesses.

In both organizations we have built relationships with local, state, and national-level clinical personnel and entities that are credible and have been providing ongoing information and guidance that we have then relayed in relevant and consumable manners for the given communities. We have had numerous successes over time as we have catered to the needs of the various communities, some of which include immigrant and refugee populations. The unique challenges we have identified with those communities in particular have been trust, language barriers, literacy challenges, and cultural nuances.

The greater successes for both organizations include COVID vaccines for qualifying children and adults through MCC has been an estimated 2,000 patrons and community members. At The Douglas Center, an estimated 98 percent of our participants, again that are individuals with special needs, have been fully vaccinated against COVID.

We aim to continue in providing support for our community members through information, conversations, and actions. Thank you again.

Mr. KRISHNAMOORTHI. Thank you, Dr. Khan.

Ms. Martinez, I now recognize you for five minutes of testimony.

Statement of Martha Martinez, Manager, Pandemic Health Navigator Program (Gail Borden Public Library District)

Ms. MARTINEZ. OK. Good afternoon and thank you for the invitation to both of you for today.

I supervise the Elgin Area Pandemic Assistance Team at the Gail Borden Library in downtown Elgin. My team consists of four community health workers: Anamaria Mora, Chas Sirridge, Luz Purcell, and Sue Tuominen. We are part of the Illinois Pandemic Health Navigator Program that is funded through a grant by the Illinois Department of Public Health and administered by the Illinois Public Health Association.

We are charged with helping those that have been impacted by COVID, specifically the underserved. That might be the elderly or others that lack access to the Internet, a computer, or a smart device. We work in a very diverse community in Elgin, with significant brown populations. Clients are relieved when they are able to come in and speak to us in Spanish. We also serve the houseless community that visits the library regularly. All of the above are residents that are in need of assistance.

We partner with the local health department to work with COVID-positive patients who may need services while they are under quarantine. We provide food deliveries, disinfectants, diapers, and we have even delivered dog food.

We can be reached in several ways. We have a published number for all to call us. We have an email address and a web page. We also staff a table in the library lobby for those that prefer to walk in and speak to someone directly. Many are looking for financial assistance, and we help to connect them with other community-based organizations that have funding for such requests.

Early in the year when vaccine appointments were hard to come by, we assisted in scheduling hundreds of appointments. As the vaccine requests dwindled, we moved to outreach work by participating in local community events and making our community aware of our services. We have also hosted many vaccine clinics at the library, and we will be hosting one this Saturday with DNA Healthcare, and we will be offering the boosters as well as the new children's vaccine.

We have helped with lost vaccine cards. We have answered questions about the vaccine, and now the boosters. Our availability via multiple channels has allowed us to keep up with the pulse of the community, both vaccinated and unvaccinated.

Gail Borden Library is a trusted entity in our community. People know to come there when they need help, and the staff is great at providing that assistance. Our pandemic team fell right into place here. We take a nonjudgmental approach with our clients and try to match them with the services that they need.

Through familiarity with our daily presence, we too have become trusted advisors in the community. We continue to promote vaccination in a respectful, non-confrontational manner. We have had many clients stop by to thank us for our help.

I would like to share some experiences.

We helped an 85-year-old man living by himself who was looking for a COVID test. Most appointments are done online, and he didn't know how to use a computer or a smart phone. We made the appointment for him close to home. He didn't use email, but he told us that he could access texting. We took a picture of his ticket and sent it to him. He was incredibly thankful for the assistance. While that was simple for us, it was challenging for him.

Another case we had was a family of eight that came to us in the 11th hour. They were desperate because they were facing an eviction notice that very same week. We worked closely with them to secure funding and to get them back on track with their rental payments. They too were happy to be able to stay in their home. Our team members have literally driven through tornadic winds to deliver medications. They have brought victims of abuse to the local crisis center. They have secured temporary shelter for a client whose utilities were turned off amid a heat wave. They have delivered food to families with empty cupboards, and they were welcomed by children peering through the window whose faces lit up when they caught a glimpse of the ice cream bars at the top of their delivery.

We know we have helped many people negatively impacted by COVID. We hope to continue with this work. We hope that we continue to be funded for this work. Special thanks to Denise Raleigh and her wonderful team at the library, for they have supported us throughout this project. Thank you.

Mr. KRISHNAMOORTHI. Thank you, Ms. Martinez.

Mr. Abram, you are now recognized for five minutes of testimony.

Statement of Don Abram, Program Manager, Interfaith Youth Core; Ben O'Donnell, Coronavirus Survivor

Mr. ABRAM. Good afternoon. Thank you for the opportunity to share my own lived and professional experiences with this committee, and for the opportunity to highlight the indispensable role that faith-based communities occupy in the local response to the ongoing COVID–19 pandemic. My name is Don Abram and I am a Black queer minister from the south side of Chicago. As a spiritual son of the Black church and a native of the far south side Roseland neighborhood, the role of faith is central to my own story. I grew up in a hand-clapping, toe-tapping Black church only minutes from my childhood home. Throughout my life, the church has served as a spiritual refugee in times of trouble and as a resource in the midst of material and financial need. In moments of both crisis and celebration, the church has proved itself to be a trustworthy, reliable, and present help to my family, my community, and I.

While the particularities of my story are unique, the powerful role of faith-based communities in the lives of everyday Americans is not. Across the city of Chicago and this country, mosques, churches, synagogues, and temples are more than houses of worship. They act as community hubs, daycare centers, food banks, and even access points for affordable housing, critical social services, and quality health care. This is especially true for low-income communities of color.

The robust safety net created by faith-inspired organizations often cultivates pathways by which marginalized communities can access life-saving resources. This is most salient in the case of the faith-based response to the COVID–19 pandemic, especially in marginalized communities wherein marginalized communities suffer disproportionately. I have seen the role that faith-based communities occupy as a program manager at Interfaith Youth Core. I have seen it up close and personal. Early on in the pandemic, as the need for vaccine education, literacy, and access ballooned, IFYC equipped Chicago-based faith leaders with the tools to launch vaccine education events and vaccine clinics in communities that needed it the most. Rabbis, preachers, imams, and spiritual teachers, from various faith traditions, came together to share best practices and to equip themselves to be vaccine Ambassadors.

Partnering with medical experts, IFYC offered a six-month train- ing program that enabled faith-based communities to maximize their impact on the ground. Leveraging decades-long relationships within their communities, faith leaders became instant trusted messengers, educating their parishioners on the efficacy of the vaccine and assuaging legitimate concerns with fact-based information. Coupling community events like block club parties and Sunday services with vaccine clinics, faith leaders were able to increase vaccination rates in their communities and ultimately helped to save lives.

As we consider effective strategies to increase vaccine uptick in the near-and long-term future, the role of faith-based leaders must be centered. Investing in a vibrant ecosystem of proximate faith leaders, in the city and across the country, will ensure that our response to the ongoing pandemic is culturally competent, contextually rooted, and grassroots focused. Over and over again, faith leaders have been proven to be effective bridge builders between local communities and health care providers, ensuring a more equitable distribution of vaccine education and vaccines themselves.

While we celebrate the progress made on vaccine adoption, particularly in marginalized communities, the need for education and the dismantling of access barriers to vaccines remains a persistent challenge. As I see it, faith leaders are best poised to craft community-based solutions and outreach strategies that target those hardest to reach. Sensitive to the particular and niche needs of their community, faith leaders are equipped to meet people where they are, and to address on-the-ground barriers to vaccine adoption.

In my capacity as a Black minister on the south side and as a faith-based organizer, I am confident in saying that faith communities are critical to us defeating the spread of COVID–19 and to us healing from the loss of friends and loved ones. It is incumbent upon us that we resource, amplify, and coordinate with faith communities across lines of difference to further our progress on vaccine uptick.

I would like to thank the committee for your time and for the consideration of my testimony. God bless you and all of those on the front lines of the ongoing pandemic.

Mr. KRISHNAMOORTHI. Thank you, Mr. Abram.

I would like to now recognize Mr. O'Donnell for your five minutes of testimony.

Statement of Ben O'Donnell, Coronavirus Survivor

Mr. O'Donnell. Thank you. I would like to thank the committee members for the invitation to this hearing today. To be able to tell part of my story to keep others safe is an honor. This pandemic and virus are still affecting so many people, and if my story and ideas can help others, I am more than happy to provide that.

My story starts in February 2020. I had a two-day physical at the Mayo Clinic to ensure I was in good health before I started my intensive training for my next Ironman, my second Ironman Triathlon. Five days later, I went on a business trip where I contracted COVID–19. I started showing symptoms on February 29. On that day there were less than 1,000 reported cases reported in the United States. I was admitted to the hospital on March 9 and spent the next 28 days in the ICU before being discharged, and over half of those days were on a ventilator. I was the first critical case in the state of Minnesota, and I was only 38 years old.

There are multiple reasons that I have the opportunity to be here today. One of those is privilege. I was able to be treated at one of the top ECMO centers in the world at M Health Fairview at the University of Minnesota. I was privileged to be the only COVID– 19 patient in the entire hospital for that first week and that all of their resources were dedicated to keeping me alive. I had the privilege to have a wife who is a Ph.D. chemist who could have data-driven discussions with the entire health care staff on what treatments they might try for me. I had the privilege to have a care team that was willing to take chances and experiment. I was also privileged to have a body strong enough to survive while they were trying to see what could be done. And I was also extremely privileged to have insurance and a job with disability pay so I was not affected financially. I did not lose my home, I did not lose any income due to this, and I know that I speak from a place of privilege when I say these words.

That is the first theme of my story. It is privilege.

The other main theme of my story is science. When I was put on ECMO or ECMO life support, it was thought that ECMO would not work for the treatment of COVID–19. However, my doctors felt that it was my only shot at survival. There was no known treatment for COVID–19 yet, so my care team searched the literature and found the best treatments that they could at that time. If my family or doctors waited until there was something 100 percent effective, I would not be here today. As it is, I was the first person in North America to be put on ECMO while suffering from COVID and survive. Now there have been thousands. Also, I was able to recover and complete another Ironman Triathlon last May.

I could spend long minutes talking about the primal fear I had when my intubation tube was blocked and needed to be removed and deprived me of oxygen for minutes before it was put back in. I could talk about the hallucinations while sedated that two years later are still crystal clear in my memory and probably will be forever. But fear will not help us in this situation. Fear will not help us to get people to get vaccinated. We cannot use it as a tactic to persuade people that vaccination is necessary.

What we need is proper discourse without fear. We need to address people's concerns with the vaccine, not their decision. We need to enter these conversations with empathy and not judgment. We should not judge people for the decision they made, but rather challenge how they came to that decision. There are many reasons for the decisions that have been made. There are those that cannot afford to take the time away from work to get vaccinated or to deal with the side effects, should they have any. When the consequence of vaccination means not being able to pay rent or mortgage or put food on your family's table, the decision is no longer a simple science and fact-based decision. These are the impossible decisions. When we bring empathy to the table, we discuss the barriers and how to overcome them. Some of these barriers have nothing to do with hesitation but rather ability. We need a way to combat this lack of privilege. Once we do that, we can discuss the next steps. And to me, the next step, which has been my message since my experience, is to follow the science.

We have plenty of information and misinformation. We have plenty of people blaming or pointing fingers at others in order to get their point across. The one phrase we throw around too much is to "do your own research." This is dangerous. My background is that of a scientist. I have a Master's degree in Organic Chemistry from the University of Notre Dame. I know science and research very well. I spent the first decade of my career developing in-vitro diagnostic tests. I even helped a colleague develop one of the tests, IL–6, that helped identify the cytokine storm that saved my life. I have spent my entire career in science, but I am not a COVID– 19 expert. I have no qualifications to do any research on this topic, and I have no capability to do my own research.

One thing my background does allow me to do is read and understand the research and to put it into a translatable format for a general audience. Too often, a single line or a research article is taken out of context and used to declare the entire article or research study really meant something contrary to its findings. The world has a large number of people that are creating and sharing misinformation. What we don't have is enough people who are translating the research in full so that it can be consumed by the general population.

In order to combat vaccine hesitancy, we cannot push the science. We need to bring empathy to the discussion to determine a way to allow everyone to follow the science.

Thank you.

Mr. KRISHNAMOORTHI. Thank you, Mr. O'Donnell.

I now recognize myself for five minutes of questions.

Dr. Gayle, you have made a tremendous number of investments during the pandemic. What would you say was the investment with the highest ROI, so to speak, especially with regard to vaccinations?

Dr. GAYLE. Yes. Well, I think this panel has spoken very eloquently to the investment in community-based efforts, and I think if I were to say where we could scale up and do more, it is in these kinds of efforts where people—again, going back to the survey that I talked about, the unvaccinated, the issue of trust is the biggest barrier. It is not anymore the access, it is not anymore the knowledge of where to get vaccinated. It really is this issue of trust. And so I think it is by investing in people who know their communities both within the health system, public health messengers, community-based care providers, but also organizations that help people when they are not just focused on COVID, these are the organizations that have stood with these populations throughout, and these are the organizations that they trust.

We talked about the role of faith institutions, for instance. We are involved with, as I mentioned, food pantries, other kinds of community-based organizations. These are the organizations that people trust. They know how to speak in ways that resonate for those populations. And I think the biggest thing is we have to realize that there is no one magic bullet and that building trust takes time. But building trust is built on meeting people where they are and making sure that we are also thinking about the broader ways in which their health, their households are affected, and being able to give them a sense that they are cared about in a holistic way I think is why these community-based efforts have made such a big difference.

Mr. KRISHNAMOORTHI. Got it.

Mr. Abram, is there something that we have learned in talking to people about taking the COVID vaccine that could be applicable in any other area where we have trouble communicating, whether it is violence prevention or any other thing? I am just curious.

Mr. ABRAM. I think so, and at the heart of what it is that we have done at IFYC is hold space for concerns and to approach the conversation with humility, recognizing that community members and those who work and live alongside them know more about the barriers that exist, know more about the particularities of concerns that come up in the community, and this is something that can be translated across issues, making sure that we create infrastructures wherein community can provide feedback to those who have resources, and we can, in real time, pivot and adjust as needed, because we created space for community partners to really show up and ask questions that they need answered.

Mr. KRISHNAMOORTHI. Got it.

Ms. Martinez, I am always impressed by Gail Borden Library. It is really a gem in terms of our library system. I am curious, in your outreach to people, have they also become more attached to the library because of your efforts with regard to getting them to take the vaccine and doing other things with the pandemic?

Ms. MARTINEZ. I believe so, because many of the people, especially early on, when people were on the fence about taking or not taking the vaccine, I think just through seeing us there day in and day out, we I think inspired some confidence in them. We would have discussions, we would answer their questions, and I think all of that contributed to getting many more people to take the vaccine. And as I mentioned earlier, just being able to speak in a language to people also gives them a sense of relief and comfort and the ability to be able to ask all their questions and get answers.

Mr. KRISHNAMOORTHI. Yes.

Dr. Khan, is there anything unique to certain minority communities—let's just take the example of the Muslim American community—that we should be aware of in terms of vaccine confidence or the lack thereof?

Dr. KHAN. Yes. Again, when speaking to a number of the barriers that we have been able to identify, language, as was mentioned, has been an important factor. When you think about some of the conservative aspects, when we created the vaccine clinics at the mosques in the gym spaces, we were aware of some individuals who may want same-sex individuals providing the vaccine for them, creating a privacy space for some individuals who may not feel comfortable lifting up their shirts or removing their shirts, things like that.

So, we have had to identify those and address those.

Again, there are the faith-based concerns, is this something permissible within our faith to get, what was used to make this, were there animal byproducts that were used, things like that. We have had to have conversations with religious leaders in collaboration with health care professionals to help disseminate some of that information.

So, it has been very important to identify, again, some of these barriers and speak to those things in particular.

Another challenge that I have come across more recently when I spoke about refugee and immigrant populations, things like that, something that we are going to have to really work hard on is a couple of weeks ago, in having a conversation with one of the community centers that we work with, we realized that there is no particular written language for one of the communities that we work with, one of the refugee communities that we work with. How is that communication happening? It is not something that they are reading online or within social media. A lot of it is that verbal communication, the literacy issues.

So, those are things that we are trying to work on, translate that via audio, simplify the language, and make sure that people are getting the information that they need.

Mr. KRISHNAMOORTHI. Thank you.

Congressman Foster?

Mr. FOSTER. Thank you. I guess I would like to start by echoing my thanks to Ms. Martinez for everything that Gail Borden Library does in the community. I have very fond memories from representing Elgin for several years, 10 years ago now. You have been a beacon of hope and assistance for people in the Elgin community for a long time.

Ms. MARTINEZ. Thank you, sir.

Mr. FOSTER. I would like to speak a little bit about vaccine hesitancy among parents of young children. Last week we achieved a significant milestone in our Nation's fight against the coronavirus when the first coronavirus vaccine was authorized for 5-to 11-year-old children. Yet, one recent study found that only three out of 10 parents of kids between 5 and 11 plan to vaccinate their children immediately. Misinformation is a problem that can harm children even if it comes through their parents.

Dr. Gayle, is there a misconception among some parents that the coronavirus is just like the flu and that their children are unlikely to be affected?

Dr. GAYLE. Well, I think a lot of the information that came out early on that suggested that children were less likely to get sick if they got the coronavirus did make parents think that this was a less serious issue for children, and I think that has persisted and in some ways remains a barrier. So, I think the reason why we have to not have parents' hesitancy multiplied through their children, get the information out, make it very clear why it is so important. We saw what happened to our educational system, where children were not able to have the kind of access to education as a result of this. This is such a huge, huge step forward to be able to now get children vaccinated safely and having the data to show that it is safe, that it is effective, and that it can make a huge impact on households.

One of the things parents sometimes are not taking into consideration is that the risk of their child is then transferred to them and the rest of their household. So, I think we have a lot of education to do and a lot of correcting of misinformation about the impact both at an individual level and, as we were talking about earlier, that this is not just about an individual, this is about our communities. This is about how do we protect our community more broadly than just the impact on the individual. Children have a huge role to play in that, and I think we have got to do it, and that is why we have dedicated November as vaccination month, to get this information out to parents so that they can be part of protecting whole communities while they protect their children's health, as well.

Mr. FOSTER. And this is not only an issue for young kids. Also, it is an issue in utero, because there is lots of evidence that it is very bad for the mother and the child to get COVID, and no evidence at all that the vaccine itself poses a risk to a child.

Dr. GAYLE. Pregnant women are going to have more serious consequences if they contract COVID. So, it is an incredibly important issue.

Mr. FOSTER. That is right. So, I understand that anecdotes are not data, but I would like to present one anecdote.

This is my grandson here. I became a grandfather on April 1. And my grandson, who shares my name, was born of a vaccinated mom, and he is healthy and happy. And not only that, he sleeps through the night.

[Laughter.]

Mr. FOSTER. So, maybe that is another reason to vaccinate here, get mothers to vaccinate their kids.

[Laughter.]

Mr. FOSTER. But, Mr. O'Donnell, as a scientist and a coronavirus survivor and a parent of a young daughter, you have an important perspective on this. What would you say to a parent who said that they didn't need a vaccine, didn't need to vaccinate their kids, because the coronavirus is less likely to be a big deal for the young and healthy?

Mr. O'Donnell. I was young and healthy when I caught COVID, and I ended up in the hospital for 28 days. I know that my five- year-old daughter is excited in asking when she can get vaccinated, as well. So for me, we can't get to a normal everyday life, and we never know what we have genetic predisposition-wise to know if we are going to be completely fine or if you will end up getting severe side effects, whether you are five years old or you are 50 years old. With that lack of knowledge out there, the only way we can combat that is that we know the vaccine works, and we have to explain how it works for people and for their children.

Mr. FOSTER. Thank you.

I guess I am out of time, so I will yield back.

Mr. KRISHNAMOORTHI. Thank you, Congressman Foster.

Mr. O'Donnell, I wanted to ask you about this ECMO treatment. Tell us a little bit about that. I think for some folks—I have heard of it but I am not terribly familiar, and I think others would want to learn more about that.

Mr. O'Donnell. So, ECMO treatment is extra-corporeal membrane oxygenation. It is where they take the blood from your body and they pump it through an external machine to put oxygen back into it because my lungs were so full of fluid that they could not oxygenate my blood itself. It is a tube probably about the size of my thumb that gets inserted into your jugular to your heart to pump blood through it. All of your blood gets pumped through it about every two minutes.

Mr. KRISHNAMOORTHI. I think this is a treatment that a lot of hospitals have provided, but a lot have not, as I understand it. Go ahead.

Mr. O'Donnell. It is a very rare treatment. Right now, I have moved to Canada, and the province that I live in only has one machine or two machines in the entire province. It is a high-risk operation and procedure, and there aren't many machines globally. The U.S. has a very large number of them, but there aren't very many of them outside of major university medical centers.

Mr. KRISHNAMOORTHI. Got it.

Mr. Abram, what is the number-one piece of misinformation that you deal with, with regard to vaccines that we should be aware of? Mr. ABRAM. Based on my experience particularly with faith-based communities, one of the primary concerns is that the side effects would be really overwhelming and could even lead to unexpected illnesses or sicknesses, and that is largely rooted in a lack of education around the vaccine and messaging that suggests it is not safe or effective, which we know goes against science. So, we have been working with faith leaders to think about creative, innovative, and ongoing ways that we can reiterate the efficacy of the vaccine.

Mr. KRISHNAMOORTHI. But don't they—I guess in that situation—at this point we are reaching 75 to 80 percent of adults 12 and over who have received the first dose, so most families have at least one person. Do they not see those folks and say, OK, that person hasn't gotten sick since they got the shot? Or is that not persuasive to them?

Mr. ABRAM. It is not persuasive, and I think that is largely because of the fact that these folks also perhaps exist outside of opportunities and spaces wherein they can ask questions around the vaccine with specificity. So, getting medical experts or folks who are knowledgeable around the efficacy of the vaccine to be in conversation with them becomes critically important. In that case, household conversations are effective. But what we see is that folks aren't always equipped with the specific medical expertise or knowledge to be able to articulate the ways in which having the vaccine affects ultimately your resistance to COVID–19.

Mr. KRISHNAMOORTHI. Within the Spanish-speaking community, Ms. Martinez, who do you think are the most trusted messengers for building vaccine confidence?

Ms. MARTINEZ. Certainly primary care doctors are.

Mr. KRISHNAMOORTHI. Who speak Spanish?

Ms. MARTINEZ. Who speak Spanish, yes, and also the clinics that they visit often, because many people don't have primary care doctors. So, the local clinics where there are Spanish speakers. For us, the VNA, the Greater Health are clinics that people trust and go to. And certainly pastors are also important in either helping move this forward or in holding people back from taking the vaccine.

Mr. KRISHNAMOORTHI. Are there some pastors who hold people back?

Ms. MARTINEZ. Well, in specific, I don't know of specific ones. I have heard that there are people or pastors that have not promoted it, and I think that is just as bad as not pushing it, when you just hold back and don't talk about it, and then it seems that it is unacceptable to go ahead and get vaccinated.

Mr. KRISHNAMOORTHI. Dr. Khan, the imams, how important are they in spreading the message; and, as Ms. Martinez said, is there a concerted effort to make sure they are vaccinated and that they spread the message?

Dr. KHAN. Yes, I think those are challenges that a number of communities have faced, as well. Not all imams, a majority of imams, have a medical or health care background to understand a lot of the specifics. So, we had challenges in the beginning as well of imams being able to share that information. But that is also our responsibility, to help educate them. As time has gone on, as we have been able to have these conversations, as we are learning more, getting more data, looking at the statistics and information, we are able to educate those community leaders.

We have Friday prayers. In Friday prayers, it is the imams that stand before the entire group that is there and speak to them and provide guidance and advice and things along those lines. It is complete silence throughout the mosque while they are listening to them. So, it has been very important to have those religious leaders and faith-based leaders speak to this and assure the individuals from a faith-based perspective that it is permissible. There are, again, a number of other challenges that come after that when we talk about safety, efficacy, and things along those lines. But, yes, it has been very important for the faith-based leaders to address this head-on.

Mr. KRISHNAMOORTHI. Got it. Thank you. Congressman Foster?

Mr. FOSTER. Thank you. I guess there is another thing that we run into from time to time that is related to the faith-based community, which is that you will be trying to convince someone to get vaccinated and at the end they say, "I will just leave it up to God." Mr. Abram or Mr. Khan, what is the answer to that? It is my understanding that there is a strong tradition in the Abrahamic religions across the world that you are supposed to take care of yourself and it is part of what God expects from you, and yet you find people using God as a reason not to get vaccinated. What is your best answer to that?

Dr. KHAN. Yes. I think that a deeper understanding of that comes with a deeper understanding of faith. We have heard those exact phrases from a number of individuals. And when you look at actual scripture, and we speak about the Prophet Mohammad, peace be upon him, and the things that he has said and shared, you see that you are meant to care for yourself and take care of yourself and those around you. It is a responsibility of ours.

We also acknowledge and realize that we have been given the intellect and opportunity to grow from an intelligence perspective, and research has helped with that. So, we are meant to acquire knowledge. When you think about the Islamic faith, when we talk about the revelations of Islam in particular, one of the first things that you look at is we believe that the angel Gabriel had come down to the Prophet Mohammad, and the first words he said to him were "Read" or "Aqra." So, to pursue knowledge has been from the inception of the conversation of faith for us.

So, it is really important that we help those individuals who say let's leave it up to God, because there are a lot of things that we don't just leave up to God, right? We take action, and then we can leave things up to God after the fact and pray for things. But it is important that we take action in protecting ourselves, protecting our family, protecting our communities, understanding that we are all one big community and things that happen overseas will affect us here as well, right? If we think about this virus in particular and where it may have originated, people are affected across the world. So, we are one big community, and it is important that we don't just think about ourselves but those around us as well.

So, yes, it is very important that we continue to gain knowledge and then take action off of the knowledge that we attain.

Mr. FOSTER. Mr. Abram, how do you respond when you encounter that?

Mr. ABRAM. So, from within my tradition in particular, but this is across religious traditions, there is a sort of theological framework that is centered on healing and treating your neighbor as you would treat yourself. There is a moral and spiritual imperative for us to care for the other, and that often is an effective theological framework that we have seen faith leaders use to advocate vaccine uptake and education, saying we have a responsibility to care for our communities, to care for ourselves, and the way that we are able to do that in this particular instance is to ensure that we are using our God-given intellect and ability and power to be able to actually encourage the vaccine adoption.

Mr. FOSTER. Thank you. This is sort of what I mentioned in my opening statement about there is a scientific question of what is best for me, all right? And a second question that has very little to do with science, which is what is my duty to the rest of humanity, and this is crucial.

Dr. Gayle, the Chicago Community Trust and its partners have worked very hard to figure out what will motivate adults to get vaccinated, but are there any transferrable lessons on how to motivate parents and guardians of children, 5 to 11 let's say, to get their children vaccinated? Is there a difference in the messaging that is best for that?

Dr. GAYLE. No. Actually, I think a lot of the same messaging. It is just really focusing it more on tackling some of the misconceptions about the importance of getting children vaccinated. A lot of it is that this is new and parents just have not had the information that they need. I think it is really the same messages in many ways, but really tailoring them so that people can understand the scientific basis for why getting children vaccinated is important as well.

If I could just go back to your last question just for a second, just to say that one of the things that I have seen is most helpful with getting clergy to address this issue is other clergy talking to their clergy peers. When faith leaders reach out to other faith leaders, they can start turning their beliefs around, and I think it is an important strategy. We saw it work with the HIV pandemic. We are seeing it work with COVID as well.

So, I think this peer-to-peer education is important not only for faith communities but it is kind of what we are all saying here, is that peer-to-peer, talking to people who you trust is the way to really shift those beliefs.

Mr. FOSTER. Thank you.

My time is up and I yield back.

Mr. KRISHNAMOORTHI. Thank you, Congressman Foster.

First of all, I would like to thank our witnesses for testifying today and coming all the way from different parts of the Chicago area. We have really benefited from your insights and your answers to our questions.

Without objection, all members will have five legislative days within which to submit additional written questions for any of the witnesses, which will be forwarded to the witnesses for their responses.

I want to say thank you again to the audience. Thank you to everybody for covering this and for your attention to this very important challenge.

Now this hearing is adjourned.

Chapter 4

COVID-19 State of Vaccine Confidence Insights Report*

Centers for Disease Control and Prevention

Summary

Major Themes

- Consumers and news outlets expressed their frustration and lack of trust in CDC.
- Continuing and Evolving Themes:
  - Consumers expressed pandemic fatigue and stated they would no longer practice prevention and mitigation strategies.
  - The public continues to have questions and concerns about pediatric COVID-19 vaccines while others eagerly await Emergency Use Authorization (EUA) for children under 5 years old.
  - Consumers continue to have questions and concerns about the safety of COVID-19 vaccine.
  - Consumers continue to discuss their support or opposition to COVID-19 boosters.

Ways to take action

Federal, state, and local partners should continue to work together to explain the rationale for updated guidance, respond to gaps in information, and confront misinformation with evidence-based messaging. These efforts aim to increase confidence in COVID-19 vaccines and expand vaccine uptake. Partners should provide regular updates on the benefits, safety, side effects and effectiveness of COVID-19 vaccines and clearly communicate what is not known. Additionally, partners should share clear, complete, and accurate messages about COVID-19 vaccines and take visible actions to build trust in the vaccine, the vaccinator, health care, and public health.

---

* This is an edited, reformatted and augmented version of Centers for Disease Control and Prevention Insights Report 25, dated May 12, 2022.

In: COVID-19 Vaccines
Editor: John Schroder
ISBN: 979-8-88697-150-7

Aims and Methods

By rapidly reviewing and analyzing numerous sources and inputs (see Appendix), the COVID-19 State of Vaccine Confidence Insights Report emphasizes major themes influencing COVID-19 vaccine hesitancy and uptake. These are characterized by the level and type of threat to vaccine confidence, degree of spread, and directionality. In addition, by examining how consumers think and feel, social processes, and the practical issues around vaccination, the Insights Report seeks to identify emerging issues of misinformation, disinformation, and places where intervention efforts can improve vaccine confidence across the United States.

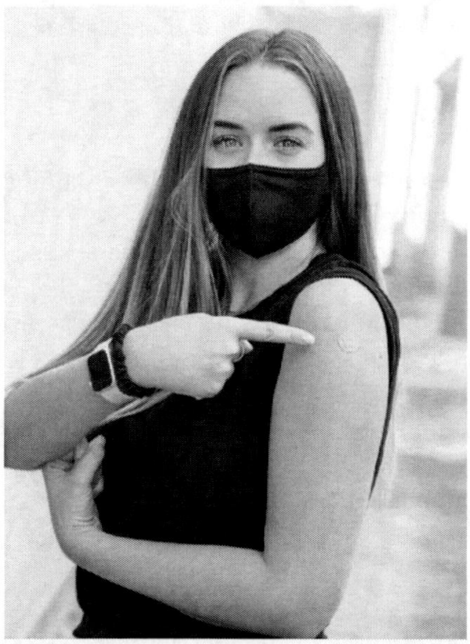

The information in this chapter is only a snapshot, and certain populations may be underrepresented. Images and quotes are illustrative examples and are not meant to comprehensively cover all content related to the highlighted themes.

How do you classify this theme/information?			
High risk	Moderate risk	Low risk	Positive sentiment
• May lead to vaccine refusals and decreased uptake • Wide reach, pervasive	• Potential to trigger hesitancy to vaccination • Moderate reach, modest dissemination	• Concerning, but low risk to vaccine confidence • Limited reach, limited dissemination	• Could increase vaccine confidence, intent, or motivation • Variable reach and dissemination

How has this theme/idea changed over time (since last report or over the course of multiple reports)?		
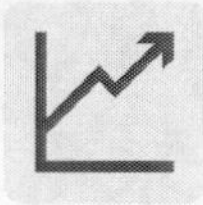 Increasing Information spreading rapidly	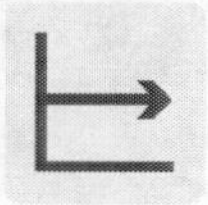 Stable Information remaining constant at prior level	 Decreasing Information is not gaining further traction and there has been no indication of additional activity

Major Themes Affecting Vaccine Confidence[a]

Consumers and News Outlets Expressed Their Frustration and Lack of Trust in CDC

On February 20, 2022, the New York Times published an article titled "The CDC Isn't Publishing Large Portions of the COVID-19 Data It Collects." Subsequently, other news and editorial outlets published articles on this topic with varying degrees of inflammatory language.[1,2,3] Google searches related to the article or news story concerning CDC's data sharing practices increased by up to 650% during this reporting period.[b] Moreover, news outlets released articles discussing the public's lack of trust in public health, science, and CDC.[4,5]

Additionally, some news outlets and social media users discussed the release of a Pfizer document, Cumulative Analysis of Post-Authorization Adverse Event Reports of Pf-07302048 (Bnt162b2) Received Through 28-Feb-2021, that presented data on reported adverse events following vaccination.[c,6,7,8] However, much like information about the Vaccine Adverse Event Reporting System (VAERS), the adverse events in the Pfizer document are an inventory of all reported events and their frequency regardless of their link to the Pfizer-BioNTech COVID-19 vaccine.[9] Some used the release of this information as evidence that the public cannot trust CDC and the media.[10, 11,12]

---

[a] Citations in this report are illustrative examples and are not the total number of instances of the corresponding themes.
[1] https://www.thedesertreview.com/news/cdc-hides-critical-safety-data/article_79520166-94f9-11ec-be01-5be1ac126d25.html.
[2] https://evolutionnews.org/2022/02/major-scandal-new-york-times-reports-cdc-withholding-massive-amounts-of-covid-19-data/.
[3] https://amac.us/the-cdc-hides-covid-data-but-says-americans-are-the-problem/.
[b] Google Trends.
[4] https://thehill.com/opinion/healthcare/597393-cdc-needs-serious-scrutiny-to-restore-americans-trust-in-science.
[5] https://www.nytimes.com/2022/03/12/opinion/public-health-trust.html.
[c] Tanaq Social Listening Report.
[6] https://twitter.com/cliff_ranger/status/1501988063043534854.
[7] https://twitter.com/Eljay2602/status/1502232928302026752.
[8] https://twitter.com/CraigKellyMP/status/1502763405622403072.
[9] https://factcheck.afp.com/http%253A%252F%252Fdoc.afp.com%252F9UC4LE.
[10] https://twitter.com/Eljay2602/status/1502232928302026752.
[11] https://twitter.com/SandraWeeden/status/1501515012225044482.
[12] https://twitter.com/JesseKellyDC/status/1496174354450853890.

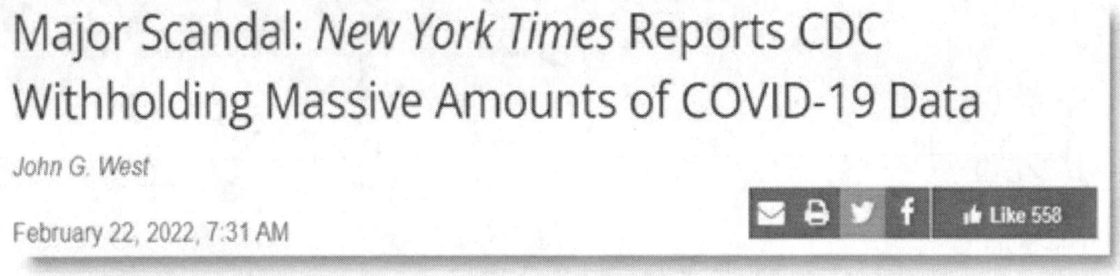

Major Scandal: *New York Times* Reports CDC Withholding Massive Amounts of COVID-19 Data

John G. West

February 22, 2022, 7:31 AM

Like 558

Perceptions, Concerns, and Threats to Vaccine Confidence

- Almost half of respondents (49%; N = 1,068) in a YouGov poll (released March 11, 2022) said their trust in CDC had gone way down or slightly down since the start of the pandemic.[13,14]
- A majority of respondents (56%; N = 2,301) in a Partnership for Public Service poll (released March 1, 2022) did not trust the federal government to do what is right.[15,16]
- Consumers expressed their beliefs that the unreleased data proves CDC lied to the public and cannot be trusted.[c,17,18,19,20]
- Some consumers believe CDC is not releasing data depicting that COVID-19 vaccines are not safe or effective, even though the unreleased data are said to be related to COVID-19 hospitalizations, booster dose uptake, and wastewater analysis.[d,21,22,23,24]
- Some online users claimed that Twitter was banning online references to vaccine deaths from the VAERS data.[25,26,27]
- Some social media users believe the recently released Pfizer document proves that the vaccines are not safe.[c,28,29,30]

---

[13] https://americansforprosperity.org/wp-content/uploads/2022/03/AFP-Civil-Liberties-Polling-Memo.pdf.
[14] https://americansforprosperity.org/covid-civil-liberties-poll/.
[15] https://ourpublicservice.org/wp-content/uploads/2022/02/Partnership-and-Freedman-Trust-Polling.pdf.
[16] https://www.politico.com/news/magazine/2022/03/01/democracy-public-crisis-trust-government-faith-00012565.
[17] https://twitter.com/JesseKellyDC/status/1496174354450853890.
[18] https://twitter.com/hamp2879/status/1497841439107010561.
[19] https://twitter.com/TheMFingCOO/status/1495971366536978442.
[20] https://twitter.com/plenalibertad2/status/1495974215400374272.
[d] CDC-INFO.
[21] https://www.facebook.com/cdc/posts/327879376040174?comment_id=327980402696738&__tn__=R
[22] https://www.instagram.com/p/CaiJpfOL9CV/c/17920788146250135/.
[23] https://www.instagram.com/p/Cak0e_qskkh/c/18027716320346322/
[24] https://rumble.com/vw6sgc-cdc-admits-to-withholding-vaccine-data-over-fears.html
[25] https://twitter.com/paranoidbull/status/1502845352562548738.
[26] https://twitter.com/gutresolution/status/1502761129759543298.
[27] https://twitter.com/RobertKennedyJr/status/1503104107787210760.
[28] https://twitter.com/toadmeister/status/1501815141964427264.
[29] https://twitter.com/xxjjkkjjkkxx/status/1499791394126188544.
[30] https://twitter.com/johncardillo/status/1499066377172402177.

- News outlets and social media users also discussed how CDC's COVID-19 guidance was confusing, untrustworthy, or unsafe for the general public.[e,31,32,33,34] Some social media users claimed CDC was changing its COVID-19 guidance for political reasons.[c,35,36,37]

Misinformation Themes

- The recently released Pfizer document proves that COVID-19 vaccines are not safe and is evidence of a conspiracy between the COVID-19 vaccine manufacturers and the government.[f,38,39]
- CDC withheld data depicting that COVID-19 vaccines are not safe or effective.[40,41]

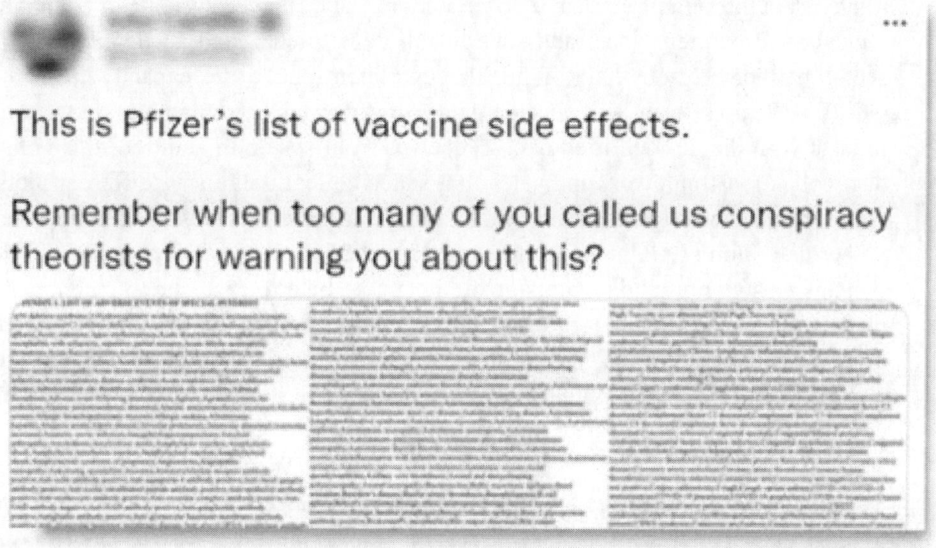

[e] CDC's Communication Surveillance Report.
[31] https://twitter.com/bc_fink/status/1501717668486791168.
[32] https://rumble.com/vx50h1-cdc-lies-completely-exposed-deadly-shots-masks-and-quarantine-extremely-dan.html.
[33] https://twitter.com/joingles/status/1502098933568389121.
[34] https://www.npr.org/sections/health-shots/2022/03/10/1085797307/cdcs-new-covid-metrics-can-leave-individuals-struggling-to-understand-their-risk.
[35] https://www.facebook.com/cdc/posts/327879376040174?comment_id=327960936032018&__tn__=R.
[36] https://www.facebook.com/cdc/posts/327879376040174?comment_id=327960452698733&__tn__=R.
[37] https://twitter.com/rTIKId/status/1498357991137058827.
[f] Project VCTR.
[38] https://twitter.com/johncardillo/status/1499066377172402177.
[39] https://twitter.com/hamp2879/status/1497841439107010561.
[40] https://twitter.com/Krommsan/status/1497824267404132353.
[41] https://www.facebook.com/cdc/posts/328697075958404?comment_id=328704485957663&__cft__%5b0%5d = AZXqRPRtVse4Df1upF5p1LraOhrmvWEgrOYnGuO7UzqBv4p86KXLPEuIqOUAvZq4ufoV1GN6gDsgpjXk1tK3vRmGWCk2RBxt2ItI7meS0C7RpVMoouRPo9Pk1TtndQf9GafreIG2Fuy5paSmZuW-G1JF&__tn__=R%5d-R.

Content Gaps and Information Voids Identified/Mentioned by Consumers and News Outlets

- Why has CDC not released all the available data on COVID-19 booster doses, hospitalizations and wastewater analyses?[42,43,444]
- CDC provides extensive publicly available summary reports plus datasets from multiple sources, including vaccine uptake, cases, deaths, and wastewater. Descriptions of data sources and FAQs are found at the websites listed - FAQ: COVID-19 Data and Surveillance | CDC and CDC COVID Data Tracker.
- CDC must balance the use of data provided with how these data may be shared, released and maintained under applicable federal laws. CDC collects COVID-19-related data through more than a dozen national surveillance systems in collaboration with federal partners, local and state health departments, and academic and private sector partners. About half of health departments have the capacity to link their COVID-19 case, death, and vaccine data. However, CDC is unable to do this type of linkage with the de-identified data it receives from states. In addition, this voluntary data collection framework indicates that states collect data using different methods, which often generate disparate, non-comparable data sets. Using this approach to gather data limits CDC's ability to aggregate and link these data on a national level. For this reason, not all data are suitable for immediate release due to incompleteness or potential inaccuracies, lack of generalizability, sample sizes that are too small for meaningful interpretation, security risks, and privacy and ethical concerns. CDC endeavors to be a responsible steward of data that are shared and to ensure accuracy, completeness, and appropriate representation.
- The National Wastewater Surveillance System (NWSS) is new (established in September 2020) and states have implemented systems at different rates. CDC waited to make data available through COVID Data Tracker until we had reasonable coverage in all 10 HHS regions. We reached that point in January 2022, and the COVID Data Tracker wastewater page went live February 2, 2022. Wastewater RNA concentrations (the raw data coming into NWSS) are not directly comparable across jurisdictions. NWSS produces three metrics to enable comparison -- percent change/trends, detection proportion, and relative level. All wastewater data, including the raw concentrations, are available through a public data request process that has been in place since early 2021.
- Has CDC released all the available data on the safety and effectiveness of COVID-19 vaccines?[45,46]
- CDC collects a significant amount of vaccine-related data. Depending on the source and type of data, sometimes it has missing data. Or it may include personally identifiable information, which hinders the interpretability of the data or the ability to share it. CDC works to communicate and publish timely and transparent information

---

[42] https://www.instagram.com/p/CaiJpfOL9CV/c/17920788146250135/.
[43] https://www.instagram.com/p/Cak0e_qskkh/c/18027716320346322/.
[44] https://rumble.com/vw6sgc-cdc-admits-to-withholding-vaccine-data-over-fears.html.
[45] https://www.instagram.com/p/Cak0e_qskkh/c/18027716320346322/.
[46] https://rumble.com/vw6sgc-cdc-admits-to-withholding-vaccine-data-over-fears.html.

about the safety of vaccines to public health officials, healthcare providers, and the public.[47]

- Data from the Vaccine Adverse Event Reporting System is publicly available and can be downloaded here: https://vaers.hhs. gov/data.html.
- Data from the Vaccine Safety Datalink (VSD) network are available by request from the National Center for Health Statistics Research Data Center (NCHS RDC). More information on the VSD data sharing program can be found here: https://www.cdc.gov/vaccinesafety/ensuringsafety/monitoring/vsd/accessing-data.html.
- Are the adverse events reported in the recently released Pfizer document proof that COVID-19 vaccines are not safe?[48,49]
- No. Multiple analyses from CDC and others have found all approved or authorized COVID-19 vaccines to be safe. Rare serious adverse events are identified and publicly reported. You may find more information by going to: Ensuring COVID-19 Vaccine Safety in the US | CDC.
- The Pfizer document is a comprehensive listing of all reported adverse events or health issues described following vaccination, regardless of whether the vaccine caused them. Tracking such events is a requirement for pharmaceutical companies, Food and Drug Administration (FDA), and CDC to identify possible safety signals, particularly rare events that may not have been possible to detect during clinical trials. An adverse event is simply an event that has occurred after vaccination — it does not mean the vaccine caused the problem. And many of these events are likely to be purely coincidental. Adverse events related to the Pfizer-BioNTech vaccine are similar to many routine vaccines. The adverse events are mild and short lasting (pain at injection site, fever). Finally, for more severe adverse events, there is a detailed process to determine whether these are related to vaccination or not. FDA and CDC use several different sources of dataa to closely monitor vaccine safety and identify events that occur more often after vaccination compared to how often they typically occur in the general population.[50] The Pfizer report did not include any comparison of adverse events in unvaccinated people.
- Why does CDC continue to update their COVID-19 vaccination and mitigation guidance?[51,52]
- CDC has continued to review isolation and quarantine recommendations for various populations throughout the COVID-19 pandemic. Recommendations take into account the societal impact (e.g., critical infrastructure and health care worker staffing shortages) and the latest science on disease severity and when and for how long a person is most infectious. CDC will continue to evaluate these recommendations as more data become available.[53]

---

[47] https://www.cdc.gov/vaccinesafety/index.html.
[48] https://twitter.com/toadmeister/status/1501815141964427264.
[49] https://twitter.com/xxjjkkjjkkxx/status/1499791394126188544.
[50] https://www.factcheck.org/2022/03/scicheck-posts-misinterpret-pfizer-covid-19-vaccine-safety-monitoring-document/.
[51] https://www.facebook.com/cdc/posts/327879376040174?comment_id=327960452698733&__tn__=R.
[52] https://twitter.com/rTIKId/status/1498357991137058827.
[53] https://www.cdc.gov/coronavirus/2019-ncov/if-you-are-sick/quarantine-isolation-background.html.

Misinformation Themes

- The recently released Pfizer document proves that COVID-19 vaccines are not safe and is evidence of a conspiracy between the COVID-19 vaccine manufacturers and the government.[g,30,54,55]
- CDC withheld data depicting that COVID-19 vaccines are not safe or effective.[56,57,58]

Ways to Take Action

- Coordinate with federal, state, local agencies, and partners to share clear, complete, and accurate messages about COVID-19 vaccines and take visible actions such as culturally appropriate messaging/education and community engagement to build trust in the vaccine, the vaccinator, and the system.
- Communicate transparently about the process for authorizing, approving, making recommendations for, monitoring the safety of, distributing, allocating, and administering COVID-19 vaccines, including data collection, analysis, and reporting.
- Provide regular updates on the benefits, safety, side effects, and effectiveness of COVID-19 vaccines and clearly communicate what is known, what isn't known, and what is being done to find out what isn't known.
- Proactively address and help stop the spread and harm of misinformation via social media platforms, partners, and trusted messengers.
- Engage communities in a sustainable, equitable, and inclusive way using two-way communication to listen, build trust, and increase collaboration.

Continuing and Evolving Themes Affecting Vaccine Confidence

The themes below have been noted in previous reports and continue to undermine vaccine confidence. The information highlighted below focuses on what is new or different from previous reports. For additional context and previous recommendations on these themes, see previous Insights Reports.

Consumers Expressed Pandemic Fatigue and Stated They Would No Longer Practice Prevention and Mitigation Strategies

Consumers continue to discuss how they are done or want to stop following COVID-19 prevention and mitigation strategies. Many online consumers expressed their elation in

---

[g] Project VCTR.

[54] https://twitter.com/hamp2879/status/1497841439107010561.

[55] https://twitter.com/MAGA_VIBES/status/1498418434031304709.

[56] https://twitter.com/Krommsan/status/1497824267404132353.

[57] https://www.facebook.com/cdc/posts/328697075958404?comment_id=328704485957663&__cft__%5b0%5d =AZXqRPRtVse4Df1upF5p1LraOhrmvWEgrOYnGuO7UzqBv4p86KXLPEuIqOUAvZq4ufoV1GN6gDsgpjXk1tK3vRmGWCk2RBxt2ItI7meS0C7RpVMoouRPo9Pk1TtndQf9GafreIG2Fuy5paSmZuW-G1JF&__tn__=R%5d-R.

[58] https://www.facebook.com/cdc/posts/328558152638963?comment_id=329491225878989&__tn__=R.

everyday occurrences with the hashtags #returntonormal[59] and #backtonormal.[60] Some online discussion verbalized concerns against prematurely lifting precautions[61] which could cause successive waves of infection.[62,63] Despite conflicting viewpoints from some consumers, the majority of online discussions have already moved from pandemic to other issues.[64,65] This shift might be due to the declining infections with the virus that causes COVID-19[66] and stalled vaccination rates for the primary series and booster doses.[h] News and other online outlets continue to publish articles discussing how the public is tired of COVID-19 and discussions around it.[67,68,69] The most recent update to the CDC Community Levels (which determines community risk levels by reviewing several indicators, such as the number of new COVID-19 cases in an area, the share of hospital beds in use, and hospital admissions) indicates more than 98% of the US population is in a location with low or medium COVID-19 Community Level, indicating to some that COVID-19 is no longer a concern.[70,71]

On March 1, the White House detailed an as-yet unfunded[72] National Preparedness Plan for COVID-19[73] comprising of four key aspects: protection against and treatment of infections with available therapies, preparation for new variants, prevention of economic and educational shutdowns, and assistance with vaccination efforts outside of the U.S.[73,74] Meanwhile, the Federal Aviation Administration's masking requirement, initially set to expire on March 18, has been extended until April 18.[75,76] These events, coupled with international conflicts,[77] domestic economic stressors,[78] and political messaging,[79] may have led to consumers expressing varying sentiments ranging from a desire to be done with prevention-related

---

[59] https://twitter.com/ernie_mourelo/status/1506475154930552836.
[60] https://twitter.com/KarlDHarrison/status/1502839667456036866.
[61] https://twitter.com/rachael_levy/status/1503000790386065410.
[62] https://twitter.com/AxelTheAussie/status/1498359122420502529.
[63] https://twitter.com/marcedavis/status/1502899098189385729.
[64] https://www.facebook.com/cdc/posts/327879376040174?comment_id=328125986015513&__tn__=R.
[65] https://twitter.com/anamdelosreyes/status/1499143665947656201.
[66] https://www.cnbc.com/2022/03/14/fauci-warns-not-to-forget-pandemics-catastrophic-experience.html.
[h] HHS Current Events Tracker.
[67] https://www.nytimes.com/2022/03/09/opinion/covid-exhaustion-the-argument.html.
[68] https://marshallparthenon.com/29050/news/two-years-into-the-pandemic-covid-fatigue-takes-its-toll/
[69] https://news.abplive.com/news/masks-off-what-is-pandemic-fatigue-and-what-experts-advise-to-tackle-this-1517896.
[70] https://www.cdc.gov/media/releases/2022/s0311-COVID-19-Community-Levels.html.
[71] https://www.facebook.com/cdc/posts/327879376040174?comment_id=328250366003075&__tn__=R.
[72] https://khn.org/news/article/podcast-khn-what-the-health-237-congress-covid-funding-march-10-2022/.
[73] https://www.whitehouse.gov/covidplan/.
[74] https://www.fiercehealthcare.com/providers/white-house-covid-19-preparedness-plan-details-4-step-plan-keep-america-open-and-prepare.
[75] https://www.npr.org/2022/03/10/1085739883/mask-mandate-planes-trains-ferries-tsa-cdc.
[76] https://www.nytimes.com/live/2022/03/10/world/covid-19-mandates-cases-vaccine/the-tsa-extends-its-mask-mandate-on-airplanes-and-public-transit-as-the-cdc-reviews-the-policys-future.
[77] https://www.instagram.com/p/Cak0e_qskkh/c/17957476678627751/.
[78] https://www.npr.org/sections/health-shots/2022/03/10/1085792118/americans-stress-is-spiking-over-inflation-war-in-ukraine-survey-finds.
[79] https://www.facebook.com/cdc/posts/328650775963034?comment_id=328682369293208&_cft__%5b0%5d=AZXOMmJcoZpkMXNtKHJb8s_la4AG3JU8w_gtcrNQ1Gx5QvEZifz0_Febs_goxXV8wlnkBTZN1cs24noGgMYllceDHgFJPIGCPyZor0d9Pr7Oa7xAUVeH0N13ZjnoQ7Tb9SeXdo0nsnAEO7uZPZ0qc2Ca&__tn__=R%5d-R.

activities[80,81] to a belief that the COVID-19 pandemic is over.[82,83] Some sources have described this as "pandemic fatigue."[84,85]

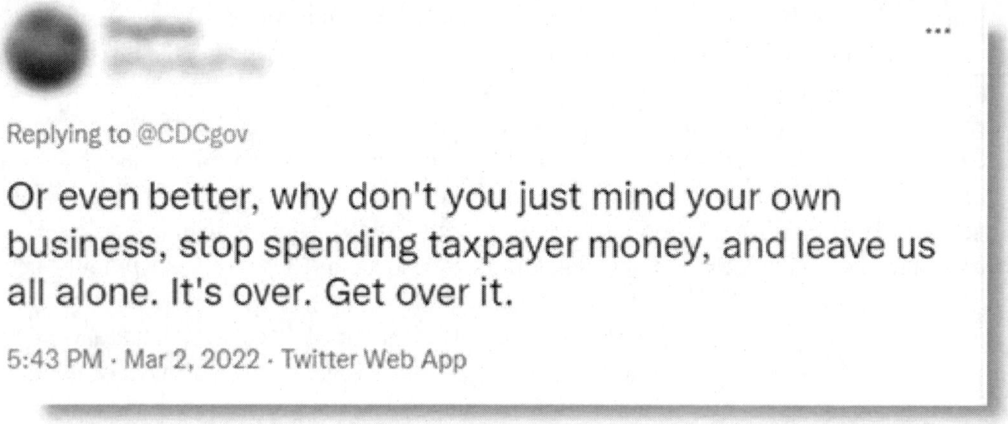
Replying to @CDCgov
Or even better, why don't you just mind your own business, stop spending taxpayer money, and leave us all alone. It's over. Get over it.
5:43 PM · Mar 2, 2022 · Twitter Web App

Perceptions, Concerns, and Threats to Vaccine Confidence

- Some consumers believe the United States may be approaching, or is already in, an endemic stage.[86,87]
- Some understand the word 'endemic' to mean that infection with the virus that causes COVID-19 is not concerning[88] or that serious COVID-19 outcomes are unpreventable.
- Online users questioned whether testing and other pandemic- related services would be available in the absence of the political will to fund these efforts.[89]

Misinformation Themes

- President Biden declared the pandemic is over.[90]
- Guidance from governmental health authorities""flip-flops"[91] or may not "follow the science."[92]
- Stalled vaccination uptake rates indicate the pandemic is over.[93,94]

---

[80] https://www.facebook.com/cdc/posts/328650775963034?comment_id=328854002609378&__cft__%5b0%5d= AZXOMmJcoZpkMXNtKHJb8s_la4AG3JU8w_gtcrNQ1Gx5QvEZifz0_Febs_goxXV8wlnkBTZN1cs24noGgMYllceDHgFJPIGCPyZor0d9Pr7Oa7xAUVeH0N13ZjnoQ7Tb9SeXdo0nsnAEO7uZPZ0qc2Ca&__tn__=R%5d-R.

[81] https://www.facebook.com/cdc/posts/327879376040174?comment_id=327953626032749&__tn__=R.

[82] https://www.instagram.com/p/CaS_tZ-sJlu/c/18194304277157358/.

[83] https://www.instagram.com/p/Camnp5HBe--/c/17999915506383735/.

[84] https://www.nytimes.com/2022/03/12/us/covid-pandemic-vaccines-mandates.html.

[85] https://twitter.com/tyler_bunch/status/1499134393054552070.

[86] https://www.facebook.com/cdc/posts/328050436023068?comment_id=328313375996774&__cft__%5b0%5d=AZUXdUIFfZcsosrMOLFOWxh04iCo-_JLbWd1E9QPQskH9V1MwQoFGusVpUz-6dAme4NIOMlj87zhJ-AgfzJLngk8dwEYgIq2EFANpg7WPJyfHBn8ikvMvNmQBBKaV4Z2vCl14oGRMDIWmhxb23cXwTBA&__tn__=R%5d-R.

[87] https://www.facebook.com/cdc/posts/327879376040174?comment_id=328777535950358&__tn__=R.

[88] https://twitter.com/anamdelosreyes/status/1499143665947656201.

[89] https://twitter.com/trudygonzales/status/1503134619364823043.

[90] https://www.facebook.com/cdc/posts/327879376040174?comment_id=328125986015513&__tn__=R

[91] https://www.facebook.com/cdc/posts/327879376040174?comment_id=327953626032749&__tn__=R.

[92] https://twitter.com/Angelasfreenews/status/1499774314131906561.

[93] https://twitter.com/Oped46/status/1499219052467679233.

[94] https://www.instagram.com/p/CaSiDqavker/c/18154872058209207/.

- CDC and government officials knew mitigation efforts like vaccines, masks, and tests would be ineffective but continued to push them for political gain.[95,96,97]

Content Gaps and Information Voids

- As the number of COVID-19 cases declines, is it still necessary to receive a primary series of COVID-19 vaccine or booster dose?[98]
  - COVID-19 vaccines are effective at protecting you from severe outcomes and death from the virus that causes COVID-19, even if you have had COVID-19 in the past. Vaccination is an important tool to help us get back to normal.[99]
- As state and local governments update their COVID-19 community mitigation recommendations, should masks still be worn in indoor public places?[100,101]
  - When making decisions about community-level and individual-level prevention strategies, health officials, stakeholders and individuals should consider CDC's COVID-19 Community Levels approaches within their local context.[102]
  - Layered prevention strategies, such as staying up to date on vaccines, screening testing, ventilation, and wearing masks, can help limit severe disease and reduce the potential for strain on the healthcare system. CDC recommends using county COVID-19 Community Levels to help determine which COVID-19 prevention measures to use for individuals and communities.[103]
  - COVID-19 Community Levels do not apply in healthcare settings like hospitals and nursing homes. Instead, healthcare settings should continue to follow CDC's infection prevention and control recommendations for healthcare workers.[104]
- Should masks and vaccines still be utilized as governments update their COVID-19 community mitigation recommendations for travel?[105,106]
  - Masks and vaccines continue to be safe and effective ways to protect against infection from the virus that causes COVID-19.
  - Everyone is recommended to stay up to date with their COVID-19 vaccines.
  - Mask use recommendations are available at: Use and Care of Mask | CDC
- Guidance from governmental health authorities"flip-flops"[91] or may not "follow the science."[92]
- Stalled vaccination uptake rates indicate the pandemic is over.[93,94]

---

95 https://www.instagram.com/p/CaiXa8YO0Lv/c/17903475053393342/.
96 https://www.instagram.com/p/CandhskM2MN/c/17960473396608350/.
97 https://www.facebook.com/cdc/posts/328558152638963?comment_id=328842375943874&__tn__=R.
98 https://www.instagram.com/p/CaIX9vulkEO/c/18280690462055345/.
99 https://www.cdc.gov/coronavirus/2019-ncov/vaccines/prepare-for-vaccination.html.
100 https://www.npr.org/2022/03/10/1085739883/mask-mandate-planes-trains-ferries-tsa-cdc.
101 https://www.nytimes.com/live/2022/03/10/world/covid-19-mandates-cases-vaccine/the-tsa-extends-its-mask-mandate-on-airplanes-and-public-transit-as-the-cdc-reviews-the-policys-future.
102 https://www.cdc.gov/coronavirus/2019-ncov/science/community-levels.html?CDC_AA_refVal=https%3A%2F%2Fwww.cdc.gov%2Fcoronavirus%2F2019-ncov%2Fmore%2Faboutcovidcountycheck%2Findex.html.
103 https://www.cdc.gov/coronavirus/2019-ncov/prevent-getting-sick/about-face-coverings.html.
104 https://cdc.sharepoint.com/teams/VaccinePlanningUnit-COVID19/Shared Documents/Clearance/Documents for Clearance/4800-4899/4839-SoVC #25/Instead, healthcare settings should continue to use community transmission rates and follow CDC's infection prevention and control recommendations for healthcare workers.
105 https://www.npr.org/2022/03/10/1085739883/mask-mandate-planes-trains-ferries-tsa-cdc.
106 https://www.nytimes.com/live/2022/03/10/world/covid-19-mandates-cases-vaccine/the-tsa-extends-its-mask-mandate-on-airplanes-and-public-transit-as-the-cdc-reviews-the-policys-future.

- CDC and government officials knew mitigation efforts like vaccines, masks, and tests would be ineffective but continued to push them for political gain.[95,96,97]

Ways to Take Action

- Develop and amplify messages explaining why vaccines and staying "up to date" on COVID-19 vaccinations are still crucial to preventing severe illness from COVID-19, including illness caused by emerging variants.
- Disseminate messages about community-level risk (CDC Community Levels) and the importance of the corresponding COVID-19 mitigation measures, such as masking, screening, testing and quarantining.
- Address new misinformation themes regarding vaccines to increase or maintain vaccine confidence in COVID-19 vaccine and booster doses.

The Public Continues to Have Questions and Concerns About Pediatric COVID-19 Vaccines While Others Eagerly Await EUA of These Vaccines for Children Under 5 Years Old

Three months after Pfizer initially submitted data to the FDA to obtain EUA for their COVID-19 vaccine in children ages under 5 years, parents eagerly await updates on the approval process while pushing to allow off-label use.[107,108,109] Also, worsening some parents' frustrations and adding to feelings of abandonment and governmental indifference, many cities and counties have lifted mask requirements.[i,j,110,111,112,113] However, many, including public health officials and political figures,[114,115,116] remain opposed to vaccination of not only this age group, but all

[107] https://www.medscape.com/viewarticle/969603.

[108] https://www.facebook.com/cdc/posts/323899369771508?comment_id=997450437841651&__cft__%5b0%5d=AZVDZg880YGghhw2ho8hedBbFGH96SarCNZWrKqqZqHtXKiLMiY63Xmj9uxrQLAtXLZRGz4ZI7AOjjAMTXVAP3e_gIrymzc_d60r5vs30Mk-k480IeXTQqWDtEYZDsrtacsgK72H6vRUxzrhHgtKRQBq&__tn__=R%5d-R.

[109] https://www.facebook.com/cdc/posts/323899369771508?comment_id=480182670326849 3&__cft__%5b0%5d=AZVDZg880YGghhw2ho8hedBbFGH96SarCNZWrKqqZqHtXKiLMiY63Xmj9uxrQLAtXLZRGz4ZI7AOjjAMTXVAP3e_gIrymzc_d60r5vs30Mk-k480IeXTQqWDtEYZDsrtacsgK72H6vRUxzrhHgtKRQBq&__tn__=R%5d-R.

[i] CDC-INFO.

[j] CDC's Communication Surveillance Report.

[110] https://twitter.com/ImmunizeUnder5s/status/1503058466390294531.

[111] https://www.facebook.com/cdc/posts/325178869643558?comment_id=326831276144984&__tn__=R.

[112] https://www.nytimes.com/2022/03/01/opinion/letters/cdc-covid-rules.html.

[113] https://www.facebook.com/cdc/posts/323899369771508?comment_id=682739286250036&__cft__%5b0%5d=AZVDZg880YGghhw2ho8hedBbFGH96SarCNZWrKqqZqHtXKiLMiY63Xmj9uxrQLAtXLZRGz4ZI7AOjjAMTXVAP3e_gIrymzc_d60r5vs30Mk-k480IeXTQqWDtEYZDsrtacsgK72H6vRUxzrhHgtKRQBq&__tn__=R%5d-R.

[114] https://abcnews.go.com/US/florida-officials-face-pushback-decision-advise-healthy-children/story?id=83324402.

[115] https://www.washingtonpost.com/health/2022/03/08/florida-releases-guidance-discouraging-covid-vaccine-most-children/.

[116] https://www.tampabay.com/news/florida-politics/2022/03/07/healthy-children-shouldnt-get-coronavirus-vaccine-florida-health-department-says/.

children.[117,118,119] Adding to this, some studies have shown decreased effectiveness or decreased antibody response in younger children, as compared to adults, further adversely affecting vaccine confidence for this age group.[120,121,122]

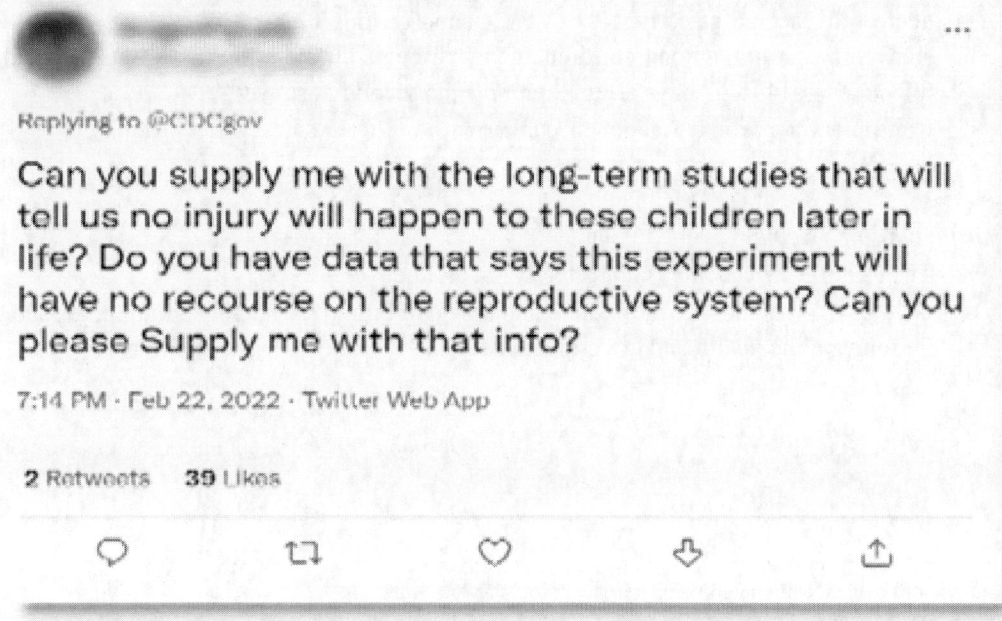

In addition, a recent online poll[123] showed that 57% of parents with children ages under 5 years reported not having enough information about COVID-19 vaccine safety and effectiveness. Moreover, 39% of this cohort said federal health agencies' information about COVID-19 vaccines was confusing.[124] Searches for "when will covid vaccine be available for kids under 5" increased by 300% during this reporting period.[k]

Perceptions, Concerns, and Threats to Vaccine Confidence

- Many parents feel they have done everything in their power to protect their children from COVID-19 and are growing impatient as a vaccine remains elusive.[125,126,127]

---

[117] https://www.instagram.com/p/CaVLPxtlVLi/c/17910811940297987/.
[118] https://www.instagram.com/p/CaVLPxtlVLi/c/17895568106536279/.
[119] https://www.instagram.com/p/CaVLPxtlVLi/c/17936502526947581/.
[120] https://www.medrxiv.org/content/10.1101/2022.02.25.22271454v1.
[121] https://www.nature.com/articles/d41586-022-00681-8/.
[122] https://www.nytimes.com/live/2022/03/01/world/covid-19-tests-cases-vaccine.
[123] https://www.kff.org/coronavirus-covid-19/poll-finding/kff-covid-19-vaccine-monitor-february-2022/.
[124] https://www.kff.org/coronavirus-covid-19/poll-finding/kff-covid-19-vaccine-monitor-february-2022/.
[125] https://twitter.com/ImmunizeUnder5s/status/1502377993993342977.
[126] https://twitter.com/AshleyRParker/status/1502336325881667593https:/twitter.com/AshleyRParker/status/1502336325881667593https:/twitter.com/AshleyRParker/status/1502336325881667593https:/twitter.com/AshleyRParker/status/1502336325881667593.
[127] https://twitter.com/cattywampusbees/status/1503019117900488706.

- The government is doing nothing to protect children ages under 5 years from COVID-19.[128,129,130]
- Parents are hesitant to vaccinate children after a study showed the Pfizer-BioNTech COVID-19 vaccine offered little protection against the Omicron variant and had decreased vaccine effectiveness (VE) against serious illness.[131,132,133] The MMWR study showed that, among children aged 5 through 11 years, the COVID-19 vaccine effectiveness14 to 67 days after receipt off the second dose was 46%.
- Consumers are worried about the unknown long-term side effects from COVID-19 vaccines.[134,135,136]

Misinformation Themes

- The COVID-19 vaccine is not effective in children·[137,138,139]
- COVID-19 vaccines are ineffective and are not required for healthy children, as touted by some public health and government officials.[140],[141]

---

128 http://vhttps/twitter.com/ImmunizeUnder5s/status/1503058466390294531

129 https://www.facebook.com/cdc/posts/323899369771508?comment_id=369129144734069&__cft__%5b0% 5d=AZVDZg880YGghhw2ho8hedBbFGH96SarCNZWrKqqZqHtXKiLMiY63Xmj9uxrQLAtXLZRGz4ZI7AOjjAMTXVAP3e_gIrymzc_d60r5vs30Mk-k480IeXTQqWDtEYZDsrtacsgK72H6vRUxzrhHgtKRQBq&__tn__=R%5d-R.

130 https://www.facebook.com/cdc/posts/323899369771508?comment_id=666191077867357&__cft__%5b0%5d=AZXlaBoas5FGo8jXLdJefA9ONxU6aqZffVBHzrFQZCvGjghtjrgH-mK9h79bl9SA1795U-ne3nJkE9KlFtx5ygA44IGmet6WaqMvAskwLsFpE6e7osRgogz9qoksUrHE-tWhSmJ34Lno366YSUuoSe2c&__tn__=R%5d-R.

131 https://www.facebook.com/cdc/posts/329443075883804?comment_id=329664045861707&__cft__%5b0%5d=AZUvqQ7NrQwsUG-41sCyfr-5BYWV9KnvvkbAxYjf-v-1BQNF5b2T-2qFXtecuTP0Ks8IuIphiQCOAcxWTR_Bak9ppjjrHuDgZ1pVw7nooJ8qFHolo4TYA5thKoqrqcqaRSIcTPiLwfUorzE1lc_ZL8Nf&__tn__=R%5d-R.

132 https://twitter.com/Lizzylasher7/status/1498745044546826244.

133 https://twitter.com/AWokeZombie/status/1498744322661011456.

134 https://www.facebook.com/cdc/posts/329443075883804?comment_id=329452232549555&__cft__%5b0%5d =AZUvqQ7NrQwsUG-41sCyfr-5BYWV9KnvvkbAxYjf-v-1BQNF5b2T-2qFXtecuTP0Ks8IuIphiQCOAcxWTR_Bak9ppjjrHuDgZ1pVw7nooJ8qFHolo4TYA5thKoqrqcqaRSIcTPiLwfUorzE1lc_ZL8Nf&__tn__=R%5d-R.

135 https://www.facebook.com/cdc/posts/328697075958404?comment_id=329223249239120&__cft__%5b0% 5d=AZXqRPRtVse4Df1upF5p1LraOhrmvWEgrOYnGuO7UzqBv4p86KXLPEuIqOUAvZq4ufoV1GN6gDsgpjXk1tK3vRmGWCk2RBxt2ItI7meS0C7RpVMoouRPo9Pk1TtndQf9GafreIG2Fuy5paSmZuW-G1JF&__tn__=R%5d-R.

136 https://www.facebook.com/cdc/posts/324589083035870?comment_id=324642703030508&__cft__%5b0% 5d=AZWpyLZpuDfAClWjYyVasorjHDbJhhz8ECo2qHhn_3Ylwmy6EL73K-7jhpgL2RozakhUKHjn4OHCKli_VYP8wi5VMdcbL1j6WQ8MPqvjOqezqdGI1WJuGhG1dBje_fqtOdm81Sy59EfQkV2F8rWTbDVa&__tn__=R%5d-R.

137 https://www.medrxiv.org/content/10.1101/2022.02.25.22271454v1.

138 https://www.nature.com/articles/d41586-022-00681-8.

139 https://twitter.com/PunchBlake/status/1499226434518278144

140 https://www.facebook.com/cdc/posts/328650775963034?comment_id=328919115936200&__cft__%5b0%5d=AZXOMmJcoZpkMXNtKHJb8s_la4AG3JU8w_gtcrNQ1Gx5QvEZifz0_Febs_goxXV8wlnkBTZN1cs24noGgMYllceDHgFJPIGCPyZor0d9Pr7Oa7xAUVeH0N13ZjnoQ7Tb9SeXdo0nsnAEO7uZPZ0qc2Ca&__tn__=R%5d-R.

141 https://twitter.com/AWokeZombie/status/1499104116047593474.

- Kids are not at risk of infection with the virus that causes COVID-19.[142,143]
- The COVID-19 vaccine is an experiment and simply a ploy by Big Pharma to make money.[144,145,146]

Content Gaps and Information Voids

- Why should children and teens get vaccinated against COVID-19?[h]
    - Children are as likely to be infected with the virus that causes COVID-19 as adults and can get very sick, have short- and long-term health complications, and spread the virus to others, including at home and school. Children infected with the virus that causes COVID-19 can also develop serious complications like multisystem inflammatory syndrome (MIS- C)—a condition where different body parts become inflamed, including the heart, lungs, kidneys, brain, skin, eyes, or gastrointestinal organs. Children with underlying medical conditions are more at risk for severe illness from COVID-19 compared to children without underlying medical conditions.[147]
- Are children eligible for a booster?[l]
    - Everyone ages 12 years and older should get a COVID-19 booster when they are eligible. Currently, a booster is not recommended for children younger than 12 years.[148]
- Is severe illness or death likely after COVID-19 vaccination in children?[k]
    - Serious adverse events after COVID-19 vaccination are rare but may occur. CDC provides timely updates on serious adverse events. Myocarditis and pericarditis after COVID-19 vaccination are rare in children. Reports of death after COVID-19 vaccination are rare.[149]
- The COVID-19 vaccine is not effective in children.[120,121,139]
- COVID-19 vaccines are ineffective and are not required for healthy children, as touted by some public health and government officials.[140,141,150,151]

Kids are not at risk of infection with the virus that causes COVID-19.[152,142]

---

[142] https://www.facebook.com/cdc/posts/328751329286312?comment_id=329385052556273&__cft__%5b0%5d=AZULoGsPMoakhEshZl_UD_F-P0V5-flO86_tXI2_P_X9dxA_P7_aE-L8cyWTlc1lVjf3v_7v2L9nO492CCDt0V3B0tbeLf8CpDD4HXtfxxZ94aI8q6kFUL1dGgtQ9X9JeWkyq5xl2AvXsjIRoBSXqKnO&__tn__=R%5d-Rhttps://www.facebook.com/cdc/posts/328751329286312?comment_id=329385052556273&__cft__%5b0%5d=AZULoGsPMoakhEshZl_UD_F-P0V5-flO86_tXI2_P_X9dxA_P7_aE-L8cyWTlc1lVjf3v_7v2L9nO492CCDt0V3B0tbeLf8CpDD4HXtfxxZ94aI8q6kFUL1dGgtQ9X9JeWkyq5xl2AvXsjIRoBSXqKnO&__tn__=R%5d-R.

[143] https://www.instagram.com/p/CanPxl4MI_S/c/17865288230646993/.

[144] https://www.instagram.com/p/CaVLPxtlVLi/c/18126214687257553/.

[145] https://www.instagram.com/p/CaVLPxtlVLi/c/17928451643109195/.

[146] https://www.instagram.com/p/CaX4Q9ZhX1r/c/17987983390452561/.

[147] https://www.cdc.gov/coronavirus/2019-ncov/vaccines/recommendations/children-teens.html.

[l] CDC-INFO.

[148] https://www.cdc.gov/coronavirus/2019-ncov/vaccines/faq-children.html.

[k] Google trends.

[149] https://www.cdc.gov/coronavirus/2019-ncov/vaccines/safety/adverse-events.html.

[150] https://twitter.com/JayReason21/status/1496222712817397760.

[151] https://twitter.com/JayReason21/status/1496222712817397760.

[152] https://www.facebook.com/cdc/posts/328650775963034?comment_id=328808169280628&__cft__%5b0%5d=AZXOMmJcoZpkMXNtKHJb8s_la4AG3JU8w_gtcrNQ1Gx5QvEZifz0_Febs_goxXV8wlnkBTZN1cs24no

Ways to Take Action

- Encourage pediatricians, public health authorities, and community leaders to describe the benefits of COVID-19 vaccination in children at eligible ages.
- Disseminate information containing accurate infection and hospitalization data in children.
- Provide up-to-date messages about the timeline for vaccination in children ages under 5 years.

Consumers Continue to Have Questions and Concerns Related to the Safety of COVID-19 Vaccines

Vaccine mis/disinformation[153,154,155] as well as reported cases of vaccine adverse events and side effects such as myocarditis,[156,157,158] encephalomyelitis,[m,159] chronic fatigue syndrome,[n] worsening migraine episodes,[160,161] sudden hearing loss,[162] menstrual and fertility disorders,[163] blood clots,[164,165] cancers,[166] and deaths[167,168,169] following COVID-19 vaccinations have continued to contribute to concerns about vaccine safety. Studies which support and reinforce COVID-19 vaccine safety were published and circulated during this reporting period, including a recent CDC study that showed myocarditis was less frequently reported as an adverse event following vaccinations with boosters as opposed to vaccinations with second primary doses among adolescents.[170] Likewise, a 6-month VAERS study conducted among people who received Pfizer-BioNTech or Moderna COVID-19 vaccines in the United States showed that

---

GgMYllceDHgFJPIGCPyZor0d9Pr7Oa7xAUVeH0N13ZjnoQ7Tb9SeXdo0nsnAEO7uZPZ0qc2Ca&__tn__=R%.

[153] https://twitter.com/Eljay2602/status/1502232928302026752.

[154] https://twitter.com/Legitscrutiny1/status/1501626151906725893.

[155] https://rumble.com/vwglmp-top-secret-pfizer-documents-leaked-pfizer-knew-that-vaxx-would-kill-thousan.html.

[156] https://twitter.com/freethought202/status/1502211661918212096/photo/1

[157] https://twitter.com/freethought202/status/1502211661918212096/photo/1

[158] https://twitter.com/RMConservative/status/1502320560386281476.

[m] WHO EARS.

[159] https://www.sciencedirect.com/science/article/pii/S2666354622000291.

[n] Google Trends.

[160] https://www.ncbi.nlm.nih.gov/pmc/articles/PMC8708794/.

[161] https://journals.sagepub.com/doi/full/10.1177/03331024211038654.

[162] https://jamanetwork.com/journals/jamaotolaryngology/fullarticle/2789496?guestAccessKey=9934d86a-9371-4c88-8f14-e96c36906e60&utm_source=For_The_Media&utm_medium=referral&utm_campaign=ftm_links&utm_content=tfl&utm_term=022422.

[163] https://twitter.com/JeanRees10/status/1497170081939398658/

[164] https://rumble.com/vw7u64-dr.-jane-ruby-warning-extremely-graphic-stop-getting-vaccinated-immediately.html.

[165] https://www.facebook.com/cdc/posts/328751329286312?comment_id=329572262537552&__cft__%5b0% 5d=AZULoGsPMoakhEshZl_UD_F-P0V5-flO86_tXI2_P_X9dxA_P7_aE-L8cyWTlc1lVjf3v_7v2L9nO492CCDt0V3B0tbeLf8CpDD4HXtfxxZ94aI8q6kFUL1dGgtQ9X9JeWkyq5xl2AvXsjIRoBSXqKnO&__tn__=R%5d-R.

[166] https://t.me/covid19vaccinevictims/4074.

[167] https://twitter.com/VacSafety/status/1501996339571265555.

[168] https://twitter.com/JennSal8/status/1502655719916511236.

[169] https://twitter.com/cliff_ranger/status/1501988063043534854.

[170] https://www.cdc.gov/mmwr/volumes/71/wr/mm7109e2.htm?s_cid=mm7109e2_w.

most adverse events were mild and transient[171,172] Also, COVID-19 mRNA vaccines were found to be safe in pregnancy[173] and to have the potential of conferring passive immunity to infants through transplacental transfer of antibodies.[174]

On WHO social listening tool, 'Pfizer' was the top hashtag, top rising hashtag, top keyword and top rising keyword.[o] Moreover, on CDC-INFO, some consumers made requests for studies focused on long-term effects of COVID-19 vaccines to be conducted.[p]

Perceptions, Concerns, and Threats to Vaccine Confidence

- Online users misrepresented the 9-page Pfizer report on adverse reactions currently circulating on social media to falsely claim that vaccines are dangerous.[175,176,177,178,179]
- Some consumers and news outlets expressed concerns about the impacts of COVID-19 vaccines causing adverse events, side effects, comorbidities and sudden deaths.[180,181,182]
- Several online consumers and websites expressed opposition to vaccines following severe allergic reactions and deaths among specific individuals (21 year old Texan,[183] NYC firefighters,[184,185] and a 5 year old from Illinois[186]) who received COVID-19 vaccines.
- Although debunked,[187] false online claims stated that a recent study proves mRNA vaccines could convert mRNA into DNA.[q,188,189,190]

Content Gaps and Information Voids

- What are the side effects of COVID-19 vaccines?[191,192]

---

[171] https://www.thelancet.com/journals/laninf/article/PIIS1473-3099(22)00123-2/fulltext.
[172] https://www.medpagetoday.com/infectiousdisease/covid19vaccine/97545.
[173] https://www.medrxiv.org/content/10.1101/2022.02.22.22271358v1.
[174] https://journals.lww.com/greenjournal/Fulltext/2022/02000/Neutralizing_Antibodies_and_Cytokines_in_ Breast.6.aspx.
[o] WHO EARS.
[p] CDC-INFO.
[175] https://twitter.com/cliff_ranger/status/1501988063043534854.
[176] https://twitter.com/CraigKellyMP/status/1502763405622403072.
[177] https://twitter.com/toadmeister/status/1501815141964427264.
[178] https://twitter.com/Eljay2602/status/1502232928302026752.
[179] https://twitter.com/imUrB00gieman/status/1502485165666230275.
[180] https://twitter.com/AmyMek/status/1466832709007798273.
[181] https://sciencebasedmedicine.org/that-latest-article-on-the-post-vaccine-myocarditis-autopsy-analysis/.
[182] https://twitter.com/JennSal8/status/1502655719916511236.
[183] https://www.caller.com/story/news/local/2022/02/24/texas-family-struggles-after-rare-severe-reaction-covid-19-vaccine-kartik-bhakta/6846156001/.
[184] https://www.nydailynews.com/coronavirus/ny-covid-fdny-union-leader-vaccine-20220220-d4dreh7sp5 hsnjqd pibkd56ulu-story.html.
[185] https://twitter.com/fynn_fan/status/1496338324230922246.
[186] https://twitter.com/JeanRees10/status/1497170081939398658/.
[187] https://healthfeedback.org/claimreview/study-lund-university-didnt-show-covid-19-mrna-vaccines-change-dna-epoch-times.
[q] Project VCTR.
[188] https://twitter.com/NguyenQLong/status/1497638565085605888.
[189] https://twitter.com/4M4NDA8ER6UER/status/1498209706174783490.
[190] https://www.mdpi.com/1467-3045/44/3/73/htm.

[191] https://twitter.com/Eljay2602/status/1502232928302026752.
[192] https://twitter.com/imUrB00gieman/status/1502485165666230275.

- Common side effects include pain, redness, swelling, tiredness, headache, muscle pain, and fever.[193,194] Severe allergic reactions and adverse effects that could cause a long-term health problem are extremely rare.[195,196]

- What is the risk of myocarditis after mRNA COVID-19 vaccination?[197]
  - The known risks of COVID-19 illness and its related, possibly severe, complications, such as long-term health problems, hospitalization, and even death, far outweigh the potential risks of having a rare adverse reaction to vaccination. This includes the possible risk of myocarditis or pericarditis.[198]
  - Most patients with myocarditis or pericarditis who received care responded well to medicine and rest and felt better quickly. Patients can usually return to their normal daily activities after their symptoms improve.[199]
  - Infection with the virus that causes COVID-19 increases the likelihood of myocarditis much more so than vaccination.[200]
- Do COVID-19 vaccines weaken the immune system?[201]
  - No studies have shown receiving COVID-19 vaccines weaken the immune system while numerous studies have documented the effectiveness of COVID-19 vaccines in preventing severe illness and death from COVID-19. For more information see: COVID-19 Vaccine Effectiveness and Safety | MMWR (cdc.gov).
- What are the effects of COVID-19 vaccines on fertility?[202]
  - Several studies have found no evidence that COVID-19 vaccines affect fertility in women or men.[203,204,205]
- What are the effects of COVID-19 vaccines on pregnancy?[206]
  - There is no evidence that COVID-19 vaccines increase the risk of preterm birth, low birth weight, or stillbirth. Infection with the virus that causes COVID-19 during pregnancy may increase the risk of severe illnesses, hospitalizations and deaths in mothers and newborns.[207] A recent MMWR found that completion of a 2-dose mRNA COVID-19 vaccination series during pregnancy might help prevent COVID-19 hospitalization among infants less than 6 months old.[208]

---

193 https://www.thelancet.com/journals/laninf/article/PIIS1473-3099(22)00054-8/fulltext.

194 https://www.cdc.gov/coronavirus/2019-ncov/vaccines/expect/after.html?s_cid=10535:%2Beffects%20%2Bof%20%2Bcovid%20%2Bvaccine:sem.b:p:RG:GM:gen:PTN:FY21.

195 https://www.cdc.gov/coronavirus/2019-ncov/vaccines/safety/allergic-reaction.html.

196 https://www.cdc.gov/mmwr/volumes/71/wr/mm7109e2.htm.

197 https://sciencebasedmedicine.org/that-latest-article-on-the-post-vaccine-myocarditis-autopsy-analysis/.

198 https://www.cdc.gov/coronavirus/2019-ncov/vaccines/safety/myocarditis.html?s_cid=10535:%2Beffects%20%2Bof%20%2Bcovid%20%2Bvaccine:sem.b:p:RG:GM:gen:PTN:FY21.

199 https://www.cdc.gov/coronavirus/2019-ncov/vaccines/safety/myocarditis.html?s_cid=11374:cdc%20covid%20vaccine%20heart%20inflammation:sem.ga:p:RG:GM:gen:PTN:FY21.

200 https://www.cdc.gov/mmwr/volumes/70/wr/mm7035e5.htm.

201 https://dailyexpose.uk/2022/02/13/the-covid-19-vaccines-cause-aids/.

202 https://twitter.com/JeanRees10/status/1497170081939398658/.

203 https://academic.oup.com/aje/advance-article/doi/10.1093/aje/kwac011/6511811?searchresult=1&login=true.

204 https://academic.oup.com/humrep/article/37/1/5/6420384?login=true.

205 https://jamanetwork.com/journals/jama/fullarticle/2781360.

206 https://www.medrxiv.org/content/10.1101/2022.02.22.22271358v1.

207 https://www.sciencedirect.com/science/article/pii/S2589750021002508?via%3Dihub.

208 https://www.cdc.gov/mmwr/volumes/71/wr/pdfs/mm7107e3-H.pdf.

- Do the mRNA COVID-19 vaccines alter DNA inside human cells?[209],[210]
- There is no evidence that the mRNA COVID-19 vaccines alter a person's DNA.[211] COVID-19 vaccines do not change or interact with your DNA. The genetic material delivered by mRNA vaccines does not enter the nucleus of your cells, which contains DNA.[191,212,213]
- Does adverse event data in the Pfizer report indicate that vaccines are dangerous?[214]
    - The Pfizer document is an inventory of adverse events, or health issues reported following vaccination, regardless of whether the vaccine caused them.[215]

Misinformation Themes

- COVID-19 vaccines cause a significant number of deaths.[216]
- For people in their twenties, the risk of death is seven times higher after vaccination than from infection with the virus that causes COVID-19.[217,218]
- COVID-19 vaccine-related myocarditis and other COVID-19-related complications caused the deaths of two teenage boys[219] and nine US soldiers.[220],[221]
- COVID-19 vaccines contain "strange life forms"[222] and can be transcribed into human DNA.[223]
- COVID-19 vaccines are not vaccines but experimental gene therapy.[224,225]
- COVID-19 vaccines cause recipients to develop vaccine-induced acquired immune deficiency syndrome (VAIDS).[226]
- Conservative news outlet claimed that athletes are either injured,[227] dead,[228] or require an EKG (heart recording)[229] following COVID-19 vaccination.

---

[209] https://twitter.com/NguyenQLong/status/1497638565085605888.

[210] https://www.reuters.com/article/factcheck-coronavirus-vaccines/fact-check-controversial-mit-study-does-not-show-that-mrna-vaccines-alter-dna-idUSL1N2PK1DC.

[211] https://www.genome.gov/about-genomics/fact-sheets/Understanding-COVID-19-mRNA-Vaccines.

[212] https://www.frontiersin.org/articles/10.3389/fimmu.2019.00594/full.

[213] https://aacrjournals.org/cancerres/article/55/7/1397/502087/Characterization-of-a-Messenger-RNA-Polynuc leo tide?msclkid=1ea30204cd6911ec894a7974061d36b0.

[214] https://twitter.com/CraigKellyMP/status/1502763405622403072.

[215] https://www.factcheck.org/2022/03/scicheck-posts-misinterpret-pfizer-covid-19-vaccine-safety-monitoring-docu ment/.

[216] https://twitter.com/JennSal8/status/1502655719916511236.

[217] https://twitter.com/AmyMek/status/1466832709007798273.

[218] https://www.usatoday.com/story/news/factcheck/2021/12/21/fact-check-covid-19-vaccines-safe-people-their-20-s/8940671002/.

[219] https://sciencebasedmedicine.org/that-latest-article-on-the-post-vaccine-myocarditis-autopsy-analysis/.

[220] https://twitter.com/VacSafety/status/1501996339571265555.

[221] https://twitter.com/sethharpesq/status/1501607223902060549.

[222] https://t.me/covid19vaccinevictims/4170.

[223] https://www.facebook.com/cdc/posts/327890212705757?comment_id=328678372626941&__tn__=R.

[224] https://www.facebook.com/cdc/posts/328558152638963?comment_id=328843105943801&__tn__=R.

[225] https://www.facebook.com/cdc/posts/327873842707394?comment_id=328033416024770&__cft__%5b0%5d=AZVcPVXA3teUYU5uw0hysUdF_t-KpRf-wv0EbkOoDPbq_VUCHCw4WcukM2-YWBqpsqISnlv V7Nomc0jGcm5uFQES2Le76YHRmfNfrYpnpGLdpL4sYsT_v6DIEJ7NMa-R2d9k-caXIw0Iw-xwvUIh4rg9&__tn__=R%5d-R.

[226] https://dailyexpose.uk/2022/02/13/the-covid-19-vaccines-cause-aids/.

[227] https://www.factcheck.org/2021/12/scicheck-article-makes-unfounded-claims-linking-athletes-injuries-deaths-to-vaccines/.

[228] https://www.factcheck.org/2021/12/scicheck-article-makes-unfounded-claims-linking-athletes-injuries-deaths-to-vaccines/.

[229] https://t.me/covid19vaccinevictims/4191.

- The World Council of Health released a guide for followers to "spike protein detox" after vaccination.[230]

Ways to Take Action

- Create and disseminate simple, clear messages about the process for authorizing, approving, making recommendations for, monitoring the safety of, distributing, allocating, and administering COVID-19 vaccines, including data handling.
- Provide regular updates on the benefits, safety, side effects and effectiveness of COVID-19 vaccines and clearly communicate what is known, what isn't known, and what is being done to find out what isn't known.

Consumers Continue to Discuss Their Support or Opposition to Booster Doses

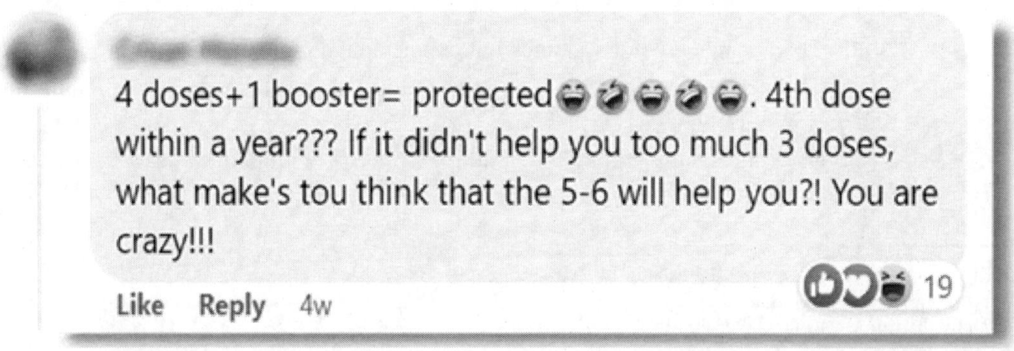

Consumers continue to question possible authorization and eligibility for a fourth dose (i.e., a second booster). Searches for "cdc booster data" rose by 400% during this reporting period.[r] On March 11, 2022, a Pfizer-BioNTech representative stated that an additional booster would be necessary due to waning immunity while supporting data would be submitted to the FDA for approval.[231,232] Moderna also believes an additional booster will be necessary.[233] However, only 38% of eligible adults report being likely to receive a booster.[s] Currently, everyone 12 years and older should get a booster when eligible. Those who are 12 years and older and are moderately/severely immunocompromised may receive a second booster. Everyone 50 years and older may also get a second booster. Although data from the CDC COVID Data Tracker show 48.2% of fully vaccinated US adults have received a booster dose, adults who have not received a booster dose yet are less likely to receive future booster doses than adults who already have.[s]

---

[230] https://www.vice.com/en/article/n7nqm7/mysterious-medical-organizations-are-calling-for-an-end-to-covid-vaccines.

[r] Google trends.

[231] https://www.nbcnews.com/health/health-news/pfizer-plans-submit-data-4th-covid-shot-fda-rcna19675.

[232] https://thehill.com/policy/healthcare/598026-pfizer-ceo-says-a-fourth-booster-shot-is-necessary.

[233] https://www.reuters.com/business/healthcare-pharmaceuticals/moderna-raises-2022-covid-vaccine-sales-forecast-19-billion-2022-02-24/.

[s] HHS Current Events Tracker.

Perceptions, Concerns, and Threats to Vaccine Confidence

- Some consumers support an additional booster of COVID-19 vaccine, comparing it to a yearly flu shot.[234,235,236] Others are uninterested in additional doses, claiming two or three doses total is their limit.[237,238,239]
- Social media users are worried the booster is causing heart and breathing problems.[240,241,242]
- Conflicting messages from global public health authorities, increased profits for vaccine companies,[243,244] and unclear data on benefit of vaccination may negatively impact vaccine uptake.[245,246,247]

Content Gaps and Information Voids

- What are the side effects of COVID-19 boosters?[t]
  - So far, reactions reported after getting a booster are similar to those after the two-dose or single-dose primary shots. Fever, headache, fatigue, and pain at the injection site were the most commonly reported side effects. Overall, most side effects were mild to moderate. However, as with the two-dose or single-dose primary shots, serious side effects are rare but can occur.[248]
- Are people who received COVID-19 vaccines abroad eligible for Moderna or Pfizer-BioNTech vaccine boosters in the United States?[t]
  - Yes. CDC has detailed guidance for COVID-19 vaccination for people who received 1 or more doses outside of the United States. Refer to Clinical Guidance for COVID-19 Vaccination CDC.[249]
- Should immunocompromised people receive a fourth dose of the COVID-19 vaccine?[u]
  - People ages 12 years and older who are moderately/severely immunocompromised should receive a total of 4 doses of mRNA COVID-19 vaccine to stay up to date. The 4 doses include a primary series of 3 doses of an Pfizer-BioNTech or Moderna COVID-19 vaccine, plus 1 booster of an Pfizer-BioNTech or Moderna COVID-19 vaccine (4th dose).
- Do people need a booster dose to be considered fully vaccinated?[u]

---

[234] https://twitter.com/100Zeus/status/1503076466510102528.
[235] https://twitter.com/LardFDorkness2/status/1503413010689187840.
[236] https://twitter.com/billiereuben21/status/1503440773940924422.
[237] https://twitter.com/gclt5/status/1503067468725641220.
[238] https://twitter.com/newsviewsbrews/status/1503411340697903115.
[239] https://twitter.com/TKiko/status/1503409089765945348.
[240] https://twitter.com/JohnRuddick2/status/1501866422636773376.
[241] https://twitter.com/DylanJamesCo/status/1503050101589262338.
[242] https://twitter.com/Bearman37908986/status/1496964524225843209.
[243] https://www.cnbc.com/2022/03/03/covid-pfizer-moderna-project-51-billion-in-combined-vaccine-sales-this-year.html.
[244] https://www.wsj.com/articles/pfizer-moderna-and-other-drugmakers-make-billions-meeting-covid-19-needs-11645811779.
[245] https://www.facebook.com/cdc/posts/328558152638963?comment_id=328824919278953&__tn__=R.
[246] https://twitter.com/SarahKr72870205/status/1498817333711802371.
[247] https://fortune.com/2022/03/03/covid-booster-fourth-dose-new-variant/.
[t] CDC-INFO.
[248] https://www.cdc.gov/coronavirus/2019-ncov/vaccines/expect/after.html.
[249] https://www.cdc.gov/coronavirus/2019-ncov/vaccines/recommendations/immuno.html.
[u] CDC-

- Fully vaccinated means a person has received all recommended doses in their primary series of COVID-19 vaccines. Up to date means a person has received all recommended doses in their primary series of COVID-19 vaccines and a booster when eligible.[250]

Misinformation Themes

- Some consumers believe the Pfizer CEO was lying about the need for a fourth dose and it is only a plan for Pfizer to make more money.[251, 252, 253]
- The first, second, and third doses did not work at preventing the spread of the virus that causes COVID-19, so neither will a fourth dose.[254, 255, 256]
- The CDC failed to release timely data, making some believe the government is hiding data showing most adults did not require an additional COVID-19 booster.[257, 258, 259]

Ways to Take Action

- Provide information to the public when data is available about the safety and benefits of an additional booster.
- Explain side effects associated with vaccination and how they compare to long-term effects and adverse events of COVID-19.
- Disseminate messages showing who is eligible and who should get an additional booster dose.

---

250 https://www.cdc.gov/coronavirus/2019-ncov/vaccines/stay-up-to-date.html?s_cid=11747:cdc%20fully%20vaccinated%20definition:sem.ga:p:RG:GM:gen:PTN:FY22.

251 https://www.instagram.com/p/CaSWK9hL_D_/c/17949550774732839/.

252 https://twitter.com/JCoulterB/status/1498764644038545410.

253 https://www.facebook.com/cdc/posts/328860049275440?comment_id=681108126658450.

254 https://www.facebook.com/cdc/posts/328860049275440?comment_id=328862992608479&__cft__%5b0%5d=AZVZpxntP2kdJxDMZN7uu-rZN0YgZ-srgH7jaeIBneYaVcH7CAgz4ZErnwjC7BN1-cI1It19_x13ZYbvgDSohr6I767f6FIEbUkpANDXJTeq7Qvzgf865mO6wo0kaOJ5n5jzD9r9k7EibPn3EPss1GO5&__tn__=R%5d-R.

255 https://www.facebook.com/cdc/posts/328860049275440?comment_id=2994617747464683&__cft__%5b0%5d=AZVZpxntP2kdJxDMZN7uu-rZN0YgZ-srgH7jaeIBneYaVcH7CAgz4ZErnwjC7BN1-cI1It19_x13ZYbvgDSohr6I767f6FIEbUkpANDXJTeq7Qvzgf865mO6wo0kaOJ5n5jzD9r9k7EibPn3EPss1GO5&__tn__=R%5d-R.

256 https://www.facebook.com/cdc/posts/328860049275440?comment_id=938954103442128&__cft__%5b0%5d=AZVZpxntP2kdJxDMZN7uu-rZN0YgZ-srgH7jaeIBneYaVcH7CAgz4ZErnwjC7BN1-cI1It19_x13ZYbvgDSohr6I767f6FIEbUkpANDXJTeq7Qvzgf865mO6wo0kaOJ5n5jzD9r9k7EibPn3EPss1GO5&__tn__=R%5d-R.

257 https://www.nytimes.com/2022/02/20/health/covid-cdc-data.html.

258 https://www.instagram.com/p/CaVTt6jlyYY/c/17923559864313033/.

259 https://www.facebook.com/cdc/posts/328860049275440?comment_id=505117204402169.

Appendix: Inputs and Sources

Type	Input	Cadence	Sources	Tactics for Utilization
Social Media Listening & Media Monitoring	Communication Surveillance Report	Daily on weekdays	• Google news • Meltwater • CrowdTangle • Native platform searches	• Share of voice topic analysis to identify themes • Emerging topics
	Meltwater	Daily	• Facebook, Twitter, Instagram • Blogs • News media • Online forums	• Share of voice topic analysis • Emerging theme topics • Identify high reach/velocity topics
	OADC (Office of the Associate Director of Communication) Channel COVID-19 Post metrics	Weekly	• Sprout Social • Native OADC account analytics	• Analyze # of posts, topics • Success of messages, # of impressions, reach, # engagements
	OADC Channel Comment Analysis	Daily on weekdays	• ·Native platform searches	• Sentiment analysis • Identify message gaps/voids
Direct Reports	CDC-INFO Metrics	Weekly	• CDC-INFO inquiry line list • Prepared response (PR) usage report	• Cross-compare PR usage with inquiry theme analysis • Sentiment analysis • Identify information gaps/voids
	VTF Media Requests	Weekly	• ·Media request line list	• Leading indicator for news coverage • Identify information gaps/voids
	Web Metrics	Weekly	• Top pages • Google search queries • Top FAQs • Referring domains	• Identify information gaps/voids, • Identify keywords/

Appendix. (Continued)

Type	Input	Cadence	Sources	Tactics for Utilization
				search terms, changes in web traffic
Research	Poll Review	Weekly	• Harris Poll, PEW research, Gallup Poll, KFF • New data related to vaccine hesitancy	• Identify socio-behavior indicators related to motivation and intention to vaccinate
	Literature Review	Weekly	• PubMed, LitCovid, ProQuest Central, Altmetric • New data related to vaccine hesitancy	• Identify current vaccination intention • Identify barriers to vaccination
Third Party Reports	Tanaq Social Listening +Media Monitoring Report	Weekly	• Meltwater • Sprout Social • First Draft • Native platform searches	• Trending topics • Demographic and geographic conversation monitoring
	CrowdTangle content insights report	Biweekly	• ·Facebook	• Top pages (voices), groups • General trends/ sentiment analysis • News analysis through posts
	First Draft News Vaccine Misinformation Insights Report	Monthly	• Proprietary methods	• Media trends analysis • Emerging threats and data deficits • Online vaccine narratives
	Project VCTR	Weekly	• Proprietary methods	• National and regional trends in negative attitudes toward vaccination • Conversations around Legislation
	Virality Project	Weekly	• · Proprietary methods	• Mis- and disinformation trends related to COVID-19 vaccines

The findings and conclusions in this chapter are those of the author(s) and do not necessarily represent the official position of the Centers for Disease Control and Prevention (CDC).

Chapter 5

Domestic Funding for COVID-19 Vaccines: An Overview*

Kavya Sekar

Federal efforts to develop, manufacture, purchase, and distribute Coronavirus Disease 2019 (COVID-19) vaccines have involved a number of agencies. Many of these efforts have thus far been funded by appropriations in COVID-19 relief acts, especially funding to the Department of Health and Human Services (HHS) U.S. Public Health Service (PHS) agencies and accounts in FY2020 and FY2021 supplemental appropriations and in the American Rescue Plan Act (ARPA, P.L. 117-2) budget reconciliation measure enacted in March 2021.

The following provides an overview of both (1) appropriations and (2) allocations and obligations for selected domestic COVID-19 vaccine related activities.

(With the exception of the mandatory funding provided by ARPA, all funding amounts discussed below are classified as discretionary.) The followingis meant to informa general understanding of relevant funding, but does not capture every federal account that can be used for vaccine- related activities. This chapter does not address financing for vaccine administration (e.g., health insurance coverage) or global vaccination funding (although some of the funding for research and development [R&D], manufacture, and purchase has flexibility for international uses).

Appropriations

The following summarizes two major categories of COVID-19 vaccine-related appropriations. Many of the below appropriations are available for broad purposes; vaccine-related activities are one potential use of funds. In general, many of the HHS appropriations mentioned are available for multiple years or until expended, and some of the funding is transferrable between accounts by the HHS Secretary.

* This is an edited, reformatted and augmented version of Congressional Research Service Publication No. IF11951, updated November 22, 2021.

In: COVID-19 Vaccines
Editor: John Schroder
ISBN: 979-8-88697-150-7

Research and Development, Manufacture, and Purchase

COVID-19 vaccine R&D, manufacture, and purchase have been largely supported by a collaboration among several federal agencies, including the National Institutes of Health (NIH) and the Biomedical Advanced Research and Development Authority (BARDA) of HHS, and DOD— formerly Operation Warp Speed (OWS) and now the Countermeasures Acceleration Group (CAG). Six vaccines were chosen for coordinated federal support under OWS. Some vaccine R&D has been supported by NIH, BARDA, and DOD separately fromthe OWS/CAGefforts.

NIH and DOD: FY2020 and FY2021 supplemental appropriations to NIH and DOD for COVID-19-related R&D can fund vaccine R&D. In the FY2020 and FY2021 supplemental appropriations acts, NIH received over $1.5 billion, available until September 30, 2024, broadly for COVID-19 related research. The CARES Act (P.L. 116- 136) provided DOD with $415 million for COVID-19 medical R&D in the Defense Health Programaccount with some flexibility to reallocate other funds toward R&D.

BARDA and Other R&D, Manufacture, and Purchase: In the FY2020 and FY2021 supplemental appropriations acts, over $50 billion in Public Health and Social Services Emergency Fund (PHSSEF) funding, available until September 30, 2024, is designated for a broad set of medical countermeasures and surge capacity purposes, including for the development, manufacture, and purchase of vaccines and related supplies. The PHSSEF account funds BARDA, the main entity that has awarded large funding agreements to pharmaceutical companies for vaccine development, manufacture, and purchase. Not less than $23.2 billion is set aside for BARDA in the FY2020 and FY2021 supplemental appropriations that can be used for vaccine-related efforts.

ARPA further provides two relevant mandatory appropriations: (1) in Section 2303, $6.05 billion, available until expended, to HHS for R&D, manufacturing, production, and purchase of vaccines and other medical products—available for COVID-19, SARS-CoV-2 or its variants, and any disease with potential for creating a pandemic; and (2) in Section 3101, $10 billion, available until September 30, 2025, for activities under the Defense Production Act(DPA) for the purchase, production and distribution of medical supplies, including vaccines and related supplies, among others. Both of these ARPA appropriations have been assignedto HHS accounts—the first to PHSSEF and the second to a new HHS DPA account.

Domestic Vaccination Programs

The Centers for Disease Control and Prevention (CDC), in collaboration with other agencies, has led efforts with state, local, tribal, and territorial (SLTT) jurisdictions to plan and implement a nationwide vaccination program. Agencies with health care programs (e.g., the Veterans Health Administration and Indian Health Service [IHS]) have separately managed vaccination programs among employees and covered populations. The Biden Administration has also expanded the role of additional agencies (e.g., the Federal Emergency Management Agency [FEMA]) in vaccination programs.

CDC: Earlier in the pandemic, before vaccines were available, CDC had received broad supplemental appropriations for its pandemic-related activities in March 2020, and used some of this funding for vaccination programgrants and planning. Since then, CDC has received several appropriations specifically for vaccine-related activities:

Vaccination Programs and SLTT Grants. For efforts to plan, promote, distribute, administer, monitor, and track COVID-19 vaccines, CDC received a total of $16.25 billion in FY2021, including $8.75 billion in the Coronavirus Response and Relief Supplemental Appropriations Act, 2021 (CRRSA), enacted in December, 2020 (P.L. 116-260, Division M), available until September 30, 2024; and $7.5 billion in ARPA Section 2301, available until expended. Of the $8.75 billion in CRRSA, at least $4.5 billion is designated for SLTT grants (or cooperative agreements), of which $210 million must be transferred to IHS, and a separate amount of not less than $300 million is designated for "high-risk and underserved populations, including racial and ethnic minority populations and rural communities."

The ARPA provision directs CDC to award supplemental funding to eligible awardees that received grants under CRRSA based on a specified alternative formula.

Vaccine Confidence. CDC also received $1 billion for vaccine confidence activities in ARPA Section 2302.

FEMA: Funding fromthe Disaster Relief Fund (DRF) has been used to support FEMA's vaccination efforts, including by reimbursing certain costs for SLTT programs and supplying direct assistance (e.g., supplies, personnel) to mass vaccination sites. ARPA Section 4005 provides additional funding of $50 billion for the DRF that can support FEMA's expanded activities.

Other Funding: Many appropriations in the supplemental appropriations acts and throughout ARPA can support domestic vaccination efforts, for example, funding for public health workforce in ARPA Section 2501, and for community health centers in ARPA Section 2601 and earlier appropriations. According to National Conference of State Legislatures data, some states and other jurisdictions have used part of the CARES Act-funded Department of the Treasury Coronavirus Relief Fund grants for vaccination efforts. For the similar ARPA-funded State and Local Fiscal Recovery Fund programs, Treasury guidance notes supporting vaccination efforts as a potential use of funds.

Allocations and Obligations

As summarized above, many appropriations can support vaccine-related activities. The following summarizes selected information on vaccine-specific allocations and obligations.

HHS: As reported by the Government Accountability Office (GAO), as of August 31,2021, HHS allocated $40.0 billion toward vaccine-related activities (those of BARDA, NIH, and CDC) for R&D, manufacture, purchase, distribution, and related activities with $31.9 billion obligated (GAO-22-105051). This does not account for activities such as some CDC SLTT vaccine-related grants. Separately, $14.8 billion of the $178 billion Provider Relief Fund was allocated for "vaccine and therapeutic development and procurement activities" as of August 2021, with $6.5 billion obligated (GAO-22-105051).

FEMA: According to FEMA, $6.1 billion had been obligated fromthe DRF for vaccination efforts as of November 10,2021.

DOD: As communicated to CRS in May 2021, DOD has allocated $534.9 million for COVID-19 vaccine R&D and had obligated $506.4 million by that time. These COVID- 19 vaccine R&D efforts are separate from OWS/CAG vaccine R&D. DOD has also been managing some

OWS/CAGvaccine-related funding on behalf of HHS, utilizing its acquisition capabilities and authorities—especially for purchase and manufacturing agreements.

Further Considerations and Outlook

Future domestic COVID-19 vaccine funding needs remain uncertain. Federally supported vaccination efforts may be underway for some time with the ongoing booster and pediatric vaccination effort; potential for additionalboosters and additionalpediatric vaccines; and a significant percentage of the population that remains unvaccinated.

Additional COVID-19 vaccine R&D may also help develop new vaccines, especially for new variants. Balances of previously appropriated funds may remain available to fund such efforts. The House-passed"Build Back Better Act" (H.R. 5376) would provide $1.3 billion in pandemic preparedness funding that could be used for vaccine R&D, production, and supply-related activities (Section 31022) in addition to broader public health funding that could support vaccine-related efforts (neither specific to COVID-19 vaccines). In the future, Congress may also consider the conditions under which domestic COVID-19 vaccination efforts could shift to routinefinancing and administration approaches—no longer requiringsole federal purchase or support of mass vaccination sites and coordinated distribution.

Chapter 6

The U.S. Government's Role in Domestic and Global COVID-19 Vaccine Supply and Distribution: Frequently Asked Questions*

Sara M. Tharakan and Taylor R. Wyatt

This chapter answers frequently asked questions regarding domestic and global vaccine supply and distribution, and U.S. spending on Coronavirus Disease 2019 (COVID-19) vaccines. Unless otherwise stated, information is current as of January 10, 2022.

Domestic Vaccine Development, Purchasing, and Distribution

Which federal agencies funded the development and manufacturing of COVID-19 vaccines? Numerous federal entities supported COVID-19 vaccine development and manufacturing, including the National Institutes of Health (NIH), the Biomedical Advanced Research and Development Authority (BARDA), the Department of Defense (DOD), and others, both within and separately from the Operation Warp Speed (OWS) initiativeThis chapter focuses on domestic BARDA efforts.

What agreements did the U.S. government enter into with vaccine manufacturers for COVID-19 vaccine development, manufacturing, and purchase? Sanofi Pasteur and GSK, ModernaTX Inc., Janssen Pharmaceuticals Inc., AstraZeneca, Novavax Inc., and Merck and IAVI entered into agreements with BARDA for the manufacturing and development of COVID-19 vaccines. In some cases, these agreements included provisions for advance purchase of completed vaccines that ensured the U.S. government would own a certain number of doses that resulted from federal investment. Pfizer Inc. accepted funding only for advance purchase of vaccines, not for development and manufacturing. Other subsequent awards were made solely for the purpose of purchasing doses from six manufacturers: Pfizer, Sanofi Pasteur and GSK, ModernaTX, Janssen Pharmaceuticals, AstraZeneca, and Novavax, Inc. Merck and

* This is an edited, reformatted and augmented version of Congressional Research Service Publication No. IF12013, dated January 10, 2022.

In: COVID-19 Vaccines
Editor: John Schroder
ISBN: 979-8-88697-150-7

IAVI received a base award for accelerating the development of a COVID-19 vaccine that did not include provision for purchase of doses.

How many COVID-19 vaccines has the U.S. government purchased for domestic use? Roughly 1.2 billion doses of COVID-19 vaccines have been purchased by the U.S. government for domestic use.

Per Pfizer, as of October 28, 2021, a total of 600 million Pfizer vaccine doses have been purchased for domestic use. (The original July 2020 agreement with BARDA and DOD included a provision for ownership of 100 million doses, with the option to purchase an additional 500 million doses. Based on public statements, additional doses purchased in 2020 and 2021 total 550 million, the majority of which were for adult/adolescent doses.) Per the Department of Health and Human Services (HHS), as of June 2021 (the most recent data available), a total of 500 million ModernaTX vaccine doses had been purchased for domestic use. As of March 2021, a total of 100 million Janssen Pharmaceuticals, Inc., vaccine doses had been purchased for domestic use. These doses were purchased in August 2020. Additionally, the U.S. government has executed contracts with Sanofi Pasteur and GSK, AstraZeneca, and Novavax Inc. that included provisions for federal ownership of a certain number of doses (100 million, 300 million, and 100 million, respectively). These vaccines currently lack an Emergency Use Authorization (EUA) or Food and Drug Administration (FDA) approval. Originally, these vaccine doses were purchased with the intent for domestic use, but they currently have an unspecified planned usage.

How much money has BARDA awarded for COVID-19 vaccine development, manufacturing, and purchasing? BARDA, in partnership with DOD, has committed about $29 billion for COVID-19 vaccine development, manufacturing, and purchasing among the seven aforementioned vaccine manufacturers. Per the BARDA COVID-19 Medical Countermeasure Portfolio website, awards include $12 billion to Pfizer; $2 billion to Sanofi Pasteur and GSK; $9.6 billion to ModernaTX; $2 billion to Janssen Pharmaceuticals; $1.6 billion to AstraZeneca; $1.6 billion to Novavax Inc; and $38 million to Merck and IAVI.

How do state and local health departments order vaccines? What systems are used to track orders and distribution, and are data regarding distribution publicly available? The U.S. government continues to determine the maximum number of COVID-19 vaccine doses per manufacturer that each of the 64 state, local, and territorial health jurisdictions can order based on their population over age 18. Additionally, federal providers (e.g., VA, DOD, HHS) and participating nongovernment entities (e.g., pharmacy chains) can place orders based on their populations of need. These jurisdictions and providers can independently determine how many doses to order, up to this threshold amount, and place their order using the Vaccine Tracking System (VTrckS). VTrckS also allows the Centers for Disease Control and Prevention (CDC) to monitor vaccine allocations, distribution, and shipments.

Roughly 639.7 million vaccine doses have been delivered domestically, of which 81.2% had been administered.

Is the U.S. government meeting its domestic vaccination goals? In December 2020, then President-elect Joseph R. Biden Jr. announced the intention of administering 100 million vaccines in his first 100 days in office; this goal was met within the first 58 days of his administration. In May 2021, the Biden Administration announced the goal of administering one dose to 70% of the eligible population by July 4, 2021; the 70% threshold was attained in August 2021. Currently, the Biden Administration is focused on vaccinating the unvaccinated and providing booster doses.

Global Vaccine Distribution and Funding

How much foreign assistance has Congress appropriated for COVID-19 vaccine distribution and related efforts? Congress has appropriated roughly $17 billion for international COVID-19 response, including $4 billion to Gavi, the Vaccine Alliance, for U.S. membership in the COVID-19 Vaccine Global Access Initiative (COVAX, the vaccines arm of the Access to COVID-19 Tools Accelerator [ACT-A], led by the World Health Organization [WHO] and others). U.S. government commitments for global vaccine readiness efforts total approximately $1.3 billion. In addition, CDC has committed $800 million for COVID-19 response and vaccine-related efforts. The remaining $11 billion is being used for a variety of foreign assistance efforts to respond to the effects of the pandemic.

Is there a central strategy and/or coordinating mechanism governing U.S. government global vaccine distribution efforts? On December 6, 2021, the United States Agency for International Development (USAID) announced the U.S. Government's Initiative for Global Vaccine Access (Global VAX) to accelerate U.S. vaccine delivery. Focus areas include bolstering cold chain supply and logistics, service delivery, vaccine confidence and demand, local planning, and vaccine safety and effectiveness in low- and middle-income countries (LMICs). Global efforts build on U.S. commitments to COVAX. Global VAX activities will be implemented using $400 million from P.L. 117-2, with a focus on safe vaccine delivery and storage, building in-country vaccine manufacturing capacity and knowledge sharing, and Rapid Response Surge Support (e.g., improving oxygen production and delivery), among other things.

How is the Biden Administration deciding how to allocate global COVID-19 vaccine dose donations? The U.S. government has promised to donate 1.2 billion vaccine doses globally. The White House stated 75% of donated doses will be shared through COVAX to maximize the number of vaccines available equitably for the largest number of countries and at-risk populations within countries. The remaining 25% will be shared directly with countries in need, those experiencing COVID-19 surges, and countries requesting immediate U.S. assistance.

Which countries have received COVID-19 vaccines from the United States? How many doses has the United States committed to donate and how many have been distributed? The U.S. government is the leading donor of COVID-19 vaccines globally, and according to the State Department, has shipped 365 million COVID-19 vaccines to 110 countries, including 103 million doses to sub- Saharan Africa; 89 million doses to East Asia and the Pacific; 60 million doses to Latin America and the Caribbean; 84 million doses to South and Central Asia; 24 million doses the Middle East and North Africa; and 4.1 million doses to Moldova, Ukraine, Kosovo, and Georgia.

What is the status of COVAX, ACT-A, and the Multilateral Leaders Task Force? COVAX has shipped 967 million COVID-19 vaccines to 144 participant countries and economies. Donors have committed $300 million toward 2022 targets. WHO reports a funding gap of $6.97 billion to reach ACT-A strategic plan targets, to achieve 70% vaccination coverage in LMICs by mid-2022. The Task Force on COVID-19 Vaccines, Therapeutics and Diagnostics for Developing Countries (the Task Force), established on May 31, 2021, by the International Monetary Fund (IMF), the World Bank Group, WHO, and the World Trade Organization (WTO), is working toward COVAX's targets, improving transparency and data sharing, and seeking $50 billion in support of COVAX and ACT-A goals.

Where is the global community in meeting these targets? The pace of vaccination in low-income countries would reportedly need to increase to nearly 20 times current levels to achieve these targets. Globally, more than 7 billion shots have been administered, the majority in high-income countries. At least 50 countries are falling short of global vaccination targets; less than 25% of their populations are fully vaccinated (defined as the number of doses in a full regimen of a specific immunization scheme; for example, two doses of the Moderna or Pfizer vaccine). It remains to be seen how the emergence of new variants (such as Omicron), and the need for booster shots for more complete protection against severe disease (in many high-income countries a three-dose regimen is becoming the norm), will affect countries' ability to meet these targets.

Which other countries/entities are top donors to COVAX, and of those that have promised COVID-19 vaccine doses, how many have been delivered? Per the Task Force, other top vaccine donors to COVAX are the European Union (464 million promised, of which 57 million have been shipped), France (120 million promised; 19 million delivered), the United Kingdom (120 million promised; 8 million delivered), and Germany (175 million promised; 15 million delivered). The United States has promised 857 million doses to COVAX, of which 131 million have been delivered.

What contracts does COVAX have with vaccine manufacturers? COVAX has formalized contracts for over 4 billion doses with nine vaccine manufacturers (AstraZeneca, Clover Biopharmaceuticals, Janssen Pharmaceuticals Inc., ModernaTX Inc., Novavax Inc., Pfizer Inc., Sanofi Pasteur and GSK, Sinopharm, and Sinovac). COVAX Advanced Market Commitment doses are capped at $3 per dose. These contracts are reportedly worth at least $12 billion.

Are there enough COVID-19 vaccines for the world's population? What factors are hindering global vaccine access? Global COVID-19 vaccine production is at approximately 1.5 billion doses per month, meaning that hypothetically there is sufficient vaccine supply to achieve global vaccination targets. Global health experts identify equitable distribution as the key current issue. WHO has called on countries to donate resources for vaccine rollout in LMICs, and for wealthy nations to swap vaccine delivery schedules with countries in need, accelerate dose sharing, and fulfill donation commitments to COVAX.

Chapter 7

Global COVID-19 Vaccine Distribution*[1]

Sara M. Tharakan and Tiaji Salaam-Blyther

Background

The Coronavirus Disease 2019 (COVID-19) pandemic has led to severe health and economic consequences across the globe, as governments work to contain the spread of the virus and its variants. In late 2020, researchers started identifying several COVID-19 variants, now driving surges in related cases and deaths across Africa and south Asia.

The United States, India, and Brazil have the highest number of confirmed COVID-19 cases, many caused by the Delta variant. Vaccines and other countermeasures play a growing role in COVID-19 control. However, insufficient access to vaccines in many low- and middle-income countries (LMICs) raises questions about how inequities may hinder pandemic control worldwide.

Congress appropriated approximately $15 billion for a range of COVID-19-related responses through supplemental appropriations (P.L. 116-123, P.L. 116-136, P.L. 116-260, and P.L. 117-2), including $4 billion for multilateral COVID-19 vaccine efforts. The Biden Administration has announced that the United States will provide over 500 million vaccine doses worldwide through direct donations and contributions via COVAX—a multilateral effort comprising nearly 200 countries, co-led by the World Health Organization (WHO), the Coalition for Epidemic Preparedness and Innovation (CEPI), and Gavi, the Vaccine Alliance. On May 31, 2021, the International Monetary Fund (IMF), the World Bank Group, WHO, and the World Trade Organization (WTO) established the Task Force on COVID-19 Vaccines, Therapeutics and Diagnostics for Developing Countries (the Task Force). The Task Force is seeking an additional $50 billion in support of COVAX and the Access to COVID-19 Tools Accelerator (ACT-A), so that at least 40% of all people worldwide could be vaccinated by the end of 2021.

* This is an edited, reformatted and augmented version of Congressional Research Service Publication No. IF11796, updated August 5, 2021.

[1] Alexandria Lee, CRS Summer Research Associate, contributed to this product.

In: COVID-19 Vaccines
Editor: John Schroder
ISBN: 979-8-88697-150-7

Global COVID-19 Vaccine Distribution

In April 2020, WHO and partners launched ACT-A to advance the development, production, and distribution of COVID-19 diagnostics, therapeutics, and vaccines. Within less than a year, multiple safe and effective COVID-19 vaccines had been developed. To date, several countries and WHO have approved eight COVID-19 vaccines for emergency use, including those made in China. WHO has not authorized emergency use for vaccines produced in Russia, though some countries that do not have sufficient access to authorized vaccines have used them. More than 200 other COVID-19 vaccine candidates are in clinical trials. Numerous therapeutics are also in development.

Although manufacturers expect to produce about 11 billion COVID-19 vaccine doses by the end of 2021, many experts assert that at current vaccine distribution rates, COVID-19 vaccines will not be widely available in LMICs until at least 2022. The vast majority of manufactured COVID-19 vaccine doses have been distributed in high-income countries (*Figure 1*).

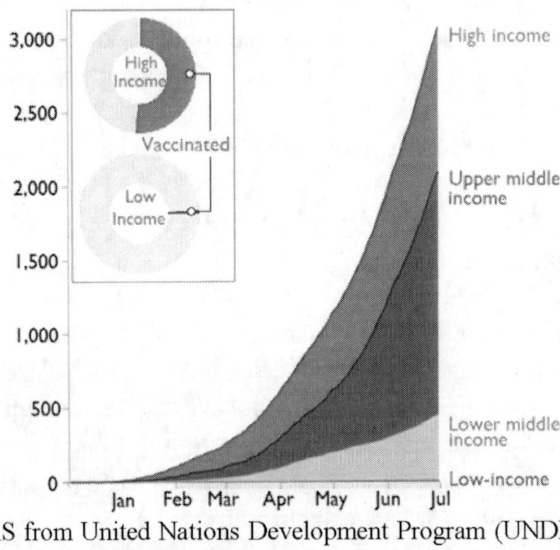

Source: Adapted by CRS from United Nations Development Program (UNDP), Global Dashboard for Vaccine Equity, accessed on August 2, 2021.

Figure 1. Global Distribution of COVID-19 Vaccines. (millions of doses, as of July 28, 2021).

Advances. By early August, donors had pledged $9.8 billion for COVAX, which had shipped more than 200 million COVID-19 vaccine doses to 138 countries worldwide. On June 11, the Group of 7 (G7) nations, at its 2021 annual meeting, committed to donate 870 million additional vaccine doses to COVAX by the end of 2022. G20 governments have also pledged $22 billion toward COVAX and ACT-A. As of June 23, 2021, the United States was the largest donor to COVAX, having pledged $3.5 billion. Other key donors include Germany ($1 billion), the United Kingdom ($733 million), Japan ($1 billion), Italy ($470 million), and Canada ($384 million).

Challenges. WHO and partners have decried the sluggish delivery of pledged vaccines and estimated that by July 31, 2021, less than 5% of vaccines that were pre-purchased by or for LMICs had been delivered. Many LMICs are expecting large donations via COVAX during the second half of 2022, but questions remain about their ability to rapidly distribute the vaccines, particularly in remote settings. The World Bank estimates an additional $35 billion in grants is needed to fund the Task Force on COVID-19 Vaccines, Therapeutics and Diagnostics for Developing Countries, and to rapidly scale up vaccine production and delivery in LMICs by 2022.

Global Vaccine Access

Insufficient vaccine supply, coupled with uneven capacity to pay for and disseminate the vaccines, has led to global vaccine-access gaps. Whereas some countries have purchased enough doses to vaccinate their populations several times over, others lack enough supply to vaccinate even their most vulnerable populations. Roughly 60% of the world's vaccine supply, according to WHO, has been purchased by rich countries whose populations account for less than 20% of all people in the world.

Each Task Force member is leveraging its resources to generate additional support for closing the equity gap. On July 26, 2021, the Task Force announced a new financing mechanism that allows certain COVAX countries to use World Bank and multilateral development bank financing to purchase advance vaccine doses in addition to their existing vaccine allotment. The IMF is also preparing a Special Drawing Rights allocation to boost the reserves and liquidity of member states toward reaching these goals.

Public health experts hope that ongoing WTO discussions over a potential waiver of certain WTO Agreements on Trade-Related Aspects of Intellectual Property Rights (TRIPS) obligations for COVID-19 vaccines and other trade policy responses to the pandemic might facilitate knowledge and technology transfers that might accelerate COVID-19 vaccine production worldwide.

U.S. Government Role

Bilateral efforts. The U.S. Agency for International Development (USAID), the Department of State, and the U.S. Centers for Disease Control and Prevention (CDC) are leveraging long-standing infectious disease control programs for the global COVID-19 response. Since March 2020, USAID and the State Department have committed more than $1.6 billion in health, humanitarian, economic, and development assistance for global COVID-19 control. CDC has committed $800 million for related efforts. These agencies are also supporting countries' efforts to implement National Deployment and Vaccination Plans, required by WHO for countries receiving vaccines through COVAX.

Multilateral efforts. In March 2021, the Biden Administration announced the United States would donate over 500 million vaccines to COVAX and other countries in need. Related pledges include

- jointly manufacturing and delivering 1 billion COVID- 19 vaccines to Southeast Asia by the end of 2022 through "the Quad," the coalition of Australia, India, Japan and the United States;

- donating 84 million vaccine doses, 75% of which will be provided through COVAX in LMICs;
- purchasing 500 million Pfizer-BioNTech COVID-19 vaccine doses for donation to COVAX; 200 million are to be delivered by the end of 2021, with the remaining 300 million to be delivered by the end of 2022.

Outlook and Issues for Congress

Many Members of Congress have demonstrated strong interest in bolstering global vaccine manufacturing and distribution capacity to support COVID-19 control. While deliberating how to balance international and domestic vaccine demand, Members may consider a variety of issues, including the following:

Vaccine manufacturing capacity in LMICs. WHO and other groups have decried the limits of current vaccine manufacturing capacity and pointed out that existing capacity cannot meet global demand for COVID-19 vaccine doses. A variety of efforts are underway, including through the U.S. International Development Finance Corporation and its partners, to scale up vaccine manufacturing capacity in LMICs. Some advocates note these efforts are vital but will likely take several years to fully operationalize and increase COVID-19 vaccine supply. In light of this discussion, Members may consider whether existing efforts are sufficient, or if efforts should be scaled up—including providing additional support for bolstering vaccine manufacturing capacity in LMICs, specifically for mRNA vaccines.

Getting shots in arms. The average cost of COVID-19 vaccines ($2-$40 per dose, depending on the type of vaccine, number of shots required, and other factors) is equivalent to the average annual per capita health spending on all health issues in many low-income countries ($41). Additional distribution costs ($3.70 per person for two doses) place further challenges on LMICs and limit the ability of their governments to reach needy populations, particularly outside major cities. The United Nations Development Program (UNDP) estimates that low-income countries would need to increase per capita health expenditure by 57% to vaccinate 70% their populations.

Three COVAX donors (Canada, Germany, and the United States) have given explicit permission to use funds for vaccine delivery, and USAID has allocated $500 million to support COVID-19 vaccine delivery in 88 countries.

Congress may consider arguments for and against using donor funds for vaccine delivery. Some argue that the limited funds should be used exclusively for vaccine purchase; others advocate using a portion of donor resources on vaccine delivery to protect the integrity of the donated commodities.

COVID-19 "vaccine passports." In January 2021, President Biden issued Executive Order 13998 to study whether the U.S. government should issue "vaccine passports" to indicate whether one has been vaccinated or recovered from COVID-19. Many health experts have endorsed the idea, citing precedents for using immunization records for various official purposes, including international travel. No federal policy has been announced, though four U.S. states have active vaccine certification apps, and 19 states have banned such systems. In July 2021, the European Union launched the EU Digital COVID Certificate Regulation to verify that a person has been vaccinated or received a negative test.

Members of Congress have not introduced legislation in support of or opposition to vaccine passports, though some bills cite key concerns. H.R. 906, for example, would prohibit the Secretary of Transportation from requiring an individual to test negative for COVID-19 to travel by air. Similarly, S. 82 calls for a joint task force, comprising the Secretaries of Transportation, Homeland Security, and Health and Human Services, to make recommendations for addressing privacy and civil liberty issues that may arise from such monitoring of air travelers' health.

Chapter 8

International COVID-19 Data and Vaccine Distribution: Selected Resources*

Hannah Fischer

The ongoing Coronavirus Disease 2019 (COVID-19) pandemic has caused millions of cases and deaths, according to the World Health Organization (WHO). The resources below provide information on tracking the international spread of the virus and global efforts to control it through vaccine distribution, diagnostic supplies, and therapeutics.

These resources are not a comprehensive list of global COVID-19 data sources. They are a starting point that may help congressional staff find resources for frequently requested data. Some links may work best with the internet browsers Chrome and Firefox.

Readers may consider using caution when comparing data across sources, time frames, and geographies, as each resource may have differing methodologies and definitions that may change over time.

International COVID-19 Access to COVID-19 Tools Accelerator

In April 2020, the WHO and partners launched the Access to COVID-19 Tools Accelerator (ACT-A) to accelerate the development, production, and distribution of COVID-19 diagnostics, therapeutics, and vaccines. Other collaborating institutions include Gavi (the Vaccine Alliance), the Coalition for Epidemic Preparedness and Innovation (CEPI), the Global Fund to Fight HIV, Tuberculosis and Malaria, the World Bank, the Bill & Melinda Gates Foundation, FIND (the Global Alliance for Diagnostics), Unitaid, and Wellcome. The ACT-A website provides more information, including

- Country Readiness and Delivery for Vaccines and
- Country Readiness and Delivery Frequently Asked Questions.

---

* This is an edited, reformatted and augmented version of Congressional Research Service Publication No. IN11732, updated December 2, 2021.

In: COVID-19 Vaccines
Editor: John Schroder
ISBN: 979-8-88697-150-7

COVAX is the vaccines pillar of the ACT-Accelerator. It aims to accelerate the development and manufacture of COVID-19 vaccines and guarantee fair and equitable access for every country in the world. COVAX is co-led by CEPI, Gavi, and WHO, alongside its key delivery partner, the United Nations Children's Fund (UNICEF). In the Americas, the Pan American Health Organization (PAHO) Revolving Fund is the recognized procurement agent for COVAX. The WHO-hosted COVAX website provides more information on COVAX, including

- COVID-19 Vaccine Introduction Toolkit and
- Guidance on developing a national deployment and vaccination plan (NDVP).

This second edition of the guidance, updated June 2021, provides new information on several topics, including

- the availability and use of the WHO-UNICEF COVID-19 Vaccine Introduction and deployment Costing (CVIC) tool;
- the COVAX Facility's humanitarian buffer that enables allocation of vaccine to cover high-risk populations in humanitarian settings;
- the use of geospatial data and digital micro plans for equitable access and delivery of COVID-19 vaccines.

International COVID-19 Tracking

The following U.S. and international organizations provide tools for tracking COVID-19 in countries and regions worldwide, including COVID-19 case and death numbers, vaccination rates, and measures of the socioeconomic and secondary impacts of COVID-19.

Centers for Disease Control and Prevention

The United States' lead public health agency collects and tracks the following international data by country using its COVID Data Tracker:

- COVID-19 cases and deaths, counts, and rates;
- Percentage change in COVID-19 cases and deaths reported in the past 7, 14, or 30 days;
- Epidemic curve trajectory classification; and
- Vaccine doses administered and people vaccinated, counts and rates.

Humanitarian Data Exchange

Run by the United Nations Office for the Coordination of Humanitarian Affairs (OCHA), the Humanitarian Data Exchange's (HDX's) COVID-19 Data Explorer: Global Humanitarian

Operations offers daily and monthly "snapshots" of global humanitarian operations relating to COVID-19, socio- economic risks, and vaccine distribution. It also provides an interactive tool for exploring international COVID-19 data in combination with other relevant humanitarian data such as

- COVID-19 Vaccine Roll-Out,
- People in need,
- School closures, and
- Vaccine Financing.

The World Bank

The World Bank's Understanding the Coronavirus (COVID-19) Pandemic through Data website offers a series of interactive datasets on the effects of COVID-19 worldwide, including, but not limited to,

- COVID-19 vs. other causes of death (see right-most tab on the chart, "Understanding the COVID-19 Pandemic through Data");
- Impacts of coronavirus on foreign remittances; and
- Financial-sector support measures in response to the coronavirus.

World Health Organization

The WHO's Coronavirus (COVID-19) Dashboard includes data on confirmed COVID-19 cases and deaths by country and region, vaccines in use by country, and persons partly or fully vaccinated by country.

International COVID-19 Vaccine Development and Distribution Tracking

The following websites provide tools focused on tracking the development, production, and distribution (i.e., shipments and deliveries) of COVID-19 vaccines in countries and regions worldwide.

Gavi, the Vaccine Alliance

Gavi is part of COVAX, the vaccines pillar of the ACT-Accelerator. Gavi's vaccine roll-out page allows users to explore vaccination status by country, including the date of the first doses received in each country, the type(s) of all vaccines received, and the number of doses allocated.

Department of State

The United States has committed to donating more than 1.1 billion doses of COVID-19 vaccines. The State Department's website tracks the status of the donation in total and by region and country.

Kaiser Family Foundation

The Kaiser Family Foundation has created a data visualizations website, using Department of State data on the United States' pledge to donate over 1.1 billion COVID-19 vaccine doses. Useful graphics include

- Recipients of U.S. COVID-19 Vaccine Donation Deliveries by Total Doses Received,
- U.S. COVID-19 Vaccine Donation Deliveries by Income,
- U.S. COVID-19 Vaccine Donation Doses Delivered by Vaccine Product, and
- Top Recipients of U.S. COVID-19 Vaccine Donation Deliveries by Total Doses Received.

UNICEF

UNICEF's Vaccine Market Dashboard provides updated information on

- COVID-19 vaccine development and progress toward vaccine approvals,
- Reported global vaccine production capacity,
- Manufacturing agreements,
- Vaccines secured and optioned through bilateral and multilateral supply agreements, and
- Reported vaccine prices.

Chapter 9

COVID-19: HHS Agencies' Planned Reviews of Vaccine Distribution and Communication Efforts Should Include Stakeholder Perspectives*

United States Government Accountability Office

Why GAO Did This Study

Vaccination remains critical in the federal response to the COVID-19 pandemic. Vaccine implementation— prioritizing, allocating, distributing, and administering doses—requires coordination among federal, state, and local levels and other stakeholders.

HHS agencies—including CDC and HRSA—set up federal vaccine distribution programs, such as CDC's retail pharmacy program that sends doses directly to pharmacies. The federal government also sends vaccine doses to states for further distribution.

The CARES Act includes a provision for GAO to report on its ongoing monitoring and oversight efforts related to the COVID-19 pandemic. This chapter examines (1) stakeholder perspectives on federal programs to distribute and administer COVID-19 vaccines, (2) efforts to inform health officials, providers, and the public about vaccination, and (3) actions HHS agencies are taking to evaluate their vaccine implementation efforts.

GAO reviewed data and documents from HHS, CDC, and HRSA, and reviewed information from and interviewed state and local health officials in four states and one city selected, in part, for geographic variation. GAO also interviewed other stakeholders, including 12 national associations representing health care providers and others.

What GAO Recommends

GAO is making four recommendations, including that CDC and HRSA obtain input from and share lessons learned with key stakeholders as they conduct their future reviews. HHS concurred with GAO's recommendations.

---

* This is an edited, reformatted and augmented version of United States Government Accountability Office, Publication No. GAO-22-104457, dated November 2021.

In: COVID-19 Vaccines
Editor: John Schroder
ISBN: 979-8-88697-150-7

What GAO Found

In late 2020 and early 2021, agencies within the Department of Health and Human Services (HHS) set up federal programs for vaccine distribution and administration. State and local health officials and other stakeholders GAO interviewed said these programs helped higher-risk populations access COVID-19 vaccination. For example, the Health Resources and Services Administration's (HRSA) health center program provided vaccinations in medically underserved areas. However, these stakeholders also cited challenges, such as initially having limited or no information on the doses federal programs were sending to pharmacies and health centers in their communities. They said this made it difficult to decide which sites, including pharmacies and health centers, to send their own allocated doses when supply was limited.

Stakeholders told GAO the Centers for Disease Control and Prevention's (CDC) education materials, such as provider toolkits, were useful to address the public's concerns about the safety of COVID-19 vaccines, but providers would have liked them sooner to be able start promoting vaccination earlier. These stakeholders, including health officials, said they had difficulty managing public expectations and responding to questions about vaccine availability when they did not receive advance notice about changes in federal priority groups for vaccination.

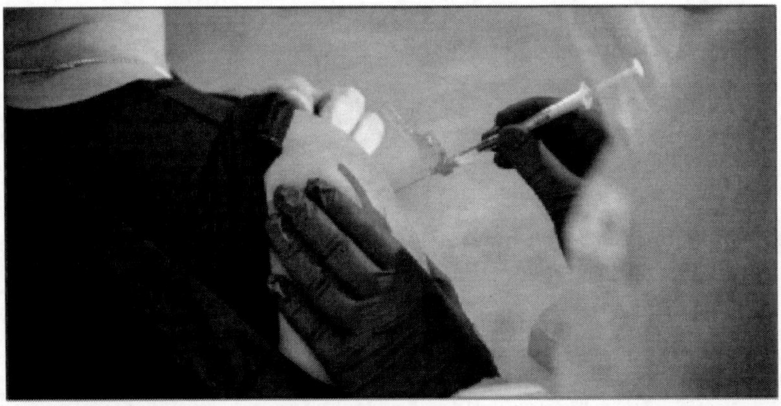

Source: Defense Visual Information Distribution Service. | GAO-22-104457.

Individual Being Vaccinated as Part of a Federal Program.

Officials from HHS agencies—CDC and HRSA—stated they intend to conduct after action reviews to identify lessons learned from their COVID-19 vaccine distribution and communication efforts. However, officials said they have not finalized their plans for conducting such reviews, nor do they plan to do so while they continue to respond to the pandemic and have ongoing programs. Thus, it is uncertain whether they will gather input, including on an ongoing basis, from key stakeholders instrumental in vaccine distribution and communication efforts, such as state and local health officials, or whether the results will be shared with those stakeholders. Doing so will help ensure CDC and HRSA learn what worked well and identify areas for improvement to inform future vaccination efforts.

Abbreviations

ACIP	Advisory Committee on Immunization Practices
CDC	Centers for Disease Control and Prevention
COVID-19	Coronavirus Disease 2019
DOD	Department of Defense
EUA	emergency use authorization
FDA	Food and Drug Administration
FEMA	Federal Emergency Management Agency
health center vaccine program	Health Center COVID-19 Vaccine Program
HHS	Department of Health and Human Services
HRSA	Health Resources and Services Administration
LTC pharmacy program	Pharmacy Partnership for Long-Term Care Program
retail pharmacy program	Federal Retail Pharmacy Program for COVID-19 Vaccination
vaccination center pilot program	Community Vaccination Center Pilot Site and Mobile Vaccination Program
VAMS	Vaccine Administration Management System

November 4, 2021
Congressional Committees:

More than a year and a half after the United States declared the Coronavirus Disease 2019 (COVID-19) pandemic a public health emergency, the nation continues to grapple with and respond to the pandemic. After an overall decline in the numbers of COVID-19 cases, hospitalizations, and deaths from their peaks in early 2021, cases began to surge again in the summer of 2021 as a new variant of the virus emerged.[1] Hospitalization and deaths attributed to COVID-19 also increased, primarily among those unvaccinated, according to federal health officials.[2] Increasing COVID-19 vaccination coverage among the public remains a critical priority for the federal government. As of October 8, 2021, about 66 percent of the U.S. population aged 12 years and older (about 187 million individuals) had been fully vaccinated, according to data from the Centers for Disease Control and Prevention (CDC).[3]

---

[1] According to the Centers for Disease Control and Prevention (CDC), viruses, such as COVID-19, constantly change through mutation, and new variants are expected to occur. Sometimes new variants emerge and disappear, while at other times, new variants persist. The Delta variant (which, as of this report, is the dominant strain) spreads much faster than previous variants and may cause more severe cases of illness than other variants.

[2] For example, one study published by CDC showed new COVID-19 hospitalization rates in New York between May and July 2021 were considerably higher among unvaccinated adults than fully vaccinated adults. See Department of Health and Human Services, Centers for Disease Control and Prevention, "New COVID-19 Cases and Hospitalizations among Adults by Vaccination Status—New York, May 3–July 25, 2021," *Morbidity and Mortality Weekly Report*, vol. 70, no. 34 (Atlanta, Ga.: Aug. 27, 2021).

[3] As of October 22, 2021, three COVID-19 vaccines were available in the United States but none of them was available for children under 12 years. Two of the three COVID-19 vaccines available for use were two-dose vaccine regimens and the third one was a single-dose vaccine. According to CDC, the count of fully vaccinated individuals

COVID-19 vaccine implementation—which includes prioritizing, allocating, distributing, and administering vaccine doses—is a highly complex undertaking, requiring coordination among multiple federal agencies, the private sector, jurisdictions, tribal officials, and health care providers.[4] At the federal level, the Department of Health and Human Services (HHS), along with its component agencies, has been a key department responsible for vaccine implementation efforts. For example, HHS, in partnership with the Department of Defense (DOD), has supported the development, manufacturing, allocation, and distribution of COVID-19 vaccine doses to states and other jurisdictions and to other federal vaccine distribution programs.

Since June 2020, we have cited the critical importance of planning for the development, manufacturing, distribution, and administration of COVID-19 vaccines.[5] In September 2020, we recommended that the Secretary of Health and Human Services, with support from the Secretary of Defense, develop a national plan for distributing and administering COVID-19 vaccines that outlines an approach for how efforts would be coordinated across federal agencies and nonfederal entities.[6] CDC issued initial planning documents in September and October 2020, and in January 2021, the White House issued a national COVID-19 response strategy that broadly outlined various programs for vaccine distribution. These documents contain general information on federally supported vaccine distribution activities, but do not provide details related to how the federal government is coordinating its efforts or information on the specific roles of the federal agencies and non-federal entities.

When COVID-19 vaccination began in December 2020, the federal government provided the majority of the limited supply of vaccine doses to the 50 states and other jurisdictions to further distribute to health care providers located in their jurisdictions. In December 2020, the federal government also began a vaccine distribution program targeting residents and staff in long-term care facilities. Then, in February 2021, it began three additional vaccine distribution programs focused on providing COVID-19 vaccine doses to pharmacies, federally supported health centers, and mass vaccination sites for administration.

For COVID-19, CDC has played a key role in informing health care providers and the public about COVID-19 vaccination. A key component of any successful vaccination effort is timely, clear, and consistent communication to stakeholders like state, territorial, and local health officials and health care providers, as well as to the public about vaccine availability, effectiveness, and safety. Communication that is responsive to the public's questions and concerns can help increase public confidence and trust in vaccines and in vaccination.

Additionally, in our 2011 review of the federal response to the H1N1 influenza pandemic, we raised the importance of capturing lessons learned from the federal government's response. We reported on the importance of identifying response actions that worked well and those that could be improved, so the nation could be better prepared when the next pandemic occurred.[7]

---

represents the number of people who have received the second dose of a two-dose COVID-19 vaccine regimen and those who received one dose of the single-dose COVID-19 vaccine.

[4] Jurisdictions include all 50 states, the District of Columbia, eight U.S. territories, and a small number of major cities.

[5] GAO, *COVID-19: Opportunities to Improve Federal Response and Recovery Efforts*, GAO-20-625 (Washington, D.C.: June 25, 2020).

[6] The Secretary neither agreed nor disagreed with our recommendation. See GAO, *COVID-19: Federal Efforts Could Be Strengthened by Timely and Concerted Actions*, GAO-20-701 (Washington, D.C.: Sept. 21, 2020).

[7] GAO, *Influenza Pandemic: Lessons from the H1N1 Pandemic Should Be Incorporated into Future Planning*, GAO-11-632 (Washington, D.C.: June 27, 2011).

The CARES Act includes a provision for GAO to report on its ongoing monitoring and oversight efforts related to the COVID-19 pandemic.[8] This report is part of our body of work in response to the CARES Act and focuses on the federal government's efforts related to the distribution and administration of and communication about COVID-19 vaccines.[9] In this chapter, we

1. describe state and local health officials' and other stakeholders' perspectives on federal efforts to distribute and administer COVID-19 vaccines, including four federal vaccine distribution programs;
2. describe state and local health officials' and other stakeholders' perspectives on federal efforts, including CDC's efforts, to inform health officials, health care providers, and the public about COVID-19 vaccination; and
3. examine actions HHS agencies are taking to evaluate their efforts to distribute and administer COVID-19 vaccines and to communicate about COVID-19 vaccination.

To address the first objective, we reviewed information from and interviewed selected state and local health officials and other stakeholders about federal efforts to distribute and administer COVID-19 vaccines, generally covering the period of December 2020 through May 2021. We focused our review on the four federal vaccine distribution programs that together distributed the most vaccine doses to the public, outside of vaccine doses distributed through states and other jurisdictions. These four programs included

- CDC's Pharmacy Partnership for Long-Term Care Program (LTC pharmacy program),
- CDC's Federal Retail Pharmacy Program for COVID-19 Vaccination (retail pharmacy program),
- the Health Resources and Services Administration's (HRSA) Health Center COVID-19 Vaccine Program (health center vaccine program),[10] and
- the Federal Emergency Management Agency's (FEMA) Community Vaccination Center Pilot Site and Mobile Vaccination Program (vaccination center pilot program).[11]

We also obtained stakeholder perspectives on federal efforts to support the administration of COVID-19 vaccines, including the use of DOD and National Guard personnel, and additional categories of individuals qualified to administer vaccines with liability protections, such as dentists and veterinarians. The selected state and local health officials and other

---

[8] Pub. L. No. 116-136, § 19010, 134 Stat. 281, 579-81 (2020).

[9] We have regularly issued government-wide reports on the federal response to COVID-19. For the latest report, see GAO, *COVID-19: Additional Actions Needed to Improve Accountability and Program Effectiveness of Federal Response,* GAO-22-105051 (Washington, D.C.: Oct. 27, 2021). Our next government-wide report will be issued in January 2022 and will be available on GAO's website at https://www.gao.gov/coronavirus. Also, see the GAO Related Products section at the end of this report for additional work we have done on COVID-19 vaccines.

[10] CDC coordinated with HRSA on the health center vaccine program, but for the purposes of this report, we refer to this program as a HRSA-operated vaccine distribution program since HRSA was the primary agency responsible for implementing the program.

[11] CDC coordinated with FEMA on the vaccination center pilot program, but for the purposes of this report, we refer to this program as a FEMA-operated vaccine distribution program since FEMA was the primary agency responsible for implementing the program.

stakeholders we spoke to are described below; the perspectives of these officials and other stakeholders are not generalizable but provided valuable insight on these issues.

- *Selected state and local health officials.* We reviewed information from and interviewed or obtained written responses from health officials from five selected jurisdictions—four states (Connecticut, Georgia, Minnesota, and Washington) and one city (Philadelphia).[12] Within each of the four states, we also interviewed health officials from one local health department that had one or more vaccination site receiving vaccine doses through one of the four federal vaccine distribution programs we examined. We conducted these interviews between late March and early May 2021.
- *Other stakeholders.* Within each of the four selected states noted above, we also interviewed representatives from the state's medical association and hospital association to obtain the perspectives of health care providers. In addition, we reviewed information from and interviewed or obtained written responses from representatives from 12 national associations who represented different stakeholder groups, including state and local health officials, tribal health organizations, health care providers involved in vaccine administration, and others.[13] We conducted these interviews between April and May 2021.

To address the second objective, we obtained information from CDC's website and from written responses on the agency's efforts to inform health officials, health care providers, and the public about COVID-19 vaccination, generally covering the period of November 2020 to August 2021. We also conducted interviews with the selected state and local health officials and other stakeholders described above to get their perspectives on CDC's efforts and about recommendations from CDC's Advisory Committee on Immunization Practices (ACIP) on which groups to initially prioritize and target when vaccine supply was limited.[14]

For both the first and second objectives, we also reviewed documentation from and interviewed officials from federal agencies involved in federal COVID-19 vaccine distribution, administration, or communication efforts. These agencies included CDC, FEMA, HRSA, and the HHS-DOD partnership tasked with supporting COVID-19 vaccine development, manufacturing, and distribution to states and other jurisdictions and selected federal entities.[15]

To address the third objective, we interviewed officials from HHS, including CDC and HRSA, and reviewed written responses from CDC and HRSA about their plans for conducting and sharing the results of after action reviews of federal COVID-19 vaccine implementation efforts. We compared CDC's and HRSA's plans for after action reviews to federal internal

---

[12] We selected jurisdictions to reflect variation in geographic location and the degree to which state public health infrastructures were centralized or decentralized. We also selected one major city that received vaccine allocations directly from the federal government and is considered a jurisdiction.

[13] We interviewed officials or obtained written responses from: American Hospital Association, American Medical Association, Association of Immunization Managers, Association of State and Territorial Health Officials, National Association of Community Health Centers, National Association of Chain Drug Stores, National Association of County and City Health Officials, National Community Pharmacists Association, National Council of Urban Indian Health, National Governors Association, National Indian Health Board, and National Rural Health Association.

[14] ACIP is comprised of medical and public health experts who make recommendations on the use of vaccines in the civilian population of the United States.

[15] This partnership was initially known as Operation Warp Speed, but since May 2021, is named the HHS-DOD COVID-19 Countermeasures Acceleration Group.

control standards regarding information and communication, and the underlying principle that management should externally communicate the necessary quality information to achieve the entity's objectives.[16] We also compared the agencies' plans with the Project Management Institute's program management standards, which similarly call for program managers to engage with key stakeholders.[17] Finally, we compared the agencies' plans to prior GAO work on lessons learned from and after action reports on the federal response to prior emergencies, including the 2009 H1N1 pandemic.[18]

Finally, we analyzed data from CDC's COVID-19 Data Tracker on the number of COVID-19 vaccine doses delivered, by distribution channel, as of August 19, 2021, and on doses administered and new cases of COVID-19 (the 7-day average of the new cases each day) as of October 8, 2021. We interviewed agency officials about the data on vaccine doses distributed and administered, and reviewed available documentation on these sources and on COVID-19 case rate data. We determined these data were sufficiently reliable for the purpose of providing context on COVID-19 vaccinations.

We conducted this performance audit from July 2020 to November 2021 in accordance with generally accepted government auditing standards. Those standards require that we plan and perform the audit to obtain sufficient, appropriate evidence to provide a reasonable basis for our findings and conclusions based on our audit objectives. We believe that the evidence obtained provides a reasonable basis for our findings and conclusions based on our audit objectives.

Background

As of October 22, 2021, three COVID-19 vaccines were available in the United States. One vaccine was licensed by the Food and Drug Administration (FDA) for individuals aged 16 years and older and was also available for individuals aged 12 to 15 years under an emergency use authorization (EUA), which allows for the temporary use of vaccines without FDA licensure, provided certain statutory criteria are met.[19] Two additional vaccines were authorized for

---

[16] GAO, *Standards for Internal Control in the Federal Government*, GAO-14-704G (Washington, D.C.: Sept. 10, 2014).

[17] Project Management Institute, Inc., *The Standard for Program Management, Fourth Edition, 2017*.

[18] GAO, *Disaster Response: HHS Should Address Deficiencies Highlighted by Recent Hurricanes in the U.S. Virgin Islands and Puerto Rico*, GAO-19-592 (Washington, D.C.: Sept. 20, 2019) and GAO-11-632.

[19] Typically, FDA must license a vaccine before it can be marketed in the United States. See 42 U.S.C. § 262. On August 23, 2021, FDA licensed the COVID-19 vaccine developed by Pfizer and BioNTech (marketed as Comirnaty) for the prevention of COVID-19 disease. For the purposes of this report, we refer to the COVID-19 vaccine that Pfizer and BioNTech developed together as the Pfizer vaccine.

The Secretary of Health and Human Services may declare that circumstances, prescribed by statute, exist justifying the emergency use of certain medical products, such as vaccines. Once a declaration of an emergency has been made, FDA may temporarily allow use of unlicensed vaccines through an EUA. For FDA to issue an EUA for a vaccine, it must be reasonable to believe that the vaccine may be effective and that the known and potential benefits of the vaccine outweigh the known and potential risks, among other statutory criteria. See 21 U.S.C. § 360bbb-3. FDA has indicated that issuance of an EUA for a COVID-19 vaccine for which there is adequate manufacturing information would require a determination by FDA that the vaccine's benefits outweigh its risks based on data from at least one well-designed phase 3 clinical trial that demonstrates the vaccine's safety and efficacy in a clear and compelling manner.

Any COVID-19 vaccine that initially receives an EUA from FDA is expected to work toward submission of a biologics license application, according to FDA guidance. See Department of Health and Human Services, Food

emergency use for individuals aged 18 years and older.[20] (See app. I for more information on COVID-19 vaccines available in the United States.) As of October 22, 2021, no vaccines had been authorized or licensed for children under 12 years, but one vaccine company (Pfizer) had requested that FDA authorize its COVID-19 vaccine for children aged 5 years to 11 years.[21]

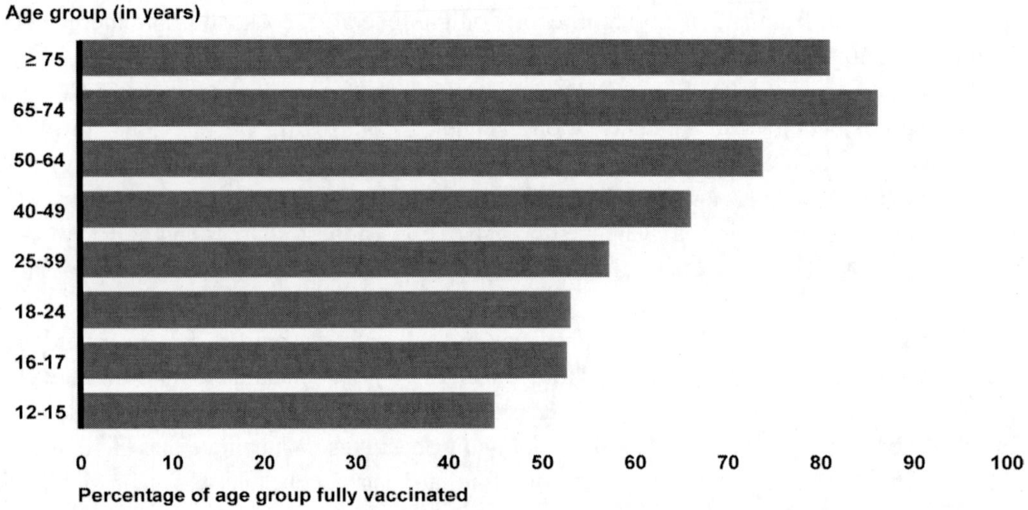

Source: GAO analysis of Centers for Disease Control and Prevention (CDC) data. | GAO-22-104457.

Notes: The figure does not include data for Texas or for individuals under age 18 years from Idaho, due to limitations in these states' reporting of demographic data to CDC. As of October 8, 2021, three COVID-19 vaccines were available in the United States. One vaccine was authorized for emergency use in individuals aged 12 years to 15 years on May 10, 2021, and was licensed for individuals aged 16 years and older. The two remaining vaccines were authorized for emergency use for individuals aged 18 years and older. As of October 8, 2021, there were no vaccines authorized or licensed for children under 12 years. In this figure, fully vaccinated refers to those individuals who have received the second dose in a two-dose COVID-19 vaccine regimen and those who received one dose of the single-dose COVID-19 vaccine.

Figure 1. Percentage of Those Fully Vaccinated in the United States, by Age Group, as of October 8, 2021.

---

and Drug Administration, *Emergency Use Authorization for Vaccines to Prevent COVID-19: Guidance for Industry*, (Silver Spring, Md.: May 2021).

[20] On June 10, 2021, one vaccine company, Moderna, requested FDA amend the EUA for its COVID-19 vaccine for use in adolescents aged 12 years to 17 years; as of October 22, 2021, FDA had not issued a decision in response. The other authorized COVID-19 vaccine was by Janssen Pharmaceutical Companies, which is part of Johnson & Johnson.

Additional or booster doses have also been authorized and recommended for fully vaccinated individuals. In August 2021, FDA authorized, and CDC recommended, the use of an additional dose of the Pfizer and Moderna COVID-19 vaccines in certain immunocompromised individuals. In September and October 2021, FDA authorized and CDC recommended that certain populations receive a booster dose of either the Pfizer, Moderna, or Janssen vaccine. In October 2021, FDA also authorized "mix and match" for the booster dose—that is, authorizing the use any available COVID-19 vaccine for use as a booster dose regardless of which COVID-19 vaccine was used as the primary series or single-dose primary series. According to CDC, an additional dose is administered when the initial immune response following a primary vaccine series is likely to be insufficient and a booster dose is administered when the initial sufficient immune response to a primary vaccine series is likely to have waned over time.

[21] As of October 22, 2021, FDA's Vaccines and Related Biological Products Advisory Committee was scheduled to meet on October 26, 2021, to discuss a request for authorization of Pfizer's COVID-19 vaccine for children aged 5 through 11 years.

As of October 8, 2021, about 66 percent of the U.S. population eligible for vaccination (i.e., those aged 12 years and older) was fully vaccinated— that is, they had received the second dose of a two-dose COVID-19 vaccine or had received the single-dose COVID-19 vaccine— but vaccination rates varied among different population groups. For example, more than 80 percent of those aged 65 years and older were fully vaccinated, compared with less than 60 percent of individuals under 40 years of age, according to CDC data. (See Figure 1).

Over time, as the number of COVID-19 vaccine doses administered increased, COVID-19 case rates fell steadily through mid-June 2021. (See Figure 2). In late June, however, the average number of cases per day began to increase as the more transmissible Delta variant was circulating. After September 2021, the average number of cases per day generally declined; as of October 8, 2021, the average number of cases per day was 93,437.

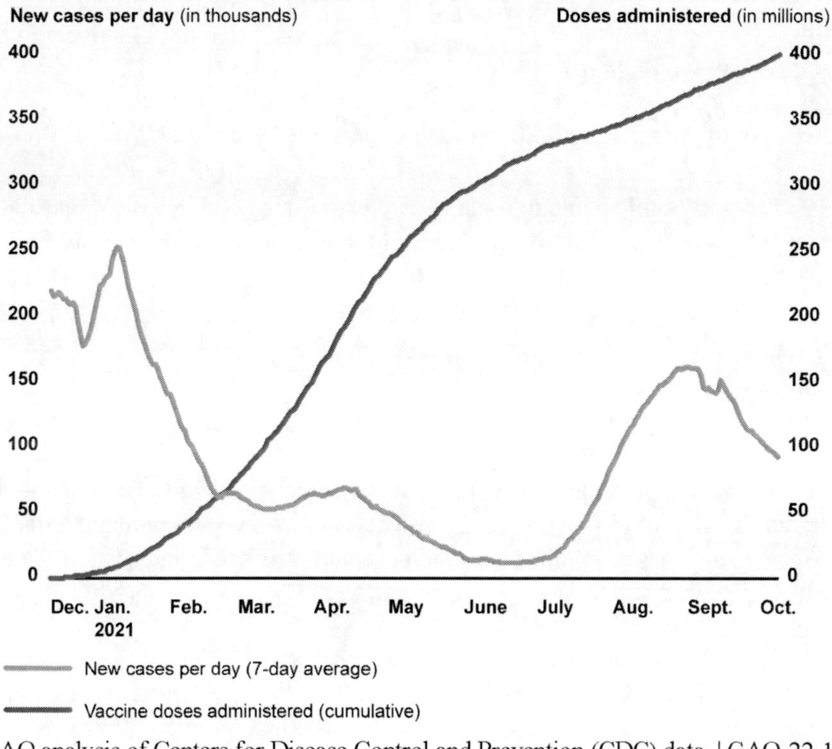

Source: GAO analysis of Centers for Disease Control and Prevention (CDC) data. | GAO-22-104457.

Notes: Data begin on December 14, 2020, when the first dose of COVID-19 vaccine was administered in the United States. Data on the number of COVID-19 vaccine doses administered reflect the cumulative number of doses administered as reported to CDC by state, local, and territorial immunization information systems and other sources. Data on COVID-19 case rates reflect the 7-day moving average for the number of new cases reported per day and are based on aggregate case reporting to CDC on probable and confirmed cases by states and jurisdictions. According to CDC, the actual number of COVID-19 cases is unknown for a variety of reasons, including that people who have been infected may not have been tested, or may not have sought medical care.

Figure 2. Number of COVID-19 Vaccine Doses Administered and Reported COVID-19 Cases per Day in the United States, December 14, 2020 to October 8, 2021.

The pace of COVID-19 vaccinations in the United States has fluctuated over time. In the first 4 months after vaccination began, as vaccine supply increased, the average number of doses administered daily climbed steadily, peaking in April 2021. In the following months, the average number of doses administered daily declined steeply and then in July 2021, began to increase once more, after COVID-19 cases had begun to surge again. As of October 8, 2021, about 34 percent of the U.S. population aged 12 years and older was not fully vaccinated.

Those unvaccinated may include people who desire to be vaccinated but face access barriers, such as lacking transportation to a vaccination site or not having the ability to take time off from work to get vaccinated.

Others may be uncertain or reluctant to be vaccinated (sometimes referred to as vaccine hesitancy) for different reasons, such as having concerns about the safety of COVID-19 vaccines or believing vaccination is unnecessary because COVID-19 is not a serious threat to their health.[22]

Federal Efforts to Allocate and Distribute COVID-19 Vaccines

COVID-19 vaccine implementation—that is, prioritizing, allocating, distributing, and administering vaccine doses—has been a key component in mitigating the disease's effect on the public's health, societal functioning, and the economy. (See text box below.) The federal government began distributing COVID-19 vaccine doses on December 12, 2020, and 2 days later, the first dose of vaccine was administered.[23]

COVID-19 vaccine implementation

COVID-19 vaccine implementation includes the prioritization, allocation, distribution, and administration of vaccine doses and relies on communication and coordination between the federal government and stakeholders, including states and other jurisdictions, local health departments, the private sector, and health care providers.

Prioritization refers to the identification of groups prioritized for vaccination when vaccine supply is limited. Within priority groups are separate target groups, which are added as vaccine supply increases. CDC's Advisory Committee on Immunization Practices issued its recommendations for priority groups and target groups for COVID-19 vaccination in December 2020.

Allocation refers to the number of vaccine doses the federal government made available through different vaccine distribution programs, such as to states and other jurisdictions. States and other jurisdictions used part of their allocations of vaccine doses from the federal government

---

[22] While different models exist for categorizing attitudes toward vaccination, a common conception is that these attitudes run along a continuum that ranges from full acceptance of vaccines on one end to full opposition to vaccines on the other. The term "vaccine hesitancy" has been used to refer to a delay in acceptance of vaccines, including the COVID-19 vaccine, despite the availability of vaccination services. An individual's level of vaccine hesitancy can vary by vaccine and over time. See National Academies of Sciences, Engineering, and Medicine, *The Critical Public Health Value of Vaccines: Tackling Issues of Access and Hesitancy: Proceedings of a Workshop* (Washington, D.C.: 2021).

[23] See app. II for a timeline of these efforts and other key events related to COVID-19 vaccine implementation.

for CDC's Pharmacy Partnership for Long-Term Care Program; the other doses were directed to health care providers within their jurisdictions. In contrast, three additional federal vaccine distribution programs—(1) CDC's Federal Retail Pharmacy Program for COVID-19 Vaccination, (2) the Health Resources and Services Administration's (HRSA) Health Center COVID-19 Vaccine Program, and (3) the Federal Emergency Management Agency's (FEMA) Community Vaccination Center Pilot Site and Mobile Vaccination Program—were implemented as separate distribution programs, and each program received a direct allocation of vaccine doses from the federal government.

Distribution refers to the delivery of COVID-19 vaccine doses to health care providers, as directed by states and other jurisdictions; federal entities, such as FEMA and HRSA; and other entities that have partnered with the federal government, such as pharmacies.

Administration refers to the administering of COVID-19 vaccine doses at various sites, including long-term care facilities, pharmacies, health centers, mass vaccination sites, and physician offices, by authorized health care providers.

Source: GAO summary of information from the Centers for Disease Control and Prevention (CDC), the Department of Health and Human Services, and the Department of Defense. | GAO-22-104457.

When COVID-19 vaccine implementation began in December 2020, the federal government allocated and distributed nearly all available vaccine doses to the 50 states and other jurisdictions.[24] Jurisdictions then decided how to further distribute their allocated vaccine doses to authorized health care providers within their boundaries, including to pharmacies, health centers, local health departments, mass vaccination sites, hospitals, physician offices, and others.[25] Initially, the vaccine supply was limited and not all health care providers that wanted to administer COVID-19 vaccines received doses, and people who wanted to be vaccinated experienced challenges doing so, according to multiple stakeholders. We previously reported that state, territorial, and local health officials and health care providers experienced multiple challenges when distribution of COVID-19 vaccines first began in mid-December 2020.[26] For example, health officials and health care providers said they lacked information on vaccine shipments, such as the number of doses being delivered, which was needed to assist their on-the-ground planning for vaccine administration.

---

[24] In December 2020, the federal government began providing allocations of COVID-19 vaccine doses to 62 jurisdictions, including all 50 states, the District of Columbia, three major cities (Chicago, New York City, and Philadelphia), and eight territories (American Samoa, the Federated States of Micronesia, Guam, the Marshall Islands, the Northern Mariana Islands, Palau, Puerto Rico, and the U.S. Virgin Islands), generally on a weekly basis. A jurisdiction could then order vaccine doses from the federal government to be distributed to authorized health care providers for administration, up to the allocated number of doses (order cap). Although there are 64 jurisdictions implementing COVID-19 vaccination and receiving federal funding for these efforts, allocations of vaccine doses were made to 62 jurisdictions because two major cities considered jurisdictions—Houston and San Antonio—had their allocations consolidated with Texas. On June 24, 2021, the federal government stopped allocating COVID-19 vaccine doses to jurisdictions and federal vaccine distribution programs because vaccine supply had increased to sufficient levels to meet the needs of jurisdictions and other federal programs, according to federal officials.

[25] As of October 22, 2021, all COVID-19 vaccines in the United States have been purchased by the U.S. Government for administration exclusively by authorized health care providers enrolled in CDC's COVID-19 Vaccination Program. Only health care providers enrolled as vaccination providers can legally store, handle, and administer COVID-19 vaccines in the United States.

[26] GAO, *COVID-19: Efforts to Increase Vaccine Availability and Perspectives on Initial Implementation*, GAO-21-443 (Washington, D.C., Apr. 14, 2021).

In December 2020, the federal government initiated CDC's LTC pharmacy program. Under this program, CDC worked with selected pharmacy partners to vaccinate residents and staff at participating nursing homes and other long-term care facilities.[27] To implement this program, pharmacies used vaccine doses from states' and other jurisdictions' allocations to conduct three on-site vaccination clinics at each participating facility.

In February 2021, as the vaccine supply began increasing, the federal government implemented three additional vaccine distribution programs.[28] These three federal programs were outlined in the White House's national strategy for the COVID-19 response and received their own allocations of vaccine doses from the federal government.[29] According to federal officials, the number of vaccine doses the federal government allocated to CDC's retail pharmacy program, HRSA's health center vaccine program, and FEMA's vaccination center pilot program were determined by the White House COVID-19 Response Team.[30] The programs were

- *CDC's retail pharmacy program,* which distributed vaccine doses directly to national pharmacy partners and independent pharmacy networks,
- *HRSA's health center vaccine program,* which distributed vaccine doses to federally supported health centers,[31] and
- *FEMA's vaccination center pilot program,* which distributed vaccine doses to federally operated community vaccination centers and to mobile vaccination units.[32]

---

[27] For the LTC pharmacy program, CDC worked with CVS, Walgreens, and Managed Health Care Associates, Inc., as pharmacy partners.

[28] In addition to allocations of vaccine doses made to states and other jurisdictions and these three federal programs, the federal government allocated and distributed vaccine doses to five federal entities (the Bureau of Prisons, DOD, Department of State, Indian Health Service, and the Veterans Health Administration). The federal government also allocated vaccine doses to HHS/National Institutes of Health for a small program managing doses allocated to federal departments and agencies for administration to critical infrastructure personnel and made a one-time allocation of 751,140 vaccine doses to the Federal Dialysis Center Program to distribute to participating dialysis centers to administer vaccines to patients and health care personnel.

[29] The *National Strategy for the COVID-19 Response and Pandemic Preparedness* includes a goal of mounting a safe, effective, and comprehensive vaccination campaign. See White House, *National Strategy for the COVID-19 Response and Pandemic Preparedness* (Washington, D.C.: Jan. 21, 2021). Earlier planning documents, including CDC's COVID-19 interim guidance for states and other jurisdictions, identified the LTC pharmacy partnership and outlined plans for direct partners such as retail pharmacy chains that would enroll directly with CDC to order and receive COVID-19 vaccines. See Department of Health and Human Services, Centers for Disease Control and Prevention, *COVID-19 Vaccination Program Interim Playbook for Jurisdiction Operations, version 2.0* (Atlanta, Ga: Oct. 29, 2020).

[30] Since January 2021, the White House COVID-19 Response Team has been responsible for coordinating across the federal government on the COVID-19 response, including COVID-19 vaccine implementation, and for communicating to the public, state, and local public health officials and other stakeholders about these efforts through regular public briefings.

[31] Federally supported health centers generally receive Health Center Program grants from HRSA under section 330 of the Public Health Service Act (42 U.S.C. § 254b) and provide primary care services in medically underserved communities. Some organizations meet all Health Center Program requirements but do not receive federal grant funding through the section 330 program. However, these centers, which are known as "look-alikes," receive other benefits, such as higher reimbursement rates from the Medicare and Medicaid programs and may receive grants through other federal programs. We use the term "federally supported health centers" to refer to both "look-alikes" and those health centers that receive grants under section 330 of the Public Health Service Act.

[32] On June 20, 2021, the last mass vaccination site under FEMA's vaccination center pilot program closed, according to federal officials. However, after that date, agency officials reported that they continued to support mobile vaccination units and community vaccination centers managed and operated by states and other jurisdictions (using doses allocated to the jurisdictions) by providing federal personnel, funding, and material, such as medical equipment and supplies.

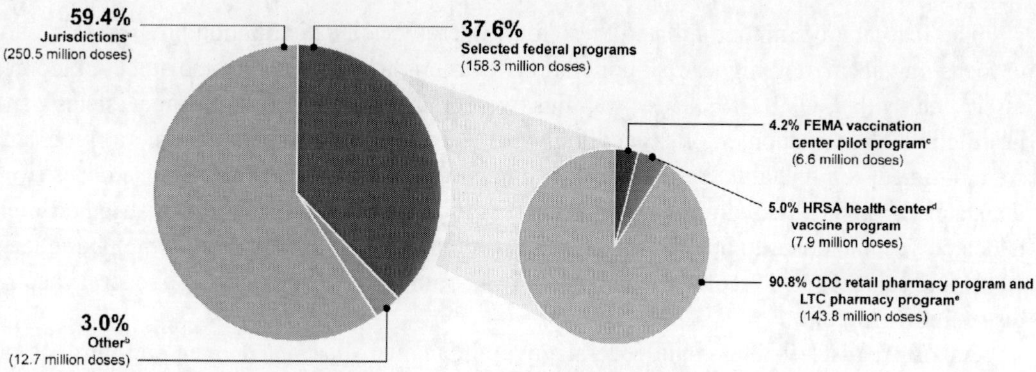

Source: GAO analysis of Centers for Disease Control and Prevention (CDC) data. | GAO-22-104457.

Notes: Figure shows cumulative number and percentage of COVID-19 vaccine doses distributed through four federal and other vaccine distribution programs from the time vaccine doses were first distributed in December 2020 to August 19, 2021.

[a]A total of 62 jurisdictions—including all 50 states, the District of Columbia, three major cities (Chicago, New York City, and Philadelphia), and eight territories (American Samoa, the Federated States of Micronesia, Guam, the Marshall Islands, the Northern Mariana Islands, Palau, Puerto Rico, and the U.S. Virgin Islands)—received allocations of COVID-19 vaccine doses, generally on a weekly basis. Although there are 64 jurisdictions implementing COVID-19 vaccination and receiving federal funding for these efforts, allocations of vaccine doses were made to 62 jurisdictions because two major cities considered jurisdictions—Houston and San Antonio—had their allocations consolidated with Texas.

[b]Other includes other federal vaccine distribution programs that received direct allocations from the federal government—(1) four federal entities (the Bureau of Prisons, Department of Defense, Indian Health Service, and the Veterans Health Administration); (2) Department of Health and Human Services/National Institutes of Health for a small program managing doses allocated to federal departments and agencies for administration to critical infrastructure personnel; and (3) a one-time allocation of vaccine doses to the Federal Dialysis Center Program to distribute to participating dialysis centers to administer vaccines to patients and health care personnel. Although the Department of State received allocations of vaccine doses from the federal government, data for this department are not included in CDC's data on distribution.

[c]CDC coordinated with the Federal Emergency Management Agency (FEMA) on the Community Vaccination Center Pilot Site and Mobile Vaccination Program (vaccination center pilot program); for the purposes of this chapter, we refer to this program as a FEMA-operated vaccine distribution program. On June 20, 2021, the last mass vaccination site under this program closed, according to agency officials.

[d]CDC coordinated with the Health Resources and Services Administration (HRSA) on the Health Center COVID-19 Vaccine Program (health center vaccine program); for the purposes of this chapter, we refer to this program as a HRSA-operated vaccine distribution program.

[e]The number of doses attributed to CDC's Federal Retail Pharmacy Program for COVID-19 Vaccination (retail pharmacy program) includes doses distributed through its Pharmacy Partnership for Long-Term Care Program (LTC pharmacy program). The LTC pharmacy program ended on April 23, 2021.

Figure 3. Percentage of COVID-19 Vaccine Doses Distributed through Four Federal Vaccine Distribution Programs Compared to the Percentage Distributed through Jurisdictions, as of August 19, 2021.

The federal government initiated these four federal vaccine distribution programs, in part, to focus on vaccinating higher-risk populations who might experience worse health outcomes associated with COVID-19. The programs were put in place to supplement states' and jurisdictions' vaccination efforts, according to federal officials. When the federal programs were initiated, some pharmacies and health centers were already receiving vaccine doses from the states or other jurisdictions in which they were located, as jurisdictions distributed their allocated vaccine doses to health care providers in their communities. Thus, some pharmacies and health centers could receive vaccine doses from both their jurisdiction and a federal vaccine distribution program.

As of August 19, 2021, the federal government had distributed over one-third of all COVID-19 vaccine doses through the four federal vaccine distribution programs, with most doses going to pharmacies (through CDC's LTC pharmacy program and its retail pharmacy program). (See Figure 3).

Although the federal government distributed the majority of vaccine doses through states and other jurisdictions when COVID-19 vaccine implementation began, this changed over time. For example, between April and July 2021, the proportion of vaccine doses distributed through states and other jurisdictions decreased from 62 percent in early April 2021, to 6 percent in mid-July 2021. During that same time, the proportion of vaccine doses distributed through CDC's retail pharmacy program increased from 29 percent to 92 percent, according to our analysis.[33]

CDC's Efforts to Inform Health Officials, Health Care Providers, and the Public about COVID-19 Vaccination

Before COVID-19 vaccine implementation began, CDC took steps to inform jurisdictional health officials, health care providers, and the public about COVID-19 vaccines. For example, CDC created its first COVID-19 Vaccine Toolkit in November 2020.[34] The agency created several other Toolkits targeted to various audiences, such as health care providers, health centers, pharmacies, and schools, which included materials for communicating about the potential and known benefits, safety, side effects, and effectiveness of COVID-19 vaccines. In addition, CDC partnered with the Ad Council to create public service announcements to encourage vaccination.[35] Providing information on safety and efficacy is important to help inform the public about COVID-19 vaccines and to address any concerns about vaccination.[36]

---

[33] Our analysis compared the proportion of vaccine doses CDC reported as distributed through the different federal vaccine distribution programs between April 1–18, 2021, and July 8–23, 2021. Our analysis began in April 2021, because this is when CDC began making data on COVID-19 vaccine doses distributed through the different federal vaccine distribution programs publicly available. Our analysis ended in July 2021, because these were the most recent data available at the time of our analysis.

[34] CDC also developed tools to help the public locate where COVID-19 vaccines were available and to schedule a vaccination appointment—VaccineFinder and the Vaccine Administration Management System (VAMS). See app. III for more information on these tools.

[35] The Ad Council is a nonprofit and nonpartisan organization that uses advertising, media, technology, and marketing to develop public service campaigns to raise awareness and to solve social issues on a national scale.

[36] For example, one survey conducted between March and May 2021 found that most people aged 18 to 39 years who responded that they probably or definitely would not get vaccinated said it was because they did not trust COVID-19 vaccines or were concerned about possible side effects. Brittney N. Baack et al., "COVID-19 Vaccination

CDC also provided guidance on which segments of the population should be prioritized for vaccination when initial vaccine supply was limited, when the agency adopted ACIP's recommendations. In December 2020, ACIP recommended that COVID-19 vaccines be allocated through a phased approach and identified broad priority groups that should be offered COVID-19 vaccines first while vaccine supply was limited.[37] ACIP recommendations generally serve as public guidance for safe use of vaccines and states and other jurisdictions may adopt different approaches.

State and Local Health Officials and Others Said Federal Programs Helped Higher-Risk Populations Gain Access to COVID-19 Vaccination, but Cited Coordination Challenges

Federal Programs Helped Higher-Risk Populations Gain Access to Vaccination, According to Selected Health Officials and Other Stakeholders

The four federal distribution programs helped higher-risk populations gain access to vaccinations and assisted with logistical aspects of administering COVID-19 vaccines, according to selected state and local health officials and other stakeholders we interviewed between late March and early May 2021. (See Figure 4 for descriptions of the four programs).

- *Helped higher-risk populations gain access to vaccinations.* The four federal vaccine programs did well in distributing vaccine doses to sites aimed at reaching populations at higher-risk for COVID-19, according to selected state and local health officials. For example,
  - CDC's LTC pharmacy program helped state health departments by facilitating the vaccination of higher-risk residents and staff of long-term care facilities, according to some state and local health officials. Some health officials said CDC's LTC pharmacy program made health care providers available to vaccinate residents and staff in long-term care facilities in their jurisdictions.[38] A few of these officials said vaccinating these higher-risk residents and staff would have otherwise been a large undertaking.
  - CDC's retail pharmacy program and FEMA's vaccination center pilot program used CDC's social vulnerability index, which measures the relative vulnerability of the populations in every Census tract. CDC's retail pharmacy program used this index when initially deciding which pharmacies to add, and FEMA's vaccination center pilot program used the index, in part, to select mass vaccination sites.[39]

Coverage and Intent among Adults Aged 18–39 Years—United States, March–May 2021," *Morbidity and Mortality Weekly Report*, vol. 70, no. 25 (2021).

[37] ACIP is comprised of medical and public health experts who make recommendations on the use of vaccines in the civilian population of the United States. To inform its policy options, the committee established a COVID-19 Vaccines Work Group in April 2020, comprised of experts in infectious diseases, vaccinology, vaccine safety, public health, and ethics. The Work Group has held numerous meetings to review data regarding vaccine candidates, COVID-19 surveillance, modeling of allocation scenarios, and vaccine implementation issues.

[38] More than 62,000 long-term care facilities participated in CDC's LTC pharmacy program, according to CDC.

[39] CDC's social vulnerability index further groups the 15 social factors into four related themes: socioeconomic status, household composition and disability, race and ethnicity and language, and housing type and transportation. Each

- Additionally, some stakeholders, including state and local health officials, noted that federally supported health centers—which provide primary care services in medically underserved areas— added vaccination access points for populations at higher risk for COVID-19 because they have limited access to care.
- HRSA's health center vaccine program and FEMA's vaccination center pilot program had flexibilities to provide more equitable access to vaccination sites. For example, HRSA's health center vaccine program was helpful because participating health centers in their area could schedule vaccination appointment times on weekends or evenings, according to health officials from one local health department. Officials from another local health department told us FEMA officials worked with them to extend operating hours to include early mornings, evenings, and Saturdays. These local health officials said the extended hours allowed them to administer up to 8,000 vaccinations a day at the FEMA site instead of the up to 6,000 vaccinations a day typically administered at this type of mass vaccination site.[40] (See Figure 5 for photos of FEMA mass vaccination sites.) Additionally, health officials from two states we interviewed told us they used FEMA's mobile vaccination units, which provided access to vaccinations by meeting individuals where they were located.

- *Assisted with logistical aspects of COVID-19 vaccinations.* Some of the federal programs supported COVID-19 vaccinations by helping jurisdictions with administrative and logistical aspects of administering vaccines, according to state and local health officials we interviewed. For example,
  - CDC's retail pharmacy program helped state health departments by allowing the federal government to enroll pharmacies as COVID-19 vaccine providers, selected state health officials told us.[41] For example, officials from one jurisdiction said CDC's retail pharmacy program enrolled as vaccine providers all 77 pharmacies located in the jurisdiction that belonged to one pharmacy partner. Thus, officials from most state health departments we interviewed said they did not have to enroll those pharmacies as individual vaccine providers, easing an administrative burden on state health departments.
  - DOD and National Guard personnel provided critical assistance and efficient administration of vaccines for FEMA's vaccination center pilot program, according to selected state health officials and other stakeholders. For example, such personnel provided traffic control and security, and helped to set up mass vaccination sites, including for FEMA's vaccination center pilot program. (See Figure 6.) Because mass vaccination sites require a large number of staff to

---

Census tract receives a ranking for each Census variable and for each of the four themes as well as an overall ranking. Census tracts are subdivisions of counties for which the Census collects statistical data.

40 Under FEMA's vaccination center pilot program, vaccination centers were available in five different types, generally depending on the approximate number of vaccinations that could be administered each day. These included type 1 (approximately 6,000 vaccinations per day), type 2 (approximately 3,000 vaccinations per day), type 3 (approximately 1,000 vaccinations per day), type 4 (approximately 250 vaccinations per day), and type 5 (approximately 250 vaccinations per day via mobile clinic).

41 Health care providers who want to administer COVID-19 vaccines have to enroll either through their jurisdictional immunization program (as part of CDC's COVID-19 Vaccination Program) or through the federal program in which they are participating. To enroll in these programs, providers have to, among other things, sign the respective program's provider agreement.

operate, the availability of DOD and National Guard personnel was critical to their operation, according to two state health officials. According to DOD, at the highest point of support by DOD active-duty personnel in the week of April 23–30, 2021, 4,731 active-duty personnel were supporting vaccination sites in over 25 states and territories. DOD reported that by June 22, 2021, active-duty personnel had administered about 5 million vaccinations.

Federal program	Description
CDC's LTC pharmacy program 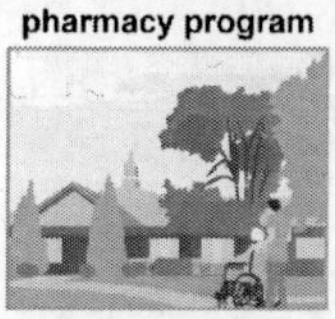	**Vaccination site:** Long-term care facilities **Description:** CDC partnered with selected pharmacy partners to conduct three vaccination clinics at each site 62,243 participating long-term care facilities, using vaccine doses the federal government directly allocated to states and other jurisdictions.[a] **Target population:** Residents and staff at long-term care facilities. **Dates active:** December 2020 – April 2021 **Number of vaccine doses administered by program end:** 8.1 million
CDC's retail pharmacy program 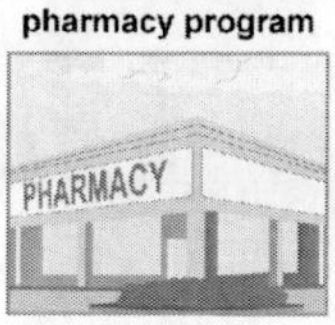	**Vaccination site:** Pharmacies **Description:** CDC partnered with 21 national pharmacy and independent pharmacy networks to distribute vaccine doses to 39,473 pharmacies, using vaccine doses directly allocated from the federal government. **Target population:** Initial pharmacy partners were selected based on several factors, including the number of stores and the ability to reach populations at risk of severe illness (e.g., elderly, socially vulnerable communities).[b] **Dates active:** February 2021 – Ongoing **Number of vaccine doses administered as of October 6, 2021:** about 133 million
HRSA's health center vaccine program 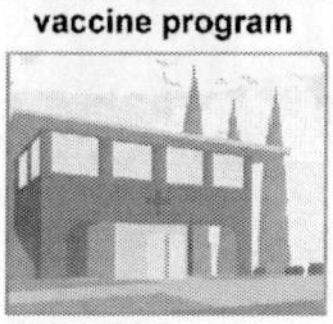	**Vaccination site:** Federally supported health centers **Description:** HRSA distributed vaccine doses to 866 participating health centers for 2,362 sites, as of September 15, 2021, using vaccine doses directly allocated from the federal government. Participating health centers could use mobile vans or help pop-up clinics or school-based clinics to administer vaccines at community-based events. **Target population:** Initial health centers were selected based on their service to disproportionately affected populations, such as migrant and seasonal agricultural workers. All federally supported health centers serve patients in medically underserved communities.[c] **Dates active:** February 2021 – Ongoing **Number of vaccine doses administered as of September 15, 2021:** 6.4 million
FEMA's vaccination center pilot program 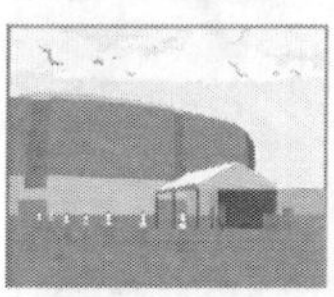	**Vaccination site:** Pilot community vaccination centers, including mass vaccination sites[d] **Description:** FEMA partnered with states to support 39 pilot community vaccination centers and 225 satellite sites across 27 states, using vaccine doses directly allocated from the federal government. These pilot community vaccination centers were managed and operated by FEMA personnel. The satellite sites brought vaccine doses to the community through mobile sites or pop-up clinics. **Target population:** Sites were selected to reach socially vulnerable communities. **Dates active:** February 2021 – June 2021 **Number of vaccine doses administered by program end:** 5.6 million

Source: GAO analysis of data and information from the Centers for Disease Control and Prevention (CDC), the Health Resources and Services Administration (HRSA), and the Federal Emergency Management Agency (FEMA). | GAO-22-104457.

Notes: This figure provides information on four federal vaccine distribution programs: (1) CDC's Pharmacy Partnership for Long-Term Care Program (LTC pharmacy program), (2) CDC's Federal Retail Pharmacy Program for COVID-19 Vaccination (retail pharmacy program), (3) HRSA's Health Center COVID-19 Vaccine Program (health center vaccine program), and (4) FEMA's Community Vaccination Center Pilot Site and Mobile Vaccination Program (vaccination center pilot program).

CDC coordinated with HRSA on the health center vaccine program and with FEMA on the vaccination center pilot program, but for the purposes of this chapter, we refer to these programs as HRSA- and FEMA-operated vaccine distribution programs since these agencies were the primary agencies responsible for implementing these programs.

Figure 4. (Continued)

In addition, the federal government allocated and distributed vaccine doses to five federal entities (the Bureau of Prisons, Department of Defense, Department of State, Indian Health Service, and the Veterans Health Administration). The federal government also allocated vaccine doses to the Department of Health and Human Services/National Institutes of Health for a small program managing doses allocated to federal departments and agencies for administration to critical infrastructure personnel and made a one-time allocation of vaccine doses to the Federal Dialysis Center Program to distribute to participating dialysis centers to administer vaccines to patients and health care personnel.

[a]A total of 62 jurisdictions—including all 50 states, the District of Columbia, three major cities (Chicago, New York City, and Philadelphia), and eight territories (American Samoa, the Federated States of Micronesia, Guam, the Marshall Islands, the Northern Mariana Islands, Palau, Puerto Rico, and the U.S. Virgin Islands)—received allocations of COVID-19 vaccine doses, generally on a weekly basis. Although there are 64 jurisdictions implementing COVID-19 vaccination and receiving federal funding for these efforts, allocations of vaccine doses were made to 62 jurisdictions because two major cities considered jurisdictions—Houston and San Antonio—had their allocations consolidated with Texas.

[b]According to CDC, social vulnerability refers to the potential negative effects on communities caused by external stresses on human health, such as natural or human-caused disasters or disease outbreaks.

[c]Federally supported health centers generally receive Health Center Program grants from HRSA under section 330 of the Public Health Service Act (42 U.S.C. § 254b) and provide primary care services in medically underserved areas. Some organizations meet all Health Center Program requirements but do not receive federal grant funding through the section 330 program. However, these centers, which are known as "look-alikes," receive other benefits, such as higher reimbursement rates from the Medicare and Medicaid programs and may receive grants through other federal programs. We use the term "federally supported health centers" to refer to both "look-alikes" and those health centers that receive grants under section 330 of the Public Health Service Act.

[d]On June 20, 2021, the last mass vaccination site under FEMA's vaccination center pilot program closed. However, after that date, the agency continued to support mobile vaccination units and community vaccination centers managed and operated by states and other jurisdictions (using doses allocated to the jurisdictions) by providing federal personnel, funding, and material, such as medical equipment and supplies, according to agency officials.

Figure 4. Four Federal Distribution Programs for COVID-19 Vaccination.

In addition, health officials from most of the states in our review reported that the National Guard supported vaccine distribution and administration efforts. Additionally, two stakeholders representing health care providers said these personnel helped to efficiently administer vaccines at FEMA sites when demand for vaccinations was high.[42] As of July 22, 2021, over 21,000 National Guard personnel had assisted with vaccine-related activities, such as distributing vaccines, providing transportation support, and administering vaccines at 721 vaccination sites, according to DOD.

---

[42] Before vaccine distribution began, stakeholders representing state and local health officials noted the importance of considering if uniformed military vaccinators would improve or undermine confidence in a COVID-19 vaccine, particularly among certain racial and ethnic groups and underserved communities where trust in government is strained. However, some stakeholders we interviewed said this concern was important to note, but did not use or experience issues with using military personnel.

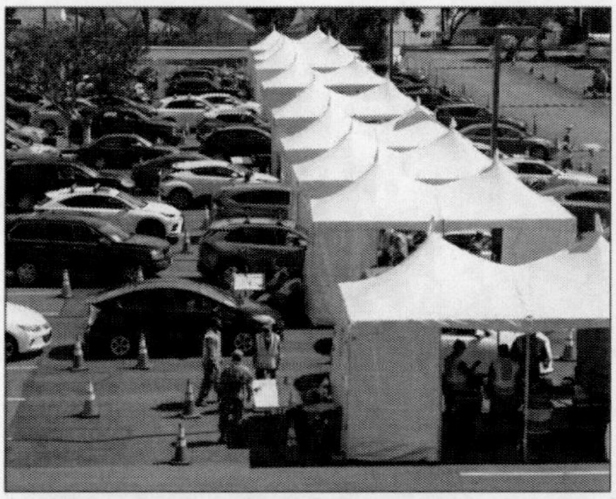

Cars in line at a mass vaccination site in Los Angeles, California, for FEMA's vaccination center pilot program. (Photo by Spc. Jacob Ward)

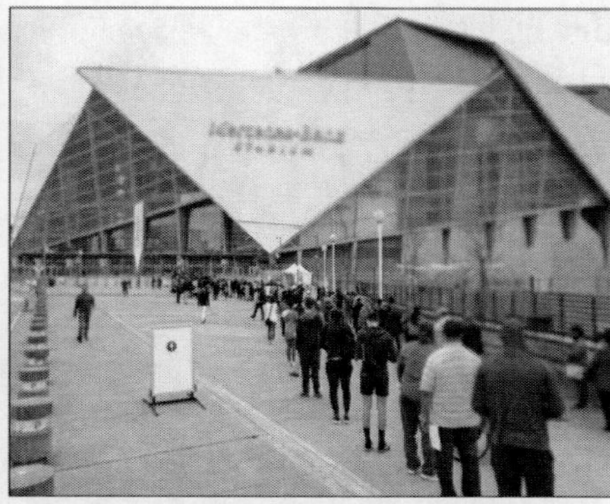

People in line at a mass vaccination site for FEMA's vaccination center pilot program in Atlanta, Georgia. (Photo by Spc. Robert P. Wormley III)

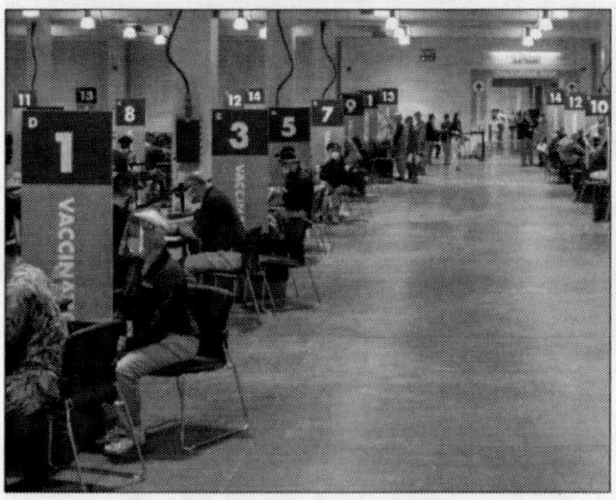

Nurses and U.S. Navy hospital corpsmen administering COVID-19 vaccine at FEMA's vaccination center pilot program in Boston, Massachusetts. (Photo by Sgt. Matthew Lumagui)

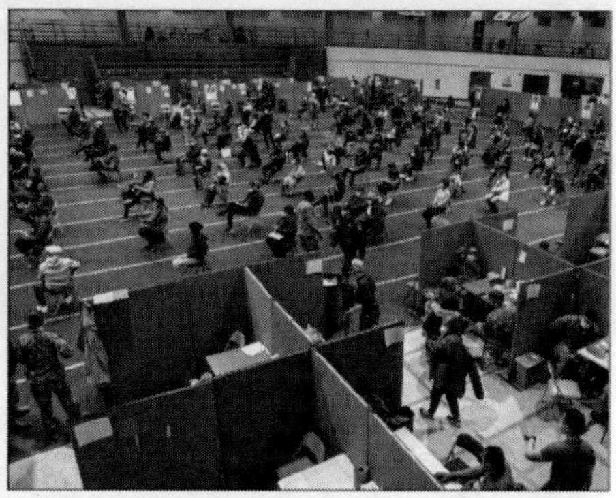

People waiting at a mass vaccination site capable of administering 3,000 doses per day as part of FEMA's vaccination center pilot program. (Photo by K.C. Wilsey)

Source: Defense Visual Information Distribution Service. | GAO-22-104457.

Note: On June 20, 2021, the last mass vaccination site under FEMA's Community Vaccination Center Pilot Site and Mobile Vaccination Program (vaccination center pilot program) closed. However, after that date, the agency continued to support mobile vaccination units and community vaccination centers managed and operated by states and other jurisdictions (using doses allocated to the jurisdictions) by providing federal personnel, funding, and material, such as medical equipment and supplies, according to agency officials.

Figure 5. FEMA Vaccination Center Pilot Program Sites.

In addition, the federal government's expansion of liability protections to additional categories of personnel for administering COVID-19 vaccines was helpful, according to some local health officials and representatives of health care providers we interviewed.[43] Specifically, in March 2021, HHS authorized additional categories of personnel to dispense and administer COVID-19 vaccines, with liability protections under the Public Readiness and Emergency Preparedness Act, including dentists, emergency medical technicians, optometrists, and others.[44] Representatives of health care providers in one state told us that it was a burden for facilities to pull nurses out of direct patient care to administer vaccines and that having the

---

[43] Some stakeholders we interviewed said additional health care providers available to administer vaccines did not address the vaccination challenge of a limited vaccine supply.

[44] Under this act, licensed health professionals and other individuals authorized to administer a countermeasure under state law are protected from liability under federal and state law for administering covered countermeasures against COVID-19, including the COVID-19 vaccines. HHS may identify additional categories of persons, known as "qualified persons," to be afforded such protections. See Pub. L. No. 109-148, div. C, 119 Stat. 2680, 2818 (2005) (codified as amended at 42 U.S.C. §§ 247d-6d et seq.). See HRSA Notice, 86 Fed. Reg. 14462 (Mar. 16, 2021).

flexibility on who could provide vaccinations was important to make sure their facilities could vaccinate as many people as possible and remain in operation.

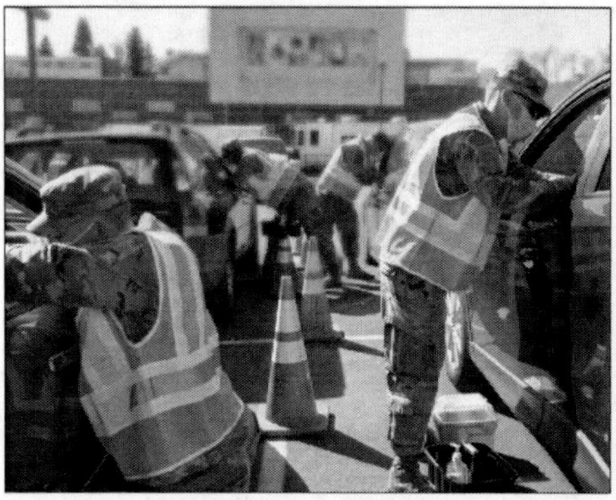

U.S. Army soldiers administering COVID-19 vaccines in Los Angeles, California. (Photo by Capt. Daniel Parker)

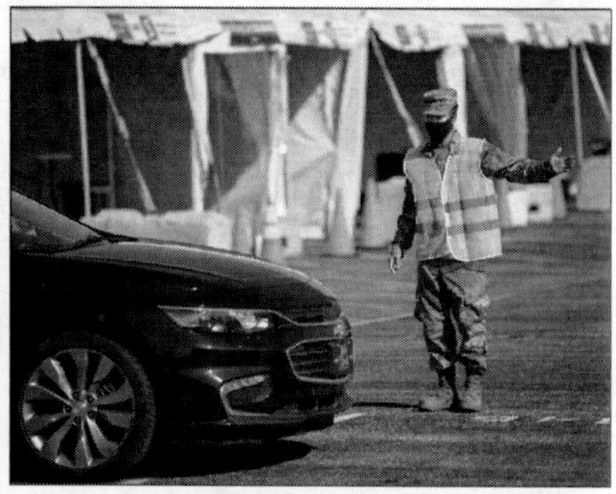

National Guard personnel assists with traffic control at a drive-through vaccine clinic in Louisville, Kentucky. (Photo by Dale Greer)

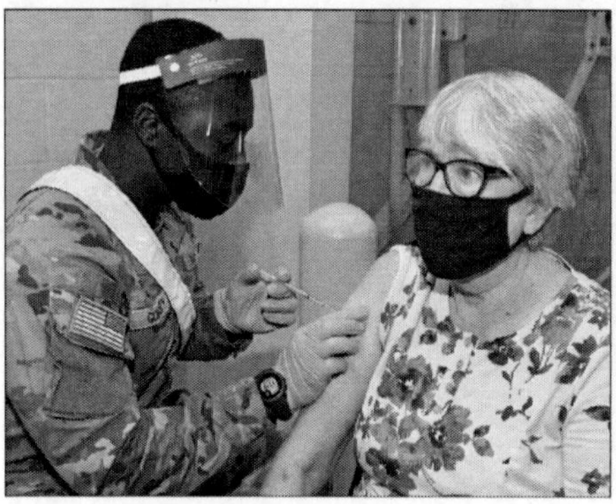

U.S. Army soldier administering COVID-19 vaccines in Houston, Texas. (Photo by Jose Rodriguez)

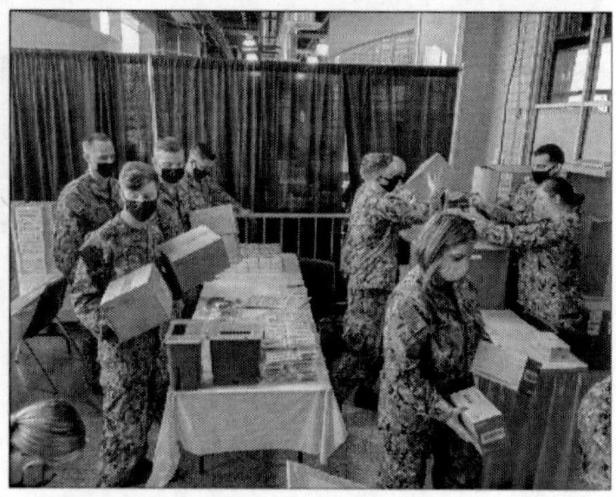

U.S. Navy sailors unpack and store medical supplies. (Photo by Steve Zumwalt)

Source: Defense Visual Information Distribution Service. | GAO-22-104457.

Figure 6. DOD and National Guard Personnel Provide Assistance at FEMA Vaccination Sites.

Stakeholders Identified Challenges Coordinating with Federal Vaccine Distribution Programs that Eased as Vaccine Supply Increased and as States and CDC Made Adjustments

Initially when vaccine supply was limited, state and local health officials faced challenges coordinating their vaccine-related efforts with the four federal vaccine programs, according to state and local health officials and other stakeholders we interviewed. Selected state and local health officials said they had to spend time and resources answering questions from the public and program participants about some of the federal programs, which officials from one state said further burdened their already limited staff and resources. However, as these vaccine distribution programs continued operating and vaccine supply increased in the spring of 2021, these coordination challenges eased. State and local health officials, representatives of health care providers, and other stakeholders we interviewed reported the following examples of the challenges they experienced coordinating with the federal programs:

- *Limited initial information on where vaccine doses were allocated and amounts allocated.* State and local health officials, health care providers, and other stakeholders said they had limited or no information about where vaccine doses were going or the amounts of doses allocated through CDC's retail pharmacy program and HRSA's health center vaccine program when these programs were initiated. Some of these officials told us the limited information on where vaccine doses were going made it difficult for states to optimally and equitably allocate and distribute their own limited supply of vaccine doses.[45] In some cases, a state's distribution of doses to a HRSA-supported health center was already high and additional federal doses provided under HRSA's health center vaccine program resulted in more doses being distributed than the health center could administer in a timely manner, according to most state health officials we interviewed.

  For CDC's retail pharmacy program, most state health officials we spoke with reported experiencing challenges with determining which pharmacy sites would receive vaccine doses from the program's pharmacy partners (i.e., the 21 national pharmacy partners and independent pharmacy networks). For example, pharmacy partners in one state chose to distribute vaccine doses to pharmacy sites the state had not identified as priorities because they were located in areas with a sufficient number of existing vaccine providers. Health officials in the state said they had to negotiate with pharmacy partners participating in CDC's retail pharmacy program to send vaccine doses to pharmacy sites in higher-need areas of their state.

  Additionally, representatives of health care providers said their members often did not know which pharmacies had received vaccine doses when CDC's retail pharmacy program was initiated, so health care providers were unable to refer their patients to pharmacies with available vaccine doses. As vaccine supply increased and there were enough vaccine doses available for all of the federal vaccine distribution programs, information on where vaccine doses were allocated and the amounts allocated became less important. On June 24, 2021, the federal government stopped its weekly allocation of COVID-19 vaccine doses to jurisdictions and federal vaccine distribution programs, including CDC's retail pharmacy program and HRSA's health center vaccine program, because vaccine supply had increased to sufficient levels to meet the needs of jurisdictions and other federal programs, according to federal officials.
- *Higher than needed vaccine allocation for LTC pharmacy program.* CDC overestimated the number of vaccine doses needed for CDC's LTC pharmacy program when vaccine supply was limited in early 2021, according to state health officials we interviewed. For example, health officials from one state said CDC set aside about 40,000 doses a week from their state's overall allocation to be allocated to the LTC pharmacy program. However, not all of the doses were used by the LTC pharmacy program because the number of residents and staff at long-term care facilities being vaccinated was not as high as CDC had expected. These officials said the inability to use those doses elsewhere affected their ability to vaccinate other residents in their state in a timely manner. According to health officials from another state, the higher-

[45] As we reported in April 2021, this information was critical for vaccination planning, especially when states were determining where to send their own allocated doses when supply was limited and demand for vaccinations was high. See GAO-21-443.

than-needed allocation of vaccine doses to the LTC pharmacy program delayed other vaccination efforts. These officials said their jurisdiction could not use the extra doses until state health officials negotiated with pharmacy partners to make the extra doses available for use by the jurisdiction instead of the LTC pharmacy program. These negotiations affected the timely availability of those vaccine doses when vaccine supply was limited.

Once states recognized the LTC pharmacy program had excess vaccine doses, some state health officials we interviewed said they worked with CDC to determine how to make available the extra vaccine doses to other populations in their areas.

- *Lack of initial planning for continuing vaccinations at long-term care facilities.* Initially, CDC did not have a plan in place to vaccinate new staff and residents of long-term care facilities who arrived after the pharmacy partners had completed their three required clinics in CDC's LTC pharmacy program, according to selected stakeholders, including jurisdictional and local health officials. Some of these stakeholders said this was a challenge because of the frequent turnover of patients and staff in long-term care facilities. For example, local health officials from one health department said there were outbreaks of COVID-19 in long-term care facilities after the LTC pharmacy program had concluded, when new patients who were not vaccinated were admitted to the facilities. In mid-March 2021, CDC began working with four pharmacy partners to provide a direct allocation of vaccine doses to long-term care pharmacies participating in CDC's retail pharmacy program.

Health Officials and Others Said Federal Efforts to Inform about Vaccination Were Helpful, but Cited Challenges Implementing Recommendations on Priority Groups

State and Local Health Officials and Other Stakeholders Said CDC's Education Materials about Vaccination Were Useful, but Would Have Liked the Information Sooner

CDC's education materials were useful in informing health officials, health care providers, and the public about COVID-19 vaccination, according to selected state and local health officials and other stakeholders. CDC's education materials included its COVID-19 Vaccine Toolkits, public service announcements, print advertisements, and other online resources that the agency released starting in late-November 2020.

State and local health officials and other stakeholders we interviewed reported the following benefits of CDC's education materials:

- **CDC's online, education materials, including its Toolkits, addressed COVID-19 vaccine safety concerns.** CDC's online, educational materials helped state and local health officials and health care providers address the public's concerns about the safety of COVID-19 vaccines, according to selected health officials and other stakeholders. For example, to inform health care providers and the public about vaccination, CDC produced several COVID-19 Vaccine Toolkits (See Table 1). These Toolkits were useful for health care providers to discuss COVID-19 vaccines with patients, according to representatives of providers from selected state hospital and medical associations we interviewed.

Table 1. COVID-19 vaccination toolkits published by CDC, November 2020 to October 2021

Toolkit title *Target audience and purpose*	Initial publication date
Recipient Education Toolkit For health care providers and workers to educate people getting vaccinated about the importance of COVID-19 vaccination	November 25, 2020
Vaccination Communication Toolkit For health centers, pharmacies, and health care providers to build confidence in COVID-19 vaccination among health care staff	December 9, 2020
Long-Term Care Facility Vaccination Toolkit For the leadership and administrators of long-term care facilities to inform staff, residents and their families about COVID-19 vaccinations in long-term care facilities	December 30, 2020
Essential Worker Vaccination Toolkit For employers of essential workers to help plan for and inform employees about COVID-19 vaccination	January 15, 2021
Community-Based Organization Vaccination Toolkit For staff of organizations serving communities to educate communities about COVID-19 vaccination and address common questions and concerns	January 15, 2021
School Settings and Childcare Programs Toolkit For education and childcare professionals to provide information about COVID-19 vaccines and increase confidence in vaccines among education and childcare staff	March 8, 2021
Health Departments and Public Health Partner Vaccination Toolkit For health departments and public health officials to educate and inform communities about COVID-19 vaccination	April 2, 2021a

Source: GAO summary of the Centers for Disease Control and Prevention (CDC) information. | GAO-22-104457.

[a]As of October 22, 2021, this Toolkit was the most recent one specific to COVID-19 vaccination published by CDC on the agency's website.

CDC also produced other materials, such as online resources, about COVID-19 vaccines' safety and effectiveness and the potential for allergic reactions, which multiple stakeholders used to inform the public about vaccination. For example, officials from one local health department said this information was helpful when answering questions from the public about health and safety concerns about receiving a vaccine while pregnant.[46] CDC also created materials to help address misinformation, which included information on how to find credible resources about COVID-19 vaccines.[47] Multiple stakeholders reported using such materials to inform hard-to-reach populations about the safety of available COVID-19 vaccines.

---

[46] On August 11, 2021, CDC recommended COVID-19 vaccination for people who are pregnant, breastfeeding, trying to become pregnant, or might become pregnant in the future. See Department of Health and Human Services, Centers for Disease Control and Prevention, "COVID-19 Vaccines While Pregnant or Breastfeeding," (Atlanta, Ga.: Aug. 11, 2021), accessed Aug. 19, 2021, https://www.cdc.gov/coronavirus/2019-ncov/vaccines/recommendations/pregnancy.html.

[47] CDC defines misinformation as false information shared by people not intending to mislead others, and disinformation as false information shared by people with the intent to mislead others. See Department of Health and Human Services, Centers for Disease Control and Prevention, "How to Address COVID-19 Vaccine Misinformation," accessed August 19, 2021, https://www.cdc.gov/vaccines/covid-19/health-departments/addressing-vaccine-misinform ation.html.

COVID-19 Vaccination Public Service Announcements

In November 2020, CDC, the Department of Health and Human Services, and other stakeholders partnered with the Ad Council to inform the public about COVID-19 vaccination by providing information about available vaccines and the benefits of vaccination. The partnership used research about the public's intentions to be vaccinated to guide its messaging, among other considerations. The public service announcements were released to the public starting in February 2021. Many announcements were available in Spanish and English to reach greater proportions of the public and were released as video ads, radio ads, print, and on other mediums.

Examples included:

- Well-known children's television characters discussing the benefits of vaccination.
- The experience of hugging loved ones again after vaccination.
- Former U.S. presidents discussing their motivations to get vaccinated.
- Information about how vaccines provide protection against COVID-19.

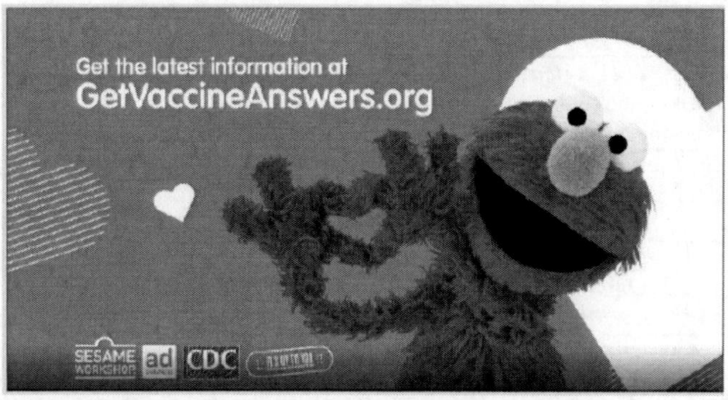
Get the latest information at
GetVaccineAnswers.org
SESAME WORKSHOP
ad
CDC

Screenshot of a televised video that are part of CDC and the Ad Council's COVID-19 vaccine education campaign.

Source: GAO summary of information from the Centers for Disease Control and Prevention (CDC) and the Ad Council. | GAO-22-104457.

- *Public service announcements promoted COVID-19 vaccination.* The public service announcements created by CDC and the Ad Council were helpful in informing the public about COVID-19 vaccination, according to state and local health officials we interviewed. (See side bar.) These announcements were particularly helpful because local governments did not always have the resources to create such messages to inform the public about vaccination, according to selected state and local health officials. These announcements targeted specific groups and provided information on the different reasons for getting vaccinated. For example, one announcement targeted those who might not consider getting vaccinated against COVID-19 as important for themselves by encouraging them to get vaccinated for others, such as their family members. Another announcement featured country music stars talking about the importance of vaccination and was directed at those who admire such celebrities.

- *CDC's materials could be tailored to reach specific communities.* CDC's education materials have been useful because they could be easily modified to meet the needs of particular communities, according to state and local health officials and other stakeholders we interviewed. For example, officials from a national association representing American Indian and Alaska Native populations reported using CDC education materials to develop culturally appropriate messages for their communities. State and local health officials we interviewed similarly reported modifying federal education materials to disseminate specific messages to encourage vaccination among specific communities in their respective areas. CDC also provided translations of various federal education materials, such as information about the different COVID-19 vaccines available and frequently asked questions, which were helpful, according to health officials from one state. (See Figure 7.) Health officials said these materials allowed their staff to provide information about COVID-19 vaccination to greater proportions of the public, including higher-risk populations.[48]

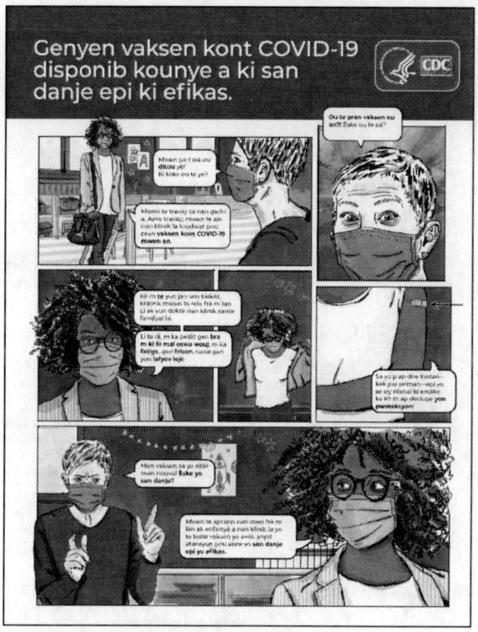
Genyen vaksen kont COVID-19 disponib kounye a ki san danje epi ki efikas.
CDC

Portion of a comic strip in Haitian Creole.

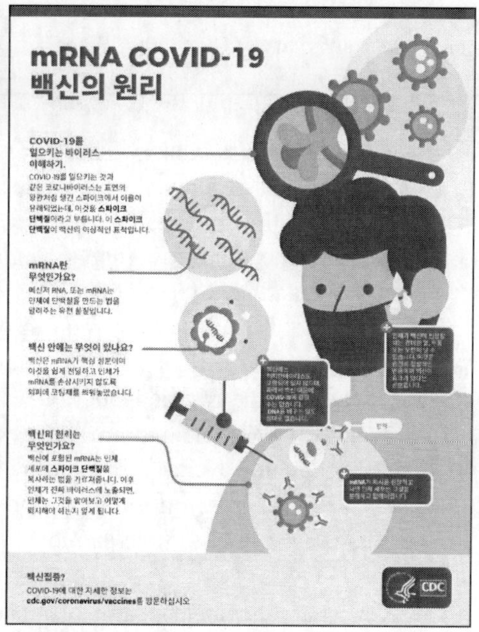
mRNA COVID-19
백신의 원리
COVID-19를 일으키는 바이러스 이해하기.
mRNA란 무엇인가요?
백신 안에는 무엇이 있나요?
CDC

Infographic in Korean.

Source: Centers for Disease Control and Prevention (CDC). | GAO-22-104457.

Figure 7. Examples of Federal Education Materials about COVID-19 Vaccines in Multiple Languages.

Vaccinate with Confidence Strategic Framework

In 2019, CDC developed its Vaccinate with Confidence strategic framework to help build confidence in vaccines generally and help prevent outbreaks of vaccine-preventable diseases in the United States. CDC explained that this was a new approach with three key priorities to increase confidence in vaccines:

[48] In our work examining the federal response to the H1N1 influenza pandemic, we found that education materials and other vaccination information were more effective when available in multiple languages in order to reach some non-English speaking populations. See GAO-11-632.

- protecting at-risk communities,
- empowering families with information about vaccines, and
- stopping myths about vaccines.

According to CDC, vaccine confidence is the trust that patients, their families, and health care providers have in recommended vaccines, providers who administer vaccines, and the processes and policies that lead to vaccine development, licensure or authorization, manufacturing, and recommendations for use.

In late 2020, CDC tailored its Vaccinate with Confidence strategic framework to provide specific information about COVID-19 vaccines to health care providers and the public. In this specific framework, CDC prioritized

- building trust in the vaccine, health care providers, and public health officials;
- promoting confidence in the vaccine among health care personnel; and
- engaging communities and individuals in equitable and inclusive ways.

Source: GAO summary of Centers for Disease Control and Prevention (CDC) information | GAO-22-104457.

- *CDC's strategic framework and consultations informed state communication strategies about COVID-19 vaccination.* Selected state health officials also reported using CDC's Vaccinate with Confidence strategic framework and consultations in developing community-specific messaging strategies to inform health care providers and the public about vaccination. (See sidebar.) As of July 2021, CDC provided 23 states with a "Confidence Consult" at the request of those states to identify potential strategies to improve vaccine confidence in their states.[49] For example, health officials from one state said they used the results from a CDC consultation to address communities' concerns about COVID-19 vaccination. These officials organized smaller community- and faith-based vaccination events after learning this was an effective way of communicating. The public tends to trust information about vaccines from local leaders and community members, according to state and local health officials we interviewed.[50]
-

However, state and local health officials and other stakeholders indicated that CDC's education materials were not always available when it would have been most helpful. CDC began releasing its COVID-19 Vaccine Toolkits in late November 2020. These Toolkits would have been more useful if CDC had released them earlier so health officials and health care providers could have used them to discuss COVID-19 vaccines with the public earlier, according to selected health officials and other stakeholders. For example, health officials from

---

[49] If requested, CDC will provide state and local health departments with Confidence Consults in which the agency examines and develops solutions to increase confidence in COVID-19 vaccine. As of July 2, 2021, CDC reported it had completed 23 Confidence Consults. CDC may offer state and local health departments additional support through rapid community assessments and Vaccine Confidence Bootcamps, both of which aim to create specific strategies to increase confidence and COVID-19 vaccinations.

[50] Experts have also suggested that some individuals may be more likely to get vaccinated if recommended by a trusted figure. See, for example, National Academies of Sciences, Engineering, and Medicine, *Strategies for Building Confidence in the COVID-19 Vaccines*, (Washington, D.C.: Feb. 3, 2021) and Scott Ratzan et al., "Missing the Point—How Primary Care Can Overcome Covid-19 Vaccine Hesitancy," *The New England Journal of Medicine*, vol. 384, no. 100 (2021).

one state health department said it would have been helpful for providers to have some materials in early fall 2020 to provide information about vaccination to their patients before COVID-19 vaccine distribution and administration began in December 2020. Having information about COVID-19 vaccines earlier, such as information on the development and authorization process, might have made some health care providers more comfortable promoting vaccinations and might have increased some individuals' comfort with the vaccines when they became available, according to some stakeholders.

According to CDC, the agency timed the release of education materials to coordinate with ACIP's December 2020 release of recommendations for priority groups and target groups and based on the vaccination rates of specific communities. For example, CDC reported it released the Toolkit for long-term care facility workers in late December 2020 because ACIP's recommendations prioritized these workers for early vaccination efforts around that time.

Health Officials and Others Reported Challenges Implementing Federal Recommendations on Vaccine Priority Groups

In December 2020, as vaccines were first becoming available, CDC adopted ACIP's recommendations on whom state and local health officials should prioritize and target with initial doses when vaccine supply was limited.[51] According to CDC, the ACIP recommendations were designed to be fluid and to allow states and local health departments to adapt the recommendations to meet their specific needs.

Selected state and local health officials told us that health care providers and the public were confused about when and where to get vaccinated in part because of federal changes regarding ACIP's recommended priority groups and differences among states and other jurisdictions on who should be prioritized and targeted for vaccination. In particular,

- *States and localities were not given advanced notice about federal changes regarding priority groups.* Selected stakeholders, including state and local health officials, reported they were not given advanced notice when the federal government made changes on prioritizing and targeting COVID-19 vaccines. (See Table 2.) Having advanced notice of federal changes would have given them time to better adjust their vaccination plans and to prepare how to answer questions from health care providers and the public. For example, officials from a state association representing health care providers reported their members did not always know whom to prioritize for vaccination after federal changes were made. Health officials from one jurisdiction stated that while they understood why eligibility changes were recommended, they would have appreciated having this information before the public was told in order to explain how these changes affected vaccine availability in their communities. For example, not having this information sooner made it challenging for health officials and health care providers to manage the public's expectations about when individuals could get vaccinated while information from the federal government about who should be eligible kept changing, according to selected stakeholders we interviewed.

[51] ACIP recommendations for COVID-19 vaccines were reviewed by the CDC Director and were published as official HHS/CDC recommendations in the *Morbidity and Mortality Weekly Report*.

Table 2. Examples of changes in information from the federal government on prioritizing and targeting COVID-19 vaccines between December 2020 and March 2021

Date	Event
December 1, 2020	CDC's Advisory Committee on Immunization Practices (ACIP) recommended that for the initial phase of vaccine implementation (phase 1a) when vaccine supply was limited, vaccines be offered to those at risk of contracting COVID-19, which included (1) health care personnel and (2) residents of long-term care facilities.[a]
December 20, 2020	CDC's ACIP recommended that after phase 1a, vaccines should be offered in phase 1b to: (1) persons aged 75 years and older and (2) frontline essential workers (non-health care) and in phase 1c to: (1) persons aged 65-74 years, (2) persons aged 16-64 years with high-risk medical conditions, and (3) other essential workers.[b] For phase 2, ACIP prioritized all people at least 16 years of age not yet recommended for vaccination in phase 1.
January 12, 2021	The Secretary of Health and Human Services announced at a press briefing that jurisdictions should open vaccination to all persons age 65 and older and all people under age 65 with a documented co-morbidity.
January 21, 2021	The White House released a national strategy for the COVID-19 response that encouraged states and other jurisdictions to open vaccination to persons age 65 years and older and essential workers.[c]
March 2, 2021	The President directed states to prioritize educators for vaccination with a goal of every educator, school staff member, and childcare worker receiving at least one shot by the end of March, using CDC's Federal Retail Pharmacy Program for COVID-19 Vaccination.
March 11, 2021	The White House announced in a press release that it was directing states, tribes, and territories to make all adults (those aged 18 years and older) in the United States eligible to receive a COVID-19 vaccine by May 1, 2021.

Source: GAO analysis of Centers for Disease Control and Prevention (CDC) information and press releases by the White House and Department of Health and Human Services. | GAO-22-104457.

[a]ACIP defines health care personnel as paid and unpaid persons serving in health care settings who have the potential for direct or indirect exposure to patients or infectious materials. Long-term care facility residents are defined as adults who reside in facilities that provide a range of services, including medical and personal care, to persons who are unable to live independently. See Kathleen Dooling et al., "The Advisory Committee on Immunization Practices' Interim Recommendation for Allocating Initial Supplies of COVID-19 Vaccine—United States, 2020," Morbidity and Mortality Weekly Report, vol. 69, no. 49 (2020).

[b]For the purposes of ACIP's recommendations, non-health care frontline essential workers include firefighters, police officers, corrections officers, food and agricultural workers, U.S. Postal Service workers, manufacturing workers, grocery story workers, public transit workers, those who are in the education sector (teachers and support staff) as well as daycare workers. According to CDC, about 49 million persons, including non-health care frontline essential workers and individuals aged 75 years and older were recommended for vaccination in phase 1b, and an additional 129 million persons were recommended for vaccination in phase 1c (including about 28 million individuals aged 65 through 74 years). See Kathleen Dooling et al., "The Advisory Committee on Immunization Practices' Updated Interim Recommendation for Allocation of COVID-19 Vaccine—United States, December 2020, "Morbidity and Mortality Weekly Report, vol. 69, no. 51-52 (2021).

[c]White House, National Strategy for the COVID-19 Response and Pandemic Preparedness (Washington, D.C.: Jan. 21, 2021).

- *Health care providers were uncertain whom to vaccinate because states and jurisdictions differed in their implementation of federal recommendations for vaccine priority groups.* Health care providers and the public were confused about who was eligible to be vaccinated, especially when vaccine supply was limited, according to selected health officials and other stakeholders. For example, stakeholders representing health care providers reported their members received conflicting information about who was eligible for vaccination, which affected their ability to vaccinate particular groups because they did not always know whom to vaccinate. Further, variation among states' target groups affected the public's confidence in COVID-19 vaccination because they received inconsistent information about when they were eligible for vaccination, according to one stakeholder we interviewed.

We previously reported similar issues regarding variation among states and who they prioritized for vaccination during the 2009 H1N1 pandemic.[52] At that time, we noted that state and local health officials appreciated the flexibility in being able to modify ACIP recommendations to meet state and local needs, but that the variation also caused confusion. Similarly, state and local health officials from one state noted their appreciation for ACIP's COVID-19 vaccine recommendations. For example, these state health officials said the recommendations were useful to communicate with the public about prioritization for vaccines. However, officials from a state association representing health care providers said there was more confusion regarding eligibility for COVID-19 vaccination because they were trying to vaccinate more people for COVID-19 and the risk for not doing so was greater compared to the 2009 H1N1 pandemic.

HHS Agencies Intend to Complete After Action Reviews to Identify Lessons Learned, but Are Uncertain about Plans to Incorporate Information from, and Share Results with, Stakeholders

Two HHS component agencies involved in COVID-19 vaccine implementation—CDC and HRSA—told us that they intend to conduct after action reviews to identify lessons learned from their COVID-19 vaccine distribution and communication efforts. Specifically,

- *CDC* noted that its Center for Preparedness and Response's Division of Emergency Operations, in collaboration with CDC subject matter experts, plans to develop an agency-wide COVID-19 after action review. Historically, such reviews have included lessons learned and recommendations for making improvements within its areas of responsibility, according to CDC. CDC indicated that its review will entail gathering information from CDC responders that participated throughout the duration of the response as well as collaborating with interagency partners, such as FEMA and the HHS/DOD partnership (formerly known as Operation Warp Speed).
  However, as of August 2021, CDC had not identified the specific topics related to vaccine distribution and communication that it intends to include in its review, or to what extent, if any, it plans to gather feedback or perspectives from external stakeholders, such as state and local health officials and providers. CDC explained that typically, its reviews are primarily focused on internal response operations and that coordinating with other departments and agencies may occur once topics are finalized. Additionally, CDC indicated that its review would result in a final report that would be vetted through leadership, but it would be for internal use only; the agency did not indicate plans to share the final report with key stakeholders outside CDC.
- *HRSA* stated that it plans to conduct an after action review and develop a final report documenting successful strategies, challenges, recommendations and considerations for future public health emergencies. HRSA noted that since the inception of its health center vaccine program, it has regularly used available data, including program survey

[52] See GAO-11-632.

> data; vaccine allocation, distribution, and administration data; and stakeholder feedback to assess and continuously improve the program's operations in real time. In conducting an after action review, HRSA stated that it anticipates that any findings would be informed by and shared as appropriate with the CDC and health center programs as well as key rural health and other stakeholders. However, as of August 2021, the agency did not specify whether state and local health officials would be included as stakeholders in this effort, how it was maintaining such feedback for the purposes of an after action review, or what specific topics would be covered related to vaccine distribution and communication.

CDC and HRSA did not provide additional details on their forthcoming after action reviews because, according to agency officials, they have yet to finalize their plans for conducting such reviews. Officials from both agencies explained that they have yet to do so, because they are still involved in the pandemic response. The agencies indicated they would initiate their reviews once the public health emergency ends or, in the case of HRSA, when the health center vaccine program and rural health clinic vaccine program end, if that occurs before the end of the public health emergency.

Federal internal control standards state that management should externally communicate the necessary quality information to achieve an entity's objectives, such as by obtaining quality information from external parties so those external parties can help the entity achieve its objectives and address related risks.[53] Additionally, as we have previously reported, *The Standard for Program Management*, produced by the Project Management Institute, Inc., states that program managers should actively engage key stakeholders throughout the life cycle of a program, which would include evaluation activities, such as completing after action reviews.[54] State and local health officials were key stakeholders in COVID-19 vaccine distribution and communication efforts as they were responsible for critical tasks, such as receiving vaccine allocations from the federal government; identifying the providers in their communities to receive and administer available doses; and communicating with health care providers and the public about vaccination.

Given the challenges state and local health officials and other stakeholders have faced throughout COVID-19 vaccine implementation, and especially early on when vaccine supply was limited, obtaining stakeholder perspectives to inform the after action review process would provide valuable information to CDC and HRSA. For example, as previously noted, when supply was limited, state and local health officials often were not aware of the number of vaccine doses being allocated to vaccination sites within their jurisdictions through federal programs, which affected the officials' ability to plan where to send their own allocated doses. Gathering perspectives from key stakeholders on challenges such as these—encompassing federal distribution and administration activities as well as efforts to inform the public about COVID-19 vaccination throughout the life cycle of the response—would provide CDC and HRSA with a more comprehensive understanding of what worked well and areas for improvement to inform future efforts. Gathering this information as the pandemic response is

---

[53] GAO-14-704G.

[54] See GAO, *Disaster Response: HHS Should Address Deficiencies Highlighted by Recent Hurricanes in the U.S. Virgin Islands and Puerto Rico*, GAO-19-592 (Washington, D.C.: Sept. 20, 2019). Project Management Institute, Inc., *The Standard for Program Management, Fourth Edition, 2017.*

ongoing is particularly important because these stakeholder perspectives could be lost or forgotten over time as vaccine implementation continues.

Moreover, given the highly complex undertaking involved with vaccine implementation spanning multiple federal agencies and key stakeholders across state and local governments and the private sector, sharing the results of after action reviews and lessons learned with stakeholders is equally imperative.[55] Any lessons learned or recommendations that CDC and HRSA identify through their reviews may also be more broadly relevant or applicable to other key stakeholders, such as state and local governments, which were also instrumental in vaccine distribution and communication activities. By sharing such information, stakeholders may also be able to learn from and adjust their related efforts, critical to ensuring an effective response for any additional vaccine efforts that may be needed related to COVID-19 or in future pandemics.

Conclusion

The administration of COVID-19 vaccines across the nation has played a vital role in the U.S. response to the pandemic. With the pandemic now well into its second year, vaccination efforts remain critically important, especially as the Delta variant has emerged and vaccines are anticipated to be made available for children. Federal agencies, including CDC and HRSA, have provided higher-risk populations access to vaccines through the implementation of several federal programs. But, state and local health officials and other stakeholders cited challenges, such as the ability to consider federal efforts when making decisions for their own vaccination programs, particularly when supply was limited.

CDC and HRSA plan to conduct after action reviews of their vaccine distribution and communication efforts, which could provide valuable information on any benefits, challenges, and lessons learned. However, the agencies indicated they do not plan to undertake such reviews until the end of the public health emergency or, in the case of HRSA, when their vaccine distribution programs end, and it is uncertain whether their plans will include gathering input from key stakeholders, such as state and local health officials, or whether the results will be shared with such stakeholders. By gathering perspectives throughout the life cycle of the response from key stakeholders—including state and local health officials—and incorporating their feedback as part of these reviews, CDC and HRSA will help ensure they obtain a more comprehensive understanding of what worked well and areas for improvement to inform future efforts.

It is particularly important to gather stakeholder perspectives on an ongoing basis, given the critical need to continue vaccination efforts, including to address threats of any new variants or to vaccinate children if those vaccines become available. Since agencies do not plan to complete after action reviews until their federal response efforts or programs end, obtaining key stakeholder perspective on an ongoing basis will help ensure those perspectives will not be lost or forgotten by the time the agencies conduct their reviews.

---

[55] We previously reported on the importance of sharing the relevant findings of after action reports with key stakeholders, such as state and local governments. GAO-11-632.

Moreover, by sharing the results of their reviews with such stakeholders, CDC and HRSA will help ensure a successful and effective response across federal, state, and local levels for any additional vaccine efforts that may be needed in the future.

Recommendations for Executive Action

We are making a total of four recommendations, including two to CDC and two to HRSA:

- As CDC finalizes its plans for an after action review related to its COVID-19 vaccine distribution and communication efforts, the Director of the Centers for Disease Control and Prevention should ensure the agency obtains feedback during the life cycle of the response from key stakeholders, including state and local health officials, and incorporates their perspectives as it conducts its review. (Recommendation 1)
- The Director of the Centers for Disease Control and Prevention should share relevant findings of its after action review related to vaccine distribution and communication with key stakeholders, such as state and local health officials, and other federal agencies, as appropriate. (Recommendation 2)
- As HRSA finalizes its plans for an after action review related to its COVID-19 vaccine distribution and communication efforts, the Administrator of the Health Resources and Services Administration should ensure the agency obtains feedback during the life cycle of the response from key stakeholders, including state and local health officials, and incorporates their perspectives as it conducts its review. (Recommendation 3)
- The Administrator of the Health Resources and Services Administration should share relevant findings of its after action review related to vaccine distribution and communication with key stakeholders, such as state and local health officials. (Recommendation 4)

Agency Comments

We provided a draft of this report to DOD, FEMA, and HHS for review and comment. In written comments provided by CDC and HRSA through HHS (reproduced in appendix IV), CDC and HRSA concurred with our recommendations. In its written comments, HHS stated that the GAO study provided valuable feedback on the implementation of CDC's and HRSA's programs and that the agencies are committed to the continuous improvement of their vaccine programs. CDC stated a timeline for an after action review had not been established as it remains involved in the COVID-19 response, and agreed the agency should share relevant findings with key stakeholders, as appropriate, from its after action review once it is completed. CDC also stated that in the meantime, it continues to incorporate continuous feedback from stakeholders. HRSA stated that it plans to incorporate feedback from key stakeholders in its after action review and anticipates sharing results as appropriate with key stakeholders, such as state and local health officials. HRSA also provided technical comments, which we incorporated as appropriate. FEMA and DOD stated they had no comments on the draft report.

Appendix I: COVID-19 Vaccines Authorized in the United States, as of October 22, 2021

As of October 22, 2021, three COVID-19 vaccines were available in the United States. One vaccine was licensed by the Food and Drug Administration (FDA) for individuals aged 16 years and older and was also available to individuals aged 12 through 15 years under an emergency use authorization (EUA).[56] An EUA allows for the temporary use of vaccines without FDA licensure, provided certain statutory criteria are met.[57] Two additional vaccines were authorized for emergency use for individuals aged 18 years and older.[58] As of October 22, 2021, no vaccines had been authorized or licensed for children under 12 years, but one vaccine company (Pfizer) had requested that FDA authorize its COVID-19 vaccine for children aged 5 years to 11 years.[59]

On August 12, 2021, FDA amended the EUAs for two COVID-19 vaccines to allow for the use of an additional dose in certain immunocompromised individuals, specifically in solid organ transplant recipients or those who are diagnosed with conditions that are considered to have an equivalent level of immunocompromise.[60] In September and October 2021, FDA authorized a booster dose of either the Pfizer, Moderna, or Janssen vaccine for certain populations.[61] In October 2021, FDA also authorized "mix and match" for the booster dose—that is, authorizing the use of any available COVID-19 vaccine for use as a booster regardless of which COVID-19 vaccine was used as the primary series or single-dose primary series.

The three available COVID-19 vaccines have varying storage requirements that may affect the setting where each vaccine can be administered. For example, some vaccine administration settings may not have equipment, such as freezers, to store vaccine doses at ultra-cold

[56] Typically, FDA must license a vaccine before it can be marketed in the United States. See 42 U.S.C. § 262. On August 23, 2021, FDA licensed the COVID-19 vaccine developed by Pfizer and BioNTech (marketed as Comirnaty) for the prevention of COVID-19 disease. For the purposes of this report, we refer to the COVID-19 vaccine that Pfizer and BioNTech developed together as the Pfizer vaccine.

[57] The Secretary of Health and Human Services may declare that circumstances, prescribed by statute, exist justifying the emergency use of certain medical products, such as vaccines. Once a declaration of an emergency has been made, FDA may temporarily allow use of unlicensed vaccines through an EUA. For FDA to issue an EUA for a vaccine, it must be reasonable to believe that the vaccine may be effective and that the known and potential benefits of the vaccine outweigh the known and potential risks, among other statutory criteria. See 21 U.S.C. § 360bbb-3. FDA has indicated that issuance of an EUA for a COVID-19 vaccine for which there is adequate manufacturing information would require a determination by FDA that the vaccine's benefits outweigh its risks based on data from at least one well-designed phase 3 clinical trial that demonstrates the vaccine's safety and efficacy in a clear and compelling manner.

Any COVID-19 vaccine that initially receives an EUA from FDA is expected to work toward submission of a biologics license application, according to FDA guidance. See FDA, *Emergency Use Authorization for Vaccines to Prevent COVID-19: Guidance for Industry*, (Silver Spring, Md.: May 2021).

[58] On June 10, 2021, one vaccine company, Moderna, requested that FDA amend the EUA for its COVID-19 vaccine for use in adolescents aged 12 years to 17 years; as of October 22, 2021, FDA had not issued a decision in response. The other authorized COVID-19 vaccine was developed by Janssen Pharmaceutical Companies, which is part of Johnson & Johnson.

[59] As of October 22, 2021, FDA's Vaccines and Related Biological Products Advisory Committee was scheduled to meet on October 26, 2021, to discuss a request for authorization of Pfizer's COVID-19 vaccine for children aged 5 through 11 years.

[60] According to CDC, an additional dose is administered when the initial immune response following a primary vaccine series is likely to be insufficient.

[61] According to CDC, a booster dose is administered when the initial sufficient immune response to a primary vaccine series is likely to have waned over time.

temperatures, the recommended storage method for the Pfizer vaccine.[62] Table 3 shows the age groups authorized for each of the three COVID-19 vaccines, as well as each vaccine's dosing schedules, and storage and handling requirements.

Table 3. COVID-19 Vaccines FDA Authorized for Emergency Use, as of October 22, 2021

Vaccine company	Date FDA initially issued or amended EUA[a]	Individuals for whom vaccine is permitted for emergency use	Dosing and schedule	Storage requirements (doses per vial and minimum lot size)
Pfizer[b]	12/11/2020 8/12/21 9/22/21	12 through 15 years[c] Certain immunocompromised individuals aged 12 years and older[e] 65 years and older; 18 through 64 years at high risk of severe COVID-19; 18 through 64 years with frequent institutional or occupational exposure to the virus that causes COVID-19[g]	2 doses, 3 weeks apart 1 dose, at least 28 days after the initial 2-dose regimen[f] 1 dose (booster) at least 6 months after the initial 2-dose regimen[h]	Stored frozen at ultra-cold temperatures[d] Once thawed and diluted, must be used within 6 hours. (6 doses per vial, minimum lot size 450 doses)
Moderna	12/18/2020 8/12/21 10/20/21	18 years and older[i] Certain immunocompromised individuals aged 18 years and older[e] 65 years and older; 18 through 64 years at high risk of severe COVID-19; 18 through 64 years with frequent institutional or occupational exposure to the virus that causes COVID-19	2 doses, 1 month apart 1 dose, at least 28 days after the initial 2-dose regimen[f] 1 dose (booster) at least 6 months after the initial 2-dose regimen[h]	Stored frozen, but may be refrigerated for up to 30 days once thawed. Once first dose is withdrawn from vial, other doses must be used within 12 hours. (2 vial sizes: maximum 11 doses per vial (range 10-11) or 15 doses per vial (range 13-15), minimum lot size 10-multi-dose vials)
Janssen[j]	2/27/2021[k] 10/20/21	18 years and older 18 years and older	1 dose 1 dose (booster) at least 2 months after completion of the single-dose primary regimen[h]	Refrigerated, but may be stored at room temperature for up to 12 hours. Once first dose is withdrawn from vial, other doses may be stored at 36 to 46 degrees Fahrenheit for up to 6 hours or at room temperature for up to 2 hours. (5 doses per vial, minimum lot size 100 doses)

Source: GAO analysis of vaccine company and Food and Drug Administration (FDA) information. | GAO-22-104457.

[a]Typically, FDA must license a vaccine before it can be marketed in the United States. See 42 U.S.C. § 262. The Secretary of Health and Human Services may declare that circumstances, prescribed by statute, exist justifying the emergency use of certain medical products, such as vaccines. Once a declaration of an emergency has been made, FDA may

[62] Alternatively, Pfizer vaccine vials may be stored frozen at a slightly higher temperatures of -13 to 5 degrees Fahrenheit for up to 2 weeks.

temporarily allow use of unlicensed vaccines through an emergency use authorization (EUA). For FDA to issue an EUA for a vaccine, it must be reasonable to believe that the vaccine may be effective and that the known and potential benefits of the vaccine outweigh the known and potential risks, among other statutory criteria. See 21 U.S.C. § 360bbb-3. FDA has indicated that issuance of an EUA for a COVID-19 vaccine for which there is adequate manufacturing information would require a determination by FDA that the vaccine's benefits outweigh its risks based on data from at least one well-designed phase 3 clinical trial that demonstrates the vaccine's safety and efficacy in a clear and compelling manner.

Any COVID-19 vaccine that initially receives an EUA from FDA is expected to work toward a submission of a biologics license application, according to FDA guidance. See Department of Health and Human Services, Food and Drug Administration, *Emergency Use Authorization for Vaccines to Prevent COVID-19: Guidance for Industry*, (Silver Spring, Md.: May 2021). On August 25, 2021, Moderna announced completion of its submission of a biologics license application to FDA. As part of the application, Moderna requested the application be given priority review.

[b]Pfizer and BioNTech developed this COVID-19 vaccine together, which for the purposes of this report we refer to as the Pfizer vaccine. On August 23, 2021, FDA licensed the two-dose Pfizer vaccine for those aged 16 years and older; this vaccine had been available for emergency use since December 11, 2020. FDA licensed the Pfizer vaccine (marketed as Comirnaty) for the prevention of COVID-19 disease. Under the authorization in effect at the time of licensure, the vaccine remains available for adolescents aged 12 through 15 years.

[c]On December 11, 2020, FDA authorized the Pfizer vaccine for emergency use in individuals aged 16 years and older, and on May 10, 2021, FDA amended the EUA to include adolescents aged 12-15 years.

[d]Alternatively, Pfizer vaccine vials may be stored frozen at a slightly higher temperatures of -13 to 5 degrees Fahrenheit for up to 2 weeks. On May 19, 2021, FDA authorized an increased storage time for thawed vials of Pfizer's COVID-19 vaccine prior to dilution. Thawed, undiluted vials can be stored in the refrigerator at 35 to 46 degrees Fahrenheit for up to 1 month. Previously, thawed, undiluted vaccine vials could be stored in the refrigerator for up to 5 days.

[e]According to FDA, immunocompromised individuals refers to solid organ transplant recipients or those who are diagnosed with conditions that are considered to have an equivalent level of immunocompromise.

[f]According to CDC, an additional dose is administered when the initial immune response following a primary vaccine series is likely to be insufficient.

[g]FDA's initial authorization included individuals18 through 64 years of age whose frequent institutional or occupational exposure to the virus that causes COVID-19 put them at high risk of serious complications, including severe COVID-19. On October 20, 2021, FDA amended the Pfizer EUA to clarify that individuals aged 18 through 64 years with frequent institutional or occupational exposure to the virus that causes COVID-19 were eligible for a booster dose, without reference to whether that exposure put them at high risk of severe COVID-19.

[h]According to CDC, a booster dose is a dose of vaccine administered when the initial sufficient immune response to a primary vaccine series is likely to have waned over time. On October 20, 2021, FDA amended the EUAs for COVID-19 vaccines to allow each of the available COVID-19 vaccines to be used "mix and match" for the booster dose—that is, authorizing the use of any available COVID-19 vaccine for use as a booster dose regardless of which COVID-19 vaccine was used as the primary series or single-dose primary series.

[i]On June 10, 2021, Moderna requested that FDA amend the EUA for its vaccine to include adolescents aged 12-17 years. As of October 22, 2021, FDA had not issued a decision in response.

[j]Janssen Pharmaceutical Companies are a part of Johnson & Johnson.

[k]On April 13, 2021, the Centers for Disease Control and Prevention (CDC) and FDA recommended a pause in the use of the Janssen vaccine so the agencies could review data involving six reported U.S. cases of a rare and severe type of blood clot in individuals after receiving this vaccine. CDC and FDA lifted the pause on April 23, 2021, following a safety review, and revised the Janssen vaccine fact sheets for health care providers and recipients and caregivers to include information about the risk.

Appendix II: Timeline of Key Events Related to COVID-19 Vaccine Implementation through October 21, 2021

Table 4. Timeline of key events related to COVID-19 vaccine implementation, November 25, 2020 through October 21, 2021

Date	Event
November 25, 2020	CDC published its first COVID-19 Vaccination Toolkit for health care providers and workers on vaccine recipient education. The Toolkit included quick references for COVID-19 vaccinators to share with those being vaccinated, including information on the mRNA COVID-19 vaccines.
December 1, 2020	CDC's Advisory Committee on Immunization Practices (ACIP) recommended that for the initial phase of vaccine implementation (phase 1a) when vaccine supply was limited, vaccines be offered to those at risk of contracting COVID-19, which included (1) health care personnel and (2) residents of long-term care facilities.[a]
December 2, 2020	CDC Director adopted ACIP's recommendation for priority groups for the initial phase of the COVID-19 vaccine implementation.
December 10, 2020	FDA's Vaccines and Related Biological Products Advisory Committee met to discuss emergency use authorization request for Pfizer vaccine. Committee voted to recommend the vaccine for emergency use.
December 11, 2020	Pfizer vaccine authorized for emergency use in individuals aged 16 years and older.[b]
December 12, 2020	Initial doses of Pfizer vaccine shipped to health care providers, as directed by states and other jurisdictions and five federal entities (the Bureau of Prisons, Department of Defense, Department of State, Indian Health Service, and the Veterans Health Administration).
December 14, 2020	First dose of COVID-19 vaccine administered; vaccine administration begins.
December 17, 2020	FDA's Vaccines and Related Biological Products Advisory Committee met to discuss emergency use authorization request for the Moderna vaccine. Committee voted to recommend the vaccine for emergency use.
December 18, 2020	Moderna vaccine authorized for emergency use in individuals aged 18 years and older.
December 20, 2020	CDC's ACIP recommended that after phase 1a, vaccines should be offered in phase 1b to: (1) persons aged 75 years and older and (2) frontline essential workers (non-health care) and in phase 1c to: (1) persons aged 65-74 years, (2) persons aged 16-64 years with high-risk medical conditions, and (3) other essential workers.[c] For phase 2, ACIP prioritized all people at least 16 years of age not yet recommended for vaccination in phase 1.
December 21, 2020	CDC Director adopted ACIP's updated recommendation for priority groups for the initial phase of the COVID-19 vaccine implementation.
Week of December 21, 2020	Vaccine doses first distributed through CDC's Pharmacy Partnership for Long-Term Care Program began.
January 11, 2021	CDC published an annex to its interim playbook for jurisdictions that provided new guidance and considerations to jurisdictions regarding when and how to transition from vaccinating initial populations of focus to increasing vaccinations among additional priority populations. It also included a framework for balancing equitable access, service delivery, and vaccine demand; tools for engaging priority populations and increasing vaccine confidence; and strategies for leveraging private-public partnerships.[d]
January 12, 2021	The Secretary of Health and Human Services announced at a press briefing that jurisdictions should open vaccination to all persons age 65 and older and all people under age 65 with a documented co-morbidity.
January 21, 2021	The White House released a national strategy for the COVID-19 response that encouraged states and other jurisdictions to open vaccination to persons age 65 years and older and essential workers.[e]
February 4, 2021	FEMA published the agency's initial guidance on community vaccination centers.[f]
February 9, 2021	Vaccine doses first distributed through CDC's Federal Retail Pharmacy Program for COVID-19 Vaccination.
February 12, 2021	DOD's announced deploying first team of 222 personnel to support FEMA's Community Vaccination Centers Pilot Site and Mobile Vaccination Program.
February 15, 2021	First FEMA Community Vaccination Centers Pilot Site and Mobile Vaccination Program sites established in Oakland and Los Angeles, California.

Date	Event
Week of February 22, 2021	Vaccine doses first distributed through HRSA's Health Center COVID-19 Vaccine Program.[g]
February 27, 2021	Janssen vaccine authorized for emergency use in individuals aged 18 years and older.[h]
March 2, 2021	The President directed states to prioritize educators for vaccination with a goal of every educator, school staff member, and childcare worker receiving at least one shot by the end of March, using CDC's Federal Retail Pharmacy Program for COVID-19 Vaccination.
March 11, 2021	The White House announced in a press release that it was directing states, tribes, and territories to make all adults (those aged 18 years and older) in the United States eligible to receive a COVID-19 vaccine by May 1, 2021.
March 12, 2021	HHS authorized additional categories of personnel to dispense and administer COVID-19 vaccines, including dentists, emergency medical technicians, optometrists, and others.[i]
March 29, 2021	The White House announced in a press release that (1) 90 percent of adults should be eligible for vaccination by April 19, 2021 and (2) 90 percent of adults should have a vaccination site within 5 miles of where they live.
April 9, 2021	Pfizer requested that FDA amend the EUA for its vaccine to include adolescents aged 12-15 years.
April 13, 2021	CDC and FDA recommended a pause in the use of Janssen vaccine so the agencies could review data involving six reported U.S. cases of a rare and severe type of blood clot in individuals after receiving this vaccine.
April 23, 2021	CDC and FDA lifted the pause in the use of Janssen vaccine following a safety review, and revised the Janssen vaccine fact sheets for health care providers and recipients and caregivers to include information about the risk.
April 23, 2021	CDC's Pharmacy Partnership for Long-Term Care Program ended.
May 1, 2021	CDC launched a national hotline (1-800-232-0233) to assist with scheduling appointments.
May 4, 2021	The White House announced efforts to make appointments for COVID-19 vaccinations more accessible. For example, the President encouraged pharmacies participating in CDC's retail pharmacy program to begin offering walk-in appointments and redirected FEMA resources to support smaller vaccination sites and more mobile clinics to meet people where they are instead of requiring them to come to a designated site to be vaccinated. The White House also announced the Vaccines.gov website to assist the public in finding vaccination appointments.
May 7, 2021	Pfizer submitted a biologics license application with FDA for its COVID-19 vaccine for those 16 years and older.
May 10, 2021	Pfizer vaccine authorized for emergency use for adolescents aged 12-15 years.
Week of May 17, 2021	HRSA's Rural Health Clinic COVID-19 Program began (vaccine doses first distributed for this program).[j]
June 1, 2021	Moderna submitted a biologics license application for its COVID-19 vaccine for those 18 years and older.
June 2, 2021	The White House announced that June 2021 would be a "National Month of Action," which included a variety of events surrounding COVID-19 vaccinations. For example, the federal government entered into partnerships with the private sector to facilitate vaccination, such as with Major League Baseball, which offered on-site vaccinations at games and gave free tickets to those who were vaccinated.
June 10, 2021	Moderna requested that FDA amend the EUA for its vaccine to include adolescents aged 12-17 years.
June 20, 2021	FEMA's Community Vaccination Centers Pilot Site and Mobile Vaccination Program ended.[k]
June 22, 2021	DOD halted deployment of active-duty servicemembers to support federal vaccination efforts.
July 1, 2021	HRSA's Rural Health Clinic Vaccine Confidence Program began supporting vaccine outreach in rural communities. Funding could be used for a variety of activities including conducting educational and outreach efforts on the benefits and safety of vaccines, providing information to rural residents about how and where to get vaccinated, and coordinating with existing vaccination sites and public health partners to identify isolated populations.

Table 4. (Continued)

Date	Event
July 6, 2021	The White House announced plans to mobilize COVID-19 surge response teams, federal personnel focused on increasing vaccination rates in communities with low rates, by, for example, filling in gaps in staffing.
July 15, 2021	U.S. Surgeon General issued advisory warning about the threat of health misinformation to the U.S. response to COVID-19, including preventing people from getting vaccinated.
July 16, 2021	FDA accepted Pfizer's application requesting licensure for its COVID-19 vaccine and granted the application priority review (meaning that FDA will aim to make a decision on the application within 6 months, compared to the 10 months for standard review).
August 11, 2021	CDC recommended COVID-19 vaccination for people who are pregnant, breastfeeding, trying to become pregnant, or might become pregnant in the future. CDC stated that there was no evidence that COVID-19 vaccines cause fertility problems in women or men.
August 12, 2021	HHS announced mandating COVID-19 vaccination for staff who serve in federally operated health care and clinical research facilities and interact with, or have the potential to come into contact, patients. HHS staff included employees, contractors, trainees, and volunteers as well as members of the U.S. Public Health Service Commissioned Corps.
August 12, 2021	FDA amended both the Pfizer and Moderna EUAs to allow for the use of an additional dose in certain immunocompromised individuals, specifically in solid organ transplant recipients or those who are diagnosed with conditions that are considered to have an equivalent level of immunocompromise.[l]
August 13, 2021	ACIP recommended using an additional dose of Pfizer and Moderna COVID-19 vaccines in certain immunocompromised individuals. CDC Director adopted ACIP's recommendations.
August 16, 2021	Pfizer submitted phase 1 data to FDA to support the evaluation of a booster dose of its COVID-19 vaccine.[m]
August 18, 2021	HHS recommended booster shots for those that have received the Pfizer or Moderna vaccines, pending an FDA review and ACIP recommendations. HHS said it was prepared to offer booster shots beginning the week of September 20 and starting 8 months after an individual's second dose.
August 18, 2021	The White House announced that HHS would develop new regulations requiring nursing homes to require that all of their workers be fully vaccinated against COVID-19 as a condition of participating in the Medicare and Medicaid programs.
August 23, 2021	FDA licensed the Pfizer vaccine for those aged 16 years and older (marketed as Comirnaty) for the prevention of COVID-19 disease. The vaccine remained available under an emergency use authorization for use in individuals aged 12 to 15 years.
August 25, 2021	Moderna submitted a completed biologics license application to FDA. As part of the application, Moderna requested the application be given priority review.
September 1, 2021	Moderna initiated its submission of data to FDA for the evaluation of a booster dose of its COVID-19 vaccine.[m]
September 9, 2021	The White House announced that • HHS would develop regulations requiring health care workers in hospitals, home health care facilities, or other medical facilities that treat Medicare and Medicaid patients be fully vaccinated; • the Department of Labor was developing an emergency rule to require all employers with 100 or more employees to ensure their workforce were fully vaccinated or showed a negative COVID-19 test at least once a week; • the Department of Labor would require employers with 100 or more workers to give those workers paid time off to get vaccinated; • the President would sign an executive order requiring all executive branch federal employees be vaccinated; and • the President would sign an executive order requiring all federal contractors be vaccinated.

Date	Event
September 17, 2021	FDA's Vaccines and Related Biological Products Advisory Committee met to discuss EUA request for a booster dose of the Pfizer vaccine. Committee voted against recommending the authorization of a booster dose for those aged 16 years and older citing data demonstrating an increased risk for adverse cardiac events, particularly among males aged 16 to 17 years, and limited data on whether this risk may be increased after a booster dose. Committee voted for recommending the authorization of a single booster dose at least 6 months after completion of the primary series for use in individuals aged 65 years and older.[m]
September 22, 2021	FDA amended the Pfizer EUA to allow for use of a single booster dose to be administered at least 6 months after completion of the primary series in • individuals aged 65 years and older; • individuals aged 18 through 64 years at high risk of severe COVID-19; and • individuals aged 18 through 64 years whose frequent institutional or occupational exposure puts them at high risk of serious complications of COVID-19 including severe illness.[m]
September 23, 2021	ACIP recommended a booster dose of the Pfizer vaccine at least 6 months after the completion of the primary series for • individuals aged 65 years and older, • residents of long-term care facilities, • individuals aged 50 through 64 years with underlying medical conditions, and • individuals aged 18 through 49 years with underlying medical conditions, based on their individual risk-benefit analysis.[m]
September 24, 2021	CDC recommended the following groups should receive a booster dose of the Pfizer vaccine at least 6 months after the completion of a primary series: • individuals aged 65 years and older, • residents in long-term care settings, and • individuals aged 50 through 64 years with underlying medical conditions. CDC also recommended the following groups may receive a booster dose of the Pfizer vaccine 6 months after the completion of a primary series, based on their individual benefits and risks: • individuals aged 18 through 49 years with underlying medical conditions and • individuals aged 18 through 64 years who are at increased risk of COVID-19 exposure and transmission because of occupational or institutional setting.[m]
October 5, 2021	Johnson & Johnson announced that it had submitted data for the Janssen COVID-19 vaccine to FDA for the evaluation of a booster dose of its COVID-19 vaccine.[m]
October 6, 2021	Pfizer submitted a request to FDA to amend its EUA for its COVID-19 vaccine to include those aged 5 through 11 years.
October 14, 2021	FDA's Vaccines and Related Biological Products Advisory Committee met to discuss EUA request for a booster dose of the Moderna vaccine. Committee voted to recommend authorizing a single booster dose to be administered at least 6 months after completion of the primary series in • individuals aged 65 years and older; • individuals aged 18 through 64 years at high risk of severe COVID-19; and • individuals aged 18 through 64 years whose frequent institutional or occupational exposure puts them at high risk of serious complications of COVID-19 including severe illness.[m]
October 15, 2021	FDA's Vaccines and Related Biological Products Advisory Committee met to discuss EUA request for a booster dose of the Janssen vaccine. Committee voted to recommend authorizing a single booster dose to be administered at least 2 months after completion of the single-dose primary regimen in individuals aged 18 years and older.[m]
October 20, 2021	The White House announced a plan for distributing and communicating about COVID-19 vaccinations for children aged 5 through 11 years, if authorized by FDA and recommended by CDC.[n]

Table 4. (Continued)

Date	Event
October 20, 2021	FDA amended the Moderna EUA to allow for use of a single booster dose to be administered at least 6 months after completion of the primary series in • individuals aged 65 years and older; • individuals aged 18 through 64 years at high risk of severe COVID-19; and • individuals aged 18 through 64 years with frequent institutional or occupational exposure to the virus that causes COVID-19.[m] FDA amended the Janssen EUA to allow for use of a single booster dose to be administered at least 2 months after completion of the single-dose primary regimen in individuals 18 years of age and older FDA authorized "mix and match" for the booster dose—that is, authorizing the use of any available COVID-19 vaccine for use as a booster dose regardless of which COVID-19 vaccine was used as the primary series or single-dose primary series. FDA amended the Pfizer EUA to clarify that individuals aged 18 through 64 years with frequent institutional or occupational exposure to the virus that causes COVID-19 were eligible for a booster dose, without reference to whether that exposure put them a high risk of severe COVID-19.
October 21, 2021	ACIP recommended a booster dose of the Moderna vaccine at least 6 months after the completion of the primary series and a booster dose of the Janssen vaccine at least 2 months after the completion of the single-dose primary regimen, as authorized by FDA.[m]
October 21, 2021	CDC adopted ACIP's recommendations, stating that individuals in the following groups who received the Pfizer vaccine or the Moderna vaccine were eligible for a booster dose 6 months or more after their the completion of a primary series: • individuals aged 65 years and older, • individuals aged 18 years and older living in long-term care settings, • individuals aged 18 years and older who have underlying medical conditions, and • individuals aged 18 years and older who work or live in high-risk settings.[m] CDC also recommended a single booster dose to be administered 2 months or more after receiving the Janssen single-dose primary regimen for individuals 18 years of age and older CDC stated its recommendations allowed for the "mix and match" of a booster dose—that is, the use of any available COVID-19 vaccine for use as a booster dose regardless of which COVID-19 vaccine was used as the primary series or single-dose primary series.

Source: GAO analysis of information from the Department of Defense (DOD), the Department of Health and Human Services (HHS), the Centers for Disease Control and Prevention (CDC), CDC's ACIP, the Federal Emergency Management Agency (FEMA), the Food and Drug Administration (FDA), the Health Resources and Services Administration (HRSA), and transcripts of press conferences by White House and HHS officials. | GAO-22-104457.

Note: The timeline represents selected events related to COVID-19 vaccine implementation— prioritizing, allocating, distributing, and administering vaccine doses—and federal communication efforts from November 2020 through October 21, 2021.

[a]ACIP defines health care personnel as paid and unpaid persons serving in health care settings who have the potential for direct or indirect exposure to patients or infectious materials. Long-term care facility residents are defined as adults who reside in facilities that provide a range of services, including medical and personal care, to persons who are unable to live independently. See Kathleen Dooling et al., "The Advisory Committee on Immunization Practices' Interim Recommendation for Allocating Initial Supplies of COVID-19 Vaccine—United States, 2020," *Morbidity and Mortality Weekly Report*, vol. 69, no. 49 (2020).

[b]Pfizer and BioNTech developed this COVID-19 vaccine together, which this report refers to as the Pfizer vaccine. The Secretary of Health and Human Services may declare that circumstances, prescribed by statute, exist justifying the emergency use of certain medical products, such as vaccines. Once a declaration of an emergency has been made, FDA may temporarily allow use of unlicensed vaccines through an emergency use authorization (EUA). For FDA to issue an EUA for a vaccine, it must be reasonable to believe that the vaccine may be effective and that the known and potential benefits of the vaccine outweigh the known and potential risks, among other statutory criteria. See 21 U.S.C. § 360bbb-3. FDA has indicated that issuance of an EUA for a COVID-19 vaccine for which there is adequate manufacturing information would require a determination by FDA that the vaccine's benefits outweigh its risks based

on data from at least one well-designed phase 3 clinical trial that demonstrates the vaccine's safety and efficacy in a clear and compelling manner.

Typically, FDA must license a vaccine before it can be marketed in the U.S. See 42 U.S.C. § 262. Any COVID-19 vaccine that initially receives an EUA from FDA is expected to work toward submission of a biologics license application, according to FDA guidance. See Department of Health and Human Services, Food and Drug Administration, *Emergency Use Authorization for Vaccines to Prevent COVID-19: Guidance for Industry*, (Silver Spring, Md.: May 2021).

[c]For the purposes of ACIP's recommendation, non-health care frontline essential workers include firefighters, police officers, corrections officers, food and agricultural workers, U.S. Postal Service workers, manufacturing workers, grocery story workers, public transit workers, those who are in the education sector (teachers and support staff) as well as daycare workers. According to CDC, about 49 million persons, including non-health care frontline essential workers and individuals aged 75 years and older were recommended for vaccination in phase 1b, and an additional 129 million persons were recommended for vaccination in phase 1c (including about 28 million individuals aged 65-74 years). See Kathleen Dooling et al., "The Advisory Committee on Immunization Practices' Updated Interim Recommendation for Allocation of COVID-19 Vaccine—United States, December 2020," Morbidity and Mortality Weekly Report, vol. 69, no. 51-52 (2021).

[d]Department of Health and Human Services, Centers for Disease Control and Prevention, *COVID-19 Vaccination Program Interim Playbook for Jurisdictions Operations Annex—Considerations for Increasing COVID-19 Vaccination: Reaching and Increasing Uptake in Priority Populations, version 1.0*, (Atlanta, Ga.: Jan.11, 2021). According to CDC, this document was a supplement to CDC's interim playbooks to assist state and other jurisdictions with COVID-19 vaccine implementation. See Department of Health and Human Services, Centers for Disease Control and Prevention, *COVID-19 Vaccination Program Interim Playbook for Jurisdiction Operations, version 1.0* (Atlanta, Ga.: Sept. 16, 2020) and *COVID-19 Vaccination Program Interim Playbook for Jurisdiction Operations, version 2.0* (Atlanta, Ga.: Oct. 29, 2020).

[e]White House, National Strategy for the COVID-19 Response and Pandemic Preparedness (Washington, D.C.: Jan. 21, 2021).

[f]In addition to its initial guidance on community vaccination centers, FEMA published five additional versions of its guidance on community vaccination centers between February 2021 and April 2021. For the final version, see Department of Homeland Security, Federal Emergency Management Agency, *Community Vaccination Centers Playbook, Final* (Washington, D.C.: April 23, 2021).

[g]Federally supported health centers generally receive Health Center Program grants from HRSA under section 330 of the Public Health Service Act (42 U.S.C § 254b) and provide primary care services in medically underserved areas. Some organizations meet all Health Center Program requirements but do not receive federal grant funding through the section 330 program. However, these centers, which are known as "look-alikes," receive other benefits, such as higher reimbursement rates from the Medicare and Medicaid programs and may receive grants through other federal programs. We use the term "federally supported health centers" to refer to both "look-alikes" and those health centers that receive grants under section 330 of the Public Health Service Act.

[h]Janssen Pharmaceutical Companies are a part of Johnson & Johnson.

[i]Under the Public Readiness and Emergency Preparedness (PREP) Act, licensed health professionals and other individuals authorized to administer a countermeasure under state law are protected from liability under federal and state law for administering covered countermeasures against COVID-19, including the COVID-19 vaccines. HHS may identify additional categories of persons, known as "qualified persons," to be afforded such protections. See Pub. L. No. 109-148, div. C, 119 Stat. 2680, 2818 (2005) (codified as amended at 42 U.S.C. §§ 247d-6d et seq.). See HRSA Notice, 86 Fed. Reg. 14462 (Mar. 16, 2021).

[j]The Rural Health Clinic COVID-19 Vaccine Distribution Program distributed 99,760 vaccine doses to 141 rural health clinics, as of September 15, 2021, according to HHS.

[k]Although FEMA's vaccination center pilot program ended, the agency continued to support community vaccination centers managed and operated by states and other jurisdictions (using doses allocated to the jurisdictions) by providing federal personnel, funding, and material, such as medical equipment and supplies, according to agency officials.

[l]According to CDC, an additional dose is administered when the initial immune response following a primary vaccine series is likely to be insufficient.

[m]According to CDC, a booster dose is a dose of vaccine administered when the initial sufficient immune response to a primary vaccine series is likely to have waned over time.

[n]As of October 21, 2021, no vaccines had been authorized or licensed for children under 12 years, but Pfizer had requested FDA to authorize its COVID-19 vaccine children aged 5 years to 11 years. FDA's Vaccines and Related Biological Products Advisory Committee was scheduled to meet on October 26, 2021, to discuss a request for authorization of Pfizer's COVID-19 vaccine for children aged 5 through 11 years.

Appendix III: Vaccine Finder and the Vaccine Administration Management System

The Centers for Disease Control and Prevention (CDC) developed tools to help the public locate where vaccines were available and to schedule a vaccination appointment. Specifically:

- *VaccineFinder* is an online tool previously developed by CDC and Boston's Children's Hospital to provide users information on the locations of providers offering vaccinations, such as for seasonal influenza. As the national supply of COVID-19 vaccine increased, CDC updated VaccineFinder to include information about COVID-19 vaccines.
  VaccineFinder, however, provided no or limited information on COVID-19 vaccines in March 2021 when vaccine demand was increasing. The public also could not schedule appointments on VaccineFinder; instead, users were given a link to a second website or a phone number to schedule appointments. When information was not available on COVID-19 vaccines on VaccineFinder, some states created their own platforms to help health care providers and the public find available vaccination appointments, according to selected health officials. In May 2021, CDC updated VaccineFinder for COVID-19 vaccines with a new website, https://www.vaccines.gov, which is dedicated specifically to COVID-19 vaccines.
- *Vaccine Administration Management System (VAMS)* is an online tool CDC developed that states or other jurisdictions, federal agencies, or other organizations could opt to use to help manage COVID-19 vaccine administration. For example, in jurisdictions that used the system, the public could use VAMS to schedule vaccination appointments. Ten jurisdictions, three federal agencies, and one multi-state health system were using VAMS as of June 2021, according to CDC officials. State health officials from one state using VAMS said health care providers reported some problems with VAMS, including difficulties completing their registration, which is needed to upload information about vaccination appointments into VAMS, and correcting record errors in a timely manner in some instances. VAMS was initially only available in English; it was made available in Spanish in April 2021, according to health officials from one state.

Appendix IV: Comments from the Department of Health & Human Services

DEPARTMENT OF HEALTH & HUMAN SERVICES OFFICE OF THE SECRETARY

Assistant Secretary for Legislation
Washington, DC 20201

October 19, 2021

Alyssa M. Hundrup
Director, Health Care
U.S. Government Accountability Office
441 G Street NW
Washington, DC 20548

Dear Ms. Hundrup:

Attached are comments on the U.S. Government Accountability Office's (GAO) report entitled, ***"COVID-19: HHS Agencies' Planned Reviews of Vaccine Distribution and Communication Efforts Should Include Stakeholder Perspectives"*** (GAO-22-104457).

The Department appreciates the opportunity to review this report prior to publication.

Sincerely,

Melanie Anne Egorin
Assistant Secretary for Legislation

GENERAL COMMENTS FROM THE DEPARTMENT OF HEALTH AND HUMAN SERVICES ON THE GOVERNMENT ACCOUNTABILITY OFFICE'S DRAFT REPORT ENTITLED — COVID-19: HHS AGENCIES' PLANNED REVIEWS OF VACCINE DISTRIBUTION AND COMMUNICATION EFFORTS SHOULD INCLUDE STAKEHOLDER PERSPECTIVES (GAO-22-104457)

The U.S. Department of Health and Human Services (HHS) appreciates the opportunity from the Government Accountability Office (GAO) to review and comment on this draft report.

The GAO study provided valuable feedback on the implementation of the Health Resources and Services Administration's (HRSA) Health Center COVID-19 Vaccine Program and the Rural Health Clinic COVID-19 Vaccine Distribution Program, as well as the Centers for Disease Control and Prevention's (CDC) Long-Term Care Partnerships Pharmacy Program and Federal Retail Pharmacy Program. HRSA and CDC are committed to continuous improvement of their vaccine programs and appreciate this opportunity to further inform those improvements.

HRSA and CDC launched the Health Center COVID-19 Vaccine Program and the Rural Health Clinic COVID-19 Vaccine Distribution Program to allocate a limited supply of COVID-19 vaccine to select health centers and rural health clinics. This was done to ensure our nation's underserved communities and those disproportionately affected by COVID-19 are equitably vaccinated against the virus and to improve vaccine access and vaccination rates to medically underserved rural communities. Additionally, starting in February of 2021, the Federal Retail Pharmacy Program was initiated and now includes over 40,000 retail and long-term care pharmacy locations nationwide and 21 national pharmacy partners and independent pharmacy networks.

To participate in the HRSA and CDC vaccine programs, participants must agree to the Conditions of Participation, which includes data reporting (i.e., required vaccine supply and administration data reported to state/other jurisdictions, as required in the CDC COVID-19 Vaccine Provider Agreement). HHS' Tiberius system is the central platform for sharing vaccine related information. Since the platform capabilities were enabled, vaccine data from these programs has been shared with jurisdictions to facilitate coordination at state and local levels through Tiberius.

HRSA and CDC are aware of the importance of continuous stakeholder engagement to ensure collaboration between vaccine programs and jurisdictions overseeing state and local immunization programs. For example, during the initial phase of the Health Center COVID-19 Vaccine Program, in order to maximize coordination, HRSA and CDC hosted weekly hour-long office hours with CDC regional coordinators and state and local immunization programs to share program updates and to address questions and solicit feedback. HRSA staff also communicated with CDC regional coordinators and state and local immunization programs on an almost daily basis to answer questions and joined regional calls with immunization programs to provide tailored opportunities for bidirectional information sharing.

As of September 15, 2021, the Health Center COVID-19 Vaccine Program distributed 6,389,574 vaccine doses to 866 participating HRSA-supported health centers for 2,362 sites. During the same time period, the Rural Health Clinic COVID-19 Vaccine Distribution Program distributed 99,760 vaccine doses to 141 rural health clinics. HRSA designed its vaccine programs as separate, direct allocations for health centers and rural health clinics and are intended to supplement – not supplant – existing vaccine distributions that health centers and rural health

Page **1** of **3**

GENERAL COMMENTS FROM THE DEPARTMENT OF HEALTH AND HUMAN SERVICES ON THE GOVERNMENT ACCOUNTABILITY OFFICE'S DRAFT REPORT ENTITLED — COVID-19: HHS AGENCIES' PLANNED REVIEWS OF VACCINE DISTRIBUTION AND COMMUNICATION EFFORTS SHOULD INCLUDE STAKEHOLDER PERSPECTIVES (GAO-22-104457)

clinics are receiving from states. As of September 29, 2021, CDC's Federal Retail Pharmacy Program distributed almost 137 million vaccine doses (including those administered through the Pharmacy Partnership for Long-term Care Program).

Recommendation 1
As CDC finalizes its plans for an after-action review related to its COVID-19 vaccine distribution and communication efforts, the Director of the Centers for Disease Control and Prevention should ensure the agency obtains feedback during the life cycle of the response from key stakeholders, including state and local health officials, and incorporates their perspectives as it conducts its review. (Recommendation 1)

HHS Response
CDC concurs with the GAO's recommendation. CDC anticipates the development of an after-action report on vaccine distribution and communication efforts. A timeline for an after-action report has not been established as CDC remains activated for the COVID-19 response. In the meantime, CDC continues to incorporate continuous feedback from stakeholders.

Recommendation 2
The Director of the Centers for Disease Control and Prevention should share relevant findings of its after action review related to vaccine distribution and communication with key stakeholders, such as state and local health officials, and other federal agencies, as appropriate. (Recommendation 2)

HHS Response
CDC concurs with the GAO's recommendation. CDC anticipates the development of an after-action report on vaccine distribution and communication efforts. A timeline for an after-action report has not been established as CDC remains activated for the COVID-19 response. In the meantime, CDC continues to incorporate continuous feedback from stakeholders.

Recommendation 3
As HRSA finalizes its plans for an after action review related to its COVID-19 vaccine distribution and communication efforts, the Administrator of HRSA should ensure the agency obtains feedback during the life cycle of the response from key stakeholders, including state and local health officials, and incorporates their perspectives as it conducts its review.

HHS Response
HRSA concurs with the GAO's recommendation. HRSA plans to conduct an after-action review and develop a final report documenting the key program accomplishments, including successful strategies, challenges, recommendations, and considerations for future public health emergencies at the conclusion of the HRSA vaccine programs. HRSA will seek to obtain feedback during the lifecycle of the response from key stakeholders to incorporate their perspectives in an after action review.

GENERAL COMMENTS FROM THE DEPARTMENT OF HEALTH AND HUMAN SERVICES ON THE GOVERNMENT ACCOUNTABILITY OFFICE'S DRAFT REPORT ENTITLED — COVID-19: HHS AGENCIES' PLANNED REVIEWS OF VACCINE DISTRIBUTION AND COMMUNICATION EFFORTS SHOULD INCLUDE STAKEHOLDER PERSPECTIVES (GAO-22-104457)

Recommendation 4

The Administrator of HRSA should share relevant findings of its after action review related to vaccine distribution and communication with key stakeholders, such as state and local health officials.

Response

HRSA concurs with GAO's recommendation. HRSA anticipates that any after action review findings would be shared as appropriate with the CDC, HRSA-supported health centers, rural health clinics, key rural health and other stakeholders, such as state and local health officials.

Chapter 10

COVID-19: HHS and DOD Transitioned Vaccine Responsibilities to HHS, but Need to Address Outstanding Issues*

United States Government Accountability Office

Abbreviations

ASPR	Office of the Assistant Secretary for Preparedness and Response
BARDA	Biomedical Advanced Research and Development Authority
CAG	HHS-DOD COVID-19 Countermeasures Acceleration Group
CAG Continuity Book	DOD's *Countermeasures Acceleration Group Continuity Book*
CDC	Centers for Disease Control and Prevention
COVID-19	Coronavirus Disease 2019
DOD	Department of Defense
DPA	Defense Production Act
EUA	emergency use authorization
FAR	Federal Acquisition Regulation
FDA	Food and Drug Administration
HHS	Department of Health and Human Services
JPEO-CBRND	Joint Program Executive Office for Chemical, Biological, Radiological, and Nuclear Defense
NIH	National Institutes of Health
OTA	other transaction agreement

Why GAO Did This Study

Vaccines have played a crucial role in battling the COVID-19 pandemic. The CAG worked with vaccine companies to develop COVID-19 vaccines, and made available a sufficient supply

* This is an edited, reformatted and augmented version of the United States Government Accountability Office Report to Congressional Addressees, Publication No. GAO-22-104453, dated January 2022.

In: COVID-19 Vaccines
Editor: John Schroder
ISBN: 979-8-88697-150-7

for all eligible people in the nation. An April 2021 memorandum of understanding between HHS and DOD called for the transfer of remaining CAG responsibilities to HHS and for identification of lessons learned.

The CARES Act includes a provision for GAO to report on its ongoing monitoring and oversight efforts related to the COVID-19 pandemic. This chapter examines, among other things, the CAG's progress on (1) transitioning its responsibilities to HHS, and (2) developing a process for a joint interagency lessons learned review.

GAO reviewed CAG transition and contracting documents and interviewed or received written responses from CAG officials, federal agencies, and representatives from the six vaccine companies that worked with the CAG.

What GAO Recommends

GAO is making five recommendations related to workforce needs, scheduling best practices for vaccine-related activities; and lessons learned from key stakeholders.

HHS did not concur with GAO's recommendation on workforce needs. GAO revised this recommendation based on updated information, but maintains that it continues to be valid, as discussed in the report.

What GAO Found

Starting in May 2020, federal efforts to accelerate the development, manufacturing, and distribution of COVID-19 vaccines had been led by a partnership between the Department of Health and Human Services (HHS) and the Department of Defense (DOD). Formerly known as Operation Warp Speed, the partnership was renamed the HHS-DOD COVID-19 Countermeasures Acceleration Group (CAG). According to HHS and DOD officials, the CAG dissolved and transitioned its responsibilities—including DOD-led vaccine activities—to HHS by December 31, 2021, as required by an April 2021 memorandum of understanding between the two departments.

Manufacturing of COVID-19 Vaccines

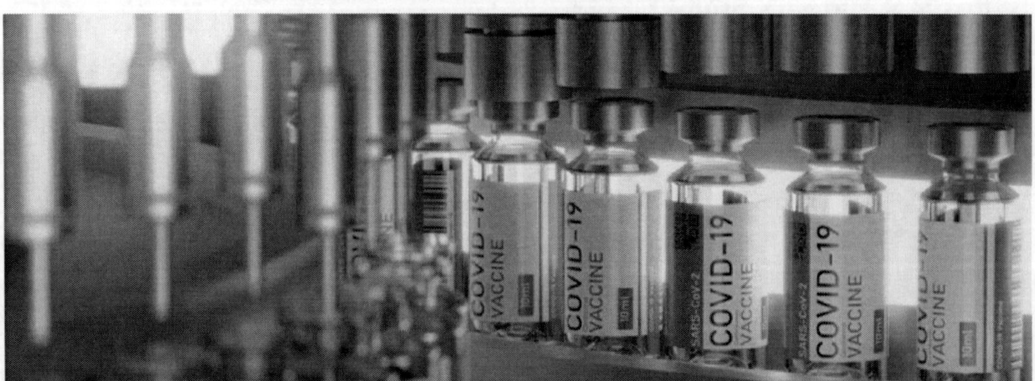

Source: Yingyaipumi/stock.adobe.com. | GAO-22-104453.

While HHS and DOD officials said they achieved transition milestones indicating that HHS is ready to assume responsibilities formerly led by DOD, it is unclear how HHS will address its workforce needs now that the CAG has dissolved.

Specifically, GAO found that HHS has assessed its workforce capabilities, but lacks strategies for addressing these workforce needs. By formally providing its support until HHS develops and implements these strategies, DOD can help ensure that HHS can continue these responsibilities uninterrupted, including responsibilities for addressing ongoing vaccine needs for boosters or for any emerging COVID-19 variants. Moreover, HHS does not have a schedule that is consistent with best practices to help it manage remaining vaccine-related activities. Such a schedule could help HHS better plan actions and mitigate delays, and be a source for identifying lessons learned for any future pandemics.

The CAG developed a plan for conducting a joint, interagency lessons-learned review. This plan outlines an approach for collecting information—such as perspectives on challenges—from CAG staff, and for sharing the plan with HHS. However, the plan misses an opportunity to gather perspectives from key external stakeholders, including vaccine companies, critical to developing vaccines. Obtaining these perspectives could provide a more comprehensive understanding of areas where the CAG was successful and opportunities for improvement, which could help inform HHS's ongoing and future vaccine work.

January 19, 2022
Congressional Addressees

Since the President declared the Coronavirus Disease 2019 (COVID-19) pandemic a national emergency on March 13, 2020, the country has reported more than 56 million confirmed cases and more than 830,000 deaths as of January 3, 2022, including a sharp increase in cases at the end of December 2021 due largely to the Omicron variant.[1] In the second year of the pandemic's catastrophic effects, the federal government's efforts to help develop and make available an adequate supply of safe and effective vaccines have been crucial to the nation's ongoing recovery. It is also critical that the federal government learn from its experiences with accelerating vaccine production so that it can be prepared to meet future vaccine needs for this pandemic—such as to counteract the emergence of new variants—or for future pandemics.[2]

To help make safe and effective vaccines available as quickly as possible, in April 2020, the federal government announced the creation of Operation Warp Speed, a partnership between the Department of Health and Human Services (HHS) and the Department of Defense (DOD). In April 2021, Operation Warp Speed was renamed the HHS-DOD COVID- 19 Countermeasures Acceleration Group (CAG), and for the purposes of this chapter, we refer to both iterations of this partnership as the CAG.

The CAG was set up to support the acceleration of vaccine development, manufacturing, and distribution to states, other jurisdictions, and federal agencies and programs for vaccine

[1] In addition to declaring a national emergency under the National Emergencies Act, the President also declared a nationwide emergency under section 501(b) of the Robert T. Stafford Disaster Relief and Emergency Assistance Act and approved major disaster declarations for all 50 states, the District of Columbia, five territories, and three federally recognized Indian tribes. On January 31, 2020, the Secretary of Health and Human Services declared a public health emergency for the United States, retroactive to January 27, 2020.

[2] As of January 2022, the Centers for Disease Control and Prevention (CDC) had listed the Delta and Omicron variants as variants of concern in the U.S. CDC had previously characterized three other variants (Alpha, Beta, and Gamma) as variants of concern but later downgraded them.

administration.[3] As a part of those efforts, HHS and DOD awarded contracts and other transaction agreements (OTA) to six vaccine companies and others for the development and manufacturing of vaccines, the purchase of vaccine doses, and the acquisition of other critical supplies and services.[4] The CAG also coordinated with other external stakeholders, including federal agencies, such as the Centers for Disease Control and Prevention (CDC), on vaccine distribution planning, according to officials.[5]

In December 2020, the first two COVID-19 vaccines—sponsored by Moderna and Pfizer—were authorized by the Food and Drug Administration (FDA) for emergency use.[6] The CAG began distributing doses of these vaccines to states and others immediately upon their authorization. As of January 2022, three COVID-19 vaccines (with the third sponsored by Janssen) were available in the United States.[7]

- Pfizer's vaccine was licensed for individuals ages 16 and older and was also available under an emergency use authorization (EUA) for individuals ages 12 to 15 years, as a lower dose for individuals ages 5 to 11 years, as a third dose for certain immunocompromised individuals ages 5 years and older, and as a booster for individuals ages 12 years and older.
- Moderna's vaccine was authorized for individuals ages 18 and older, as a third dose for certain immunocompromised individuals ages 18 an older, and as a booster for individuals ages 18 and older.
- Janssen's vaccine was authorized for individuals ages 18 and older and as a booster for the same population.[8]

By September 2021, the federal government had acquired over 673 million doses of these three vaccines, sufficient to fully vaccinate 373 million people, in line with the CAG's overall goal of having sufficient adult vaccines for the American public.[9]

An April 2021 memorandum of understanding between HHS and DOD called for the two departments to coordinate plans to transition the CAG's responsibilities to HHS, including activities that had been led by DOD. The memorandum also called for HHS and DOD to

---

[3] Jurisdictions include all 50 states, the District of Columbia, eight U.S. territories, and a small number of major cities.

[4] OTAs are flexible agreements that allow the parties to negotiate terms and conditions without requiring parties to comply with certain federal procurement laws and regulations. See 10 U.S.C. § 2371b. For more information on the accelerated COVID-19 vaccine development process, see GAO, *Operation Warp Speed: Accelerated COVID-19 Vaccine Development Status and Efforts to Address Manufacturing Challenges.* GAO-21-319, (Washington, D.C.: Feb. 11, 2021).

[5] For more information about the CAG, see our April 2021 report on the federal government's vaccine efforts. GAO, *COVID-19: Efforts to Increase Vaccine Availability and Perspectives on Initial Implementation.* GAO-21-443 (Washington, D.C.: Apr. 14, 2021).

[6] The Secretary of Health and Human Services may declare that circumstances, prescribed by statute, exist justifying the emergency use of certain medical products, such as vaccines. Once a declaration has been made, FDA may temporarily allow use of unlicensed vaccines through an emergency use authorization (EUA). For FDA to issue an EUA for a vaccine, it must be reasonable to believe that the vaccine may be effective and that the known and potential benefits of the vaccine outweigh the known and potential risks, among other statutory criteria. See 21 U.S.C. § 360bbb-3. Pfizer developed its COVID-19 vaccine in collaboration with BioNTech.

[7] Janssen Pharmaceutical Companies are a part of Johnson & Johnson.

[8] All three vaccines (Janssen, Moderna, and Pfizer) were also authorized for use as a heterologous (or "mix and match") booster for individuals ages 18 years and older, as of January 2022.

[9] According to CDC, as of October 2021, people were considered "fully vaccinated" 2 weeks after their second dose in a two-dose series, such as the Pfizer or Moderna vaccine, or 2 weeks after a single-dose vaccine, such as the Janssen vaccine. As of January 11, 2022, the term "fully vaccinated" did not include boosters.

develop a joint interagency process for incorporating lessons learned from the CAG's work into HHS's continued operations, and to dissolve the CAG by December 31, 2021.

The CARES Act includes a provision for us to report on the federal response to the COVID-19 pandemic. Specifically, the act requires us to monitor and oversee the federal government's efforts to prepare for, respond to, and recover from the pandemic.[10] This report is part of our body of work in response to the CARES Act and focuses on the activities of the CAG.[11]

In this chapter, we

1. examine the CAG's progress on transitioning responsibilities to HHS for developing, manufacturing, and distributing COVID-19 vaccines;
2. examine the CAG's progress on developing a joint interagency review process to identify lessons learned from its COVID-19 vaccine development, manufacturing, and distribution efforts; and
3. describe preliminary lessons learned we obtained from the CAG, selected federal departments, and vaccine company representatives who coordinated with the CAG on COVID-19 vaccine development, manufacturing, and distribution.

To address the first objective, we reviewed documents pertaining to the CAG's transition efforts, including the April 2021 memorandum between HHS and DOD, and the CAG's July 2021 transition plan. Specifically, we reviewed the CAG's transition readiness, including its efforts to establish milestones to gauge its progress towards transition readiness, as required by the April 2021 memorandum, and compared these efforts to selected leading practices for agency reforms, including transitions, which we identified in prior work.[12] We also reviewed the CAG's efforts to assess HHS's workforce capacity to assume the CAG's responsibilities and to develop workforce strategies to address any workforce capacity gaps. We also then compared these efforts to selected leading practices for both agency reforms and strategic workforce planning.[13] We also obtained information on the CAG's plans to assess the need for continued use of certain tools for tracking and managing remaining vaccine development, manufacturing, and distribution activities. We compared HHS's plans to manage the scheduling

---

[10] Pub. L. No. 116-136, § 19010, 134 Stat. 281, 579-81 (2020). This report also responds, in part, to a bipartisan request from the House Select Subcommittee on the Coronavirus Crisis for GAO to examine Operation Warp Speed (renamed the CAG in April 2021).

[11] We have regularly issued government-wide reports on the federal response to COVID-19. For the latest report, see GAO, *COVID-19: Additional Actions Needed to Improve Accountability and Program Effectiveness of Federal Response*, GAO-22-105051 (Washington, D.C.: Oct. 27, 2021). Our next government-wide report will be issued in January 2022 and will be available on GAO's website at https://www.gao.gov/coronavirus. Also, see the GAO Related Products section at the end of this report for additional work we have done on COVID-19 vaccines.

[12] Specifically, we assessed HHS's transition readiness efforts against the following selected agency reform leading practices: (1) developing an implementation plan with key milestones and deliverables to track implementation progress; (2) establishing a dedicated implementation team to manage the reform process; and (3) designating leaders to be responsible for the implementation of the proposed reforms. See GAO, *Government Reorganization: Key Questions to Assess Agency Reform Efforts*, GAO-18-427 (Washington, D.C., June 13, 2018).

[13] Specifically, we assessed HHS's efforts to assess its workforce capacity against the leading practice for agency reform that agencies conduct strategic workforce planning to determine whether they will have the needed resources and capacity, including the skills and competencies, in place for the proposed reforms or reorganization. See GAO-18-427. In addition, we also assessed these efforts against selected leading practices for strategic workforce planning, including that agencies should determine the critical skills and competencies needed to achieve programmatic results and develop strategies to address gaps in critical skills and competencies. See GAO, *Human Capital: Key Principles for Effective Strategic Workforce Planning,* GAO-04-39 (Washington, D.C., Dec. 11, 2003).

of vaccine development, manufacturing, and distribution activities to best practices for scheduling, as outlined in the GAO *Schedule Assessment Guide.*[14] In addition, we conducted an abridged assessment of the CAG's schedule as of May 11, 2021.[15]

To address the second objective, we reviewed documentation on the progress the CAG had made as of October 2021 to develop a joint interagency review process to identify lessons learned from its COVID-19 vaccine efforts. We interviewed CAG officials about its joint, interagency plan to develop a lessons-learned process. We compared the CAG's lessons-learned plan to leading practices we and others have previously identified for conducting a lessons-learned process, such as collecting and disseminating lessons learned.[16] We also compared the departments' plans with the Project Management Institute's program management standards, which call for program managers to engage with key stakeholders.[17]

To address the third objective, we reviewed DOD's *Countermeasures Acceleration Group Continuity Book* (CAG Continuity Book), which highlighted information about lessons learned that DOD officials within the CAG documented over the course of the CAG's COVID-19 response efforts as of May 2021.[18] In June and July 2021, we also obtained written responses or interviewed representatives from the six vaccine companies that were awarded contracts or OTAs under the CAG—AstraZeneca, Janssen, Moderna, Novavax, Pfizer, and Sanofi—about their experiences working with the CAG on vaccine development, manufacturing, and distribution. We also interviewed officials from the CAG and component offices and agencies of HHS and DOD about their perspectives on activities that worked well and any challenges they identified with the CAG's COVID-19 vaccine response efforts in June and July 2021. Within HHS, we interviewed or obtained written responses from officials from the Office of the Assistant Secretary for Preparedness and Response (ASPR), Biomedical Advanced Research and Development Authority (BARDA), CDC, FDA, and the National Institutes of Health (NIH). Within DOD, our interviews included officials from the Joint Program Executive Office for Chemical, Biological, Radiological, and Nuclear Defense (JPEO-CBRND) and the Army Contracting Command. We selected these offices and agencies because the CAG indicated that they were integral to the CAG's vaccine efforts.

---

[14] See GAO, *Schedule Assessment Guide: Best Practices for Project Schedules*, GAO-16 89G (Washington, D.C.: Dec. 22, 2015).

[15] Our abridged assessment of the CAG's schedule focused on the extent to which it was "well-constructed," as defined in the GAO *Schedule Assessment Guide*. The "well- constructed" characteristic is one of four general characteristics associated with high- quality schedules, according to the guide, and we focused on it for this abridged assessment because it reflects basic quality measures of a schedule.

[16] 16See GAO, *Federal Real Property Security: Interagency Security Committee Should Implement a Lessons-Learned Process*, GAO-12-901 (Washington, D.C.: Sept. 10, 2012); and *Project Management: DOE and NNSA Should Improve Their Lessons Learned Process for Capital Asset Projects*, GAO-19-25 (Washington, D.C.: Dec. 21, 2018). Department of the Army, Combined Arms Center, Center for Army LessonsLearned, *Establishing a Lessons Learned Program: Observations, Insights, and Lessons* (Fort Leavenworth, KS: June 2011).

[17] Project Management Institute, Inc., *A Guide to the Project Management Body of Knowledge (PMBOK® Guide)*, Sixth Edition, 2017; Project Management Institute, Inc., *Implementing Organizational Project Management: A Practice Guide*, First Edition, 2014. *PMBOK* is a trademark of Project Management Institute, Inc. The *PMBOK® Guide.* provides guidelines for managing individual projects, including collecting requirements and defining the project's scope. The Project Management Institute is a not-for-profit association that provides global standards for, among other things, project and program management. These standards are utilized worldwide and provide guidance on how to manage various aspects of projects, programs, and portfolios.

[18] CAG officials from DOD said they provided the CAG Continuity Book to incoming CAG personnel when they joined the partnership. DOD officials developed it to capture key personnel's mission, work streams, and lessons learned.

We conducted this performance audit from July 2020 to January 2022 in accordance with generally accepted government auditing standards.

Those standards require that we plan and perform the audit to obtain sufficient, appropriate evidence to provide a reasonable basis for our findings and conclusions based on our audit objectives. We believe that the evidence obtained provides a reasonable basis for our findings and conclusions based on our audit objectives.

Background

A June 2020 memorandum of understanding between HHS and DOD established the CAG, then called Operation Warp Speed, with the primary purpose of accelerating the development, production, and distribution of COVID-19 vaccines. (See appendix I for information on the status of vaccine candidates and obligations made under the CAG.)

The CAG was co-chaired by the Secretaries of Health and Human Services and Defense, who appointed HHS and DOD officials to lead five key initiatives: (1) vaccine development; (2) therapeutics; (3) supply, production, and distribution; (4) security and assurance; and (5) research, development, acquisition, and contracting.[19] In addition, the CAG had an HHS Chief Advisor, an HHS Chief Operating Officer, and a DOD Chief of Staff.[20]

As of September 2021, DOD had assigned 76 officials from the Army, the Navy, the Air Force, and the Marine Corps to work on the CAG's five key initiatives. HHS officials told us that the department generally did not assign a specific number of staff to work directly on the CAG, but stated that hundreds of officials from various HHS agencies, such as ASPR, CDC, and NIH, have worked on CAG-related efforts.

DOD Designated Lead for Most Vaccine-Related CAG Activities

The April 2021 memorandum of understanding between HHS and DOD designated DOD as the lead for implementing most vaccine-related initiatives within the CAG, with HHS to provide support. In particular, the memorandum tasked DOD with designating DOD officials to serve in the following roles, leading three of the five key initiatives:

- Director of vaccine development—directed and oversaw development and testing of vaccines in coordination with the six vaccine companies that were part of the CAG;
- Director of supply, production, and distribution—implemented and oversaw acquisition of supplies and vaccines, including having DOD officials embedded in vaccine production factories to assist with supply chain management and development of a federal governmental plan to distribute these items to the jurisdictions and other federal agencies and programs; and

[19] This report focuses primarily on the CAG's vaccine-related responsibilities.

[20] The Chief Advisor was responsible for providing technical advice regarding vaccine development and manufacturing and coordinated CAG activities with other federal departments. The Chief Operating Officer was responsible for coordinating the logistics, supply chain, development, production, and delivery of vaccines, as well as supporting HHS efforts under the CAG. The Chief of Staff supported the Chief Operating Officer in leading the CAG.

- Director of security and assurance—developed security measures for the CAG, and a security plan to support production and distribution of vaccines and supplies from the development phase to distribution.

The April 2021 memorandum also identified lead roles for DOD and HHS on the two other key initiatives. The memorandum indicated that officials from both departments shared responsibility for overseeing and supporting the research, development, acquisition, and contracting initiative, and it tasked HHS with designating a director to lead the therapeutics initiative.

Plans to Transition CAG Responsibilities to HHS

The April 2021 memorandum between HHS and DOD tasked HHS and DOD to jointly develop a plan to transition all CAG responsibilities to HHS and fully dissolve the CAG by December 31, 2021, with transition activities to begin in the fall of 2021.[21] The April 2021 memorandum stated that the transition plan was to include

- a cross-walk plan that transfers DOD activities to HHS,
- key milestones that must be achieved to ensure successful transition,
- synchronization of transition planning to ensure uninterrupted support, communications, and decision-making related to ongoing vaccine- related activities, and
- full incorporation of current efforts and lessons learned into the U.S. National Vaccine Program.[22]

Leading Practices for Agency Reforms

Reforming and reorganizing the federal government is a major endeavor that can include refocusing, realigning, or enhancing agency missions, including transitions. We have previously identified leading practices for federal agencies to follow when planning and implementing agency reforms.[23] Examples of these leading reform practices include

- identifying leaders to be responsible for the implementation of the proposed reform;
- establishing a dedicated implementation team that has the capacity, including staffing, resources, and change management, to manage the reform process;

---

[21] The original June 2020 memorandum between HHS and DOD specified that their partnership would be in place until January 31, 2021. However, on January 14, 2021,HHS and DOD extended their partnership until May 2021. Then, through their April 2021 memorandum, HHS and DOD further extended their partnership until the end of December 2021, and renamed it the CAG.

[22] The U.S. National Vaccine Program is located in the Office of the Assistant Secretary for Health within HHS. The program was established in 1986 and is responsible for the research, development, and testing of all types of vaccines, such as for the influenza and other infectious diseases, as well as the production, procurement, and distribution of vaccines to the public, among others.

[23] See GAO-18-427.

- developing an implementation plan with key milestones and deliverables to track implementation progress; and
- conducting strategic workforce planning to determine whether the new agency will have the needed resources and capacity, including the skills and competencies, in place for the proposed reform.

CAG Transitioned to HHS, but HHS Readiness to Assume All Responsibilities Unclear

The CAG Completed its Transition to HHS in December 2021

In July 2021, the CAG established a team led by co-chairs from DOD and HHS for transitioning all of the CAG's responsibilities—particularly those led by DOD—to HHS. The CAG also developed a transition plan, as called for in the April 2021 memorandum of understanding between HHS and DOD. These steps are consistent with selected leading reform practices identified in our prior work, which highlight the importance of establishing a dedicated implementation team and plan when an agency undergoes an agency reform, such as a transition.

As part of the transition plan, CAG officials developed a crosswalk—as required by the April 2021 memorandum—to guide the incremental transfer of DOD-led responsibilities to HHS. Specifically, the crosswalk organized the transition of responsibilities from DOD to HHS into nine lines of effort.[24] These lines of effort identified DOD-led responsibilities across the CAG's five key initiatives that HHS was to assume as part of the transition (see table 1). According to CAG officials, ASPR was the HHS office in charge of leading the transition of CAG responsibilities, including those led by DOD, to HHS.[25] In addition, CAG officials told us that a new office within ASPR, called the HHS Coordination Operations and Response Element, would be responsible for continuing all of the CAG's responsibilities. CAG officials told us in July 2021 that this new office would remain in place at least during the COVID-19 pandemic, but did not indicate whether it would be permanent.

Transition activities for each of the nine lines of effort began by October 15, 2021, according to CAG officials. For example, for each line of effort, CAG officials said HHS and DOD started what they refer to as "left-seat, right-seat" training, in which DOD officials trained their HHS counterparts on activities they led for about 1 month, followed by HHS officials leading activities with DOD officials assisting. CAG officials told us that the goal of this "left-seat, right seat" training is to ensure that HHS is ready to continue all of the CAG's responsibilities using HHS's own capabilities.

According to DOD and HHS officials, HHS completed its planned transition activities and the CAG dissolved on December 31, 2021, as called for in the April 2021 memorandum.

---

[24] CAG officials told us in October 2021 that DOD officials led all nine lines of effort. However, HHS officials told us in January 2022 that the Legal line of effort and the Research and Clinical Trials for Vaccines and Therapeutics line of effort were already supported by HHS officials and therefore were not transitioned from DOD to HHS.

[25] ASPR serves as the principal advisor to the Secretary of Health and Human Services on all matters related to federal public health and medical preparedness and responses for public health emergencies, among other things. 42 U.S.C. § 300hh-10(b)(1).

Table 1. Nine lines of effort for transitioning DOD responsibilities in the CAG to HHS

Line of Effort	Description
Vaccine and Therapeutics Development and Manufacturing	Coordinates the management of private-sector vaccine and therapeutic manufacturing capacity, assesses potential areas of vaccine and therapeutics supply risk and recommends mitigation options, and supports the acquisition of equipment and materials for delivery of vaccine doses.
Distribution and Administration of Therapeutics	Supports HHS's efforts to distribute COVID-19 therapeutics.
Analytics and Information Technology	Coordinates the requirements, design, and implementation of information networks. Additionally, it is responsible for leading collaborative analysis of production forecast models used by CAG leadership for decision-making.
Research and Clinical Trials for Vaccines and Therapeutics	Provides advice and alignment of all aspects of research and clinical trials for COVID-19 vaccine and therapeutics, including supporting project coordination team efforts—such as reviewing clinical trial protocol documents.
Comptroller	Oversees budget efforts and provides executive budget analysis to senior CAG officials. It also acts as the financial liaison between HHS and DOD.
External Affairs	Provides public and legislative affairs support to CAG leadership and executive staff. Specifically, it works to maintain an open and transparent dialogue with federal, state, and local government, as well as interagency partners such as the Centers for Disease Control and Prevention (CDC) and Biomedical Advanced Research and Development Authority (BARDA).
Security and Assurance	Coordinates the programs designed to safeguard the development, manufacture, and distribution of vaccines and therapeutics, and to prevent disruption across the vaccine supply chain. Additionally, it provides industrial security for companies' supply chains to identify and mitigate foreign influence or threats.
Legal	Provides legal guidance, and serves as the designated ethics counsel for personnel that are part of the CAG.
Supply, Production, and Distribution	Coordinates supply chain management, distribution, operations, and administration: Supply chain management recommends the use and administration of Defense Production Act ratings. Distribution is responsible for monitoring and enabling the movement of vaccine products from the distributor's location to the administration site. Operations is responsible overseeing vaccine production capacity, national and international distribution, and administration of COVID-19 vaccines. Administration is responsible for coordination activities and disseminating guidance to states and federal partners to ensure timely and efficient distribution and administration of COVID-19 vaccines.

Source: GAO analysis of information from the Department of Health and Human Services (HHS)-Department of Defense (DOD) COVID-19 Countermeasures Acceleration Group (CAG). | GAO-22-104453.

Notes: The lines of effort outlined in this table represent all of the CAG's responsibilities, according to documentation we reviewed and interviews with CAG officials; however, our review was primarily focused on the CAG's vaccine-related responsibilities. CAG officials told us in October 2021 that DOD officials led all nine lines of effort. However, HHS officials told us in January 2022 that the Legal line of effort and the Research and Clinical Trials for Vaccines and Therapeutics line of effort were already supported by HHS officials and therefore were not transitioned from DOD to HHS.

Additionally, CAG officials said HHS and DOD determined that DOD would provide acquisition support to HHS through at least September 2023, based on a May 2021 memorandum regarding the need for ongoing acquisition services related to vaccines, such as continued purchases of vaccine doses and other supplies. DOD's acquisition support has played a significant role in fulfilling the CAG's vaccine-related responsibilities, such as by helping to enable increases in manufacturing capacity and the purchase of vaccine doses and related supplies. DOD's contracting techniques, including solicitation approaches like broad agency announcements and commercial solutions openings, allowed DOD to obtain company input related to vaccine requirements, facility expansion, and related supplies.[26] In addition, DOD used prototype OTA and technology investment agreements to attract companies the government does not normally do business with, including vaccine companies, and to obtain vaccine-related items such as vials.[27]

For more information on these and other contracting techniques used for vaccine-related acquisitions under the CAG, see appendix II. DOD acquisition officials told us they used some of these techniques for the first time to address the COVID-19 pandemic, and doing so required a high level of acquisition expertise and staff investment.

According to DOD officials, HHS and DOD are developing plans to incrementally reduce DOD acquisition responsibilities and transition them to HHS after September 2023. DOD officials told us that as of September 15, 2021, they did not have an estimated date for when they would complete their acquisition transition plans, but the extension of DOD support through September 2023 would allow sufficient time to complete them.

It Is Unclear If HHS Is Ready to Fully Assume the CAG's Responsibilities

Neither the CAG nor HHS have completed all the tasks necessary to ensure that HHS is in a position to fully assume all of the CAG's responsibilities beginning January 1, 2022. In particular, HHS and DOD officials indicated that they developed and completed transition milestones showing HHS's readiness to assume the CAG's responsibilities without a loss of capabilities. However, the documentation HHS provided to us in January 2022 does not identify or describe such milestones for all lines of effort or show how the milestones were achieved. Similarly, although HHS conducted workforce assessments to evaluate its workforce capacity for leading the lines of effort, it has not developed and implemented strategies to address identified workforce needs for some lines of effort. Further, HHS has not developed a schedule to manage the remaining vaccine development, manufacturing, and distribution activities.

Documentation Does Not Identify Transition Milestones or How They Were Achieved

The April 2021 memorandum between HHS and DOD and the CAG's July 2021 transition plan specify that the CAG would develop milestones, by August 2021, to gauge the progress of the transition and indicate when it is ready to transfer responsibilities for each of the nine lines of

[26] A broad agency announcement is a notice from the government that requests scientific or research and development proposals from private firms concerning certain areas of interest to the government. See Federal Acquisition Regulation (FAR) § 35.016. The commercial solutions opening pilot program allows DOD to mirror the contracting practices that commercial companies normally use, enabling DOD to design projects, and negotiate payment milestones, intellectual property rights, and other terms and conditions for a desired completion period of within 60 days. See National Defense Authorization Act for Fiscal Year 2017, Pub. L. No. 114-328, § 879, 130 Stat. 2000, 2312-13 (2016) (codified at 10 U.S.C. § 2303 note).

[27] Technology investment agreements are used to stimulate or support research to foster the best technologies for future defense needs. See 32 C.F.R. Part 37 (2020).

effort to HHS.[28] Developing such milestones is consistent with leading practices we identified for agency reform practices.[29] In documentation HHS and DOD provided to us in January 2022, the departments indicated that they developed and achieved transition milestones for the lines of effort by December 2021.

While the transition is now complete, and responsibilities have been transferred to HHS, the documentation the departments provided to us in January 2022 did not identify or describe such milestones for all lines of effort, or show how they were achieved. Specifically, CAG officials provided finalized milestones for two lines of effort—the External Affairs and the Comptroller lines of effort. For these lines of effort, the CAG developed specific milestones to be achieved—such as the reconciliation and handoff of CAG financial documents to HHS for the Comptroller line of effort—in its transition progress assessment documentation. For five other lines of effort, HHS provided documentation that a senior official reviewed transition milestones and associated tasks and approved HHS to assume responsibilities, but the documentation does not identify specific milestones or show how they were achieved. For example, documentation for the Supply, Production, and Distribution and Analytics and Information Technology lines of effort identified transition tasks that had not yet been completed, without an indication of when or by whom those tasks would be finalized. According to HHS officials, milestones were continuously adjusted based on a variety of factors as the transition progressed. Without documentation of specific milestones and how they were achieved, it is unclear how HHS determined its readiness to assume the CAG's responsibilities.

HHS Has Not Finalized Strategic Workforce Planning

As of January 2022 HHS had conducted assessments of HHS's workforce capacity for seven lines of effort.[30] For two of these— Comptroller and Vaccine and Therapeutics Development and Manufacturing—HHS determined that it had a sufficient amount of personnel in place with the required skills to continue the lines of effort's responsibilities. For another line of effort—External Affairs—HHS completed a workforce assessment that showed it identified and filled a position for a communication specialist. This action resulted in sufficient capacity for that line of effort, according to HHS. However, for the remaining four lines of effort, the transition documentation we reviewed did not indicate that HHS had developed and implemented a workforce strategy to resolve identified personnel gaps resulting from DOD's departure. For instance, activities under the Security and Assurance line of effort include coordinating programs designed to safeguard the development, manufacture, and distribution of vaccines, and to provide industrial security for vaccine companies' supply chains. The CAG's transition document for this line of effort indicated that the workforce assessment found that HHS did not

---

[28] The transition included nine lines of effort. In providing comments on a draft of this report, HHS stated that two lines of effort—the Legal line of effort and the Research and Clinical Trials for Vaccines and Therapeutics line of effort—were already supported by existing staff within HHS and therefore did not require transition milestones.

[29] See GAO-18-427. One leading agency reform practice is that agencies should develop and implement a plan with key milestones and deliverables to track progress for the reform, such as a transition.

[30] The transition included nine lines of effort. In providing comments on a draft of this report, HHS stated that two lines of effort—the Legal line of effort and the Research and Clinical Trials for Vaccines and Therapeutics line of effort—were already supported by existing staff within HHS and therefore did not require workforce assessments as part of the transition from CAG to HHS.

have the necessary staff to continue the CAG's responsibilities, and identified a need for multiple additional contractors to maintain the line of effort's capabilities. However, the documentation did not identify a strategy for addressing this need.

In another example, activities under the Supply, Production, and Distribution line of effort included providing assistance to vaccine companies, such as through detailing DOD personnel to serve as temporary quality control staff at vaccine manufacturing sites. According to CAG officials, additional activities for this Supply, Production, and Distribution line of effort included managing the supply of manufacturing items and the allocation and distribution of vaccine doses to jurisdictions and other entities. CAG officials' assessment of this line of effort found that HHS did not have the staff with the necessary specialized skills and competencies—including communication and logistic expertise—to continue the CAG's responsibilities, according to officials. As a result, officials stated that HHS awarded a contract on October 15, 2021 to bring in personnel to help resolve those skill gaps. However, the transition document we reviewed noted that as of December 1, 2021, HHS was awaiting contractor personnel for the Supply, Production, and Distribution line of effort while managing the limited availability of existing contracting support, and that none of that particular line of effort's responsibilities had transitioned to HHS, raising questions about HHS's readiness to take on such work.[31]

Our prior work shows that delays in developing and implementing workforce strategies to address identified personnel gaps may be problematic. For example, in our September 2020 report describing, in part, medical supply management responsibility shifting to HHS related to the COVID-19 pandemic, we found that it could be hard to hire the acquisition staff with expertise in Defense Production Act (DPA) contracting that ASPR had determined they would need to further support COVID-19 vaccine and related supply acquisitions.[32] This misalignment of staff needs with available resources could lead to skill gaps within HHS's workforce, and put HHS in jeopardy of successfully assuming all of the CAG's responsibilities. Determining critical workforce skills and capabilities—and developing strategies to address any needs—also follows selected leading practices identified by our prior work.[33]

Given that DOD has specialized skills and competencies and had been leading many of the CAG's vaccine-related responsibilities before the CAG dissolved, addressing workforce capacity needs is particularly important, so that HHS can continue these responsibilities uninterrupted. Without doing so, there is a risk that HHS may not have some of the capabilities necessary to continue critical vaccine-related activities going forward.

HHS Indicated It Will Continue Using a Key Information System, but Has Not Developed a Schedule to Manage Activities

As HHS was assuming the CAG's responsibilities, HHS officials indicated they planned to continue utilizing a key information system—Tiberius—for tracking their ongoing COVID-19

---

[31] Our review of the transition document for the Supply, Production, and Distribution line of effort indicated that DOD personnel would continue their responsibilities for this line of effort, beyond December 31, 2021.

[32] See GAO, *COVID-19: Federal Efforts Could be Strengthened by Timely and Concerted Actions*, GAO-20-701 (Washington, D.C., Sept. 21, 2020). The DPA facilitates the supply and timely delivery of products, materials, and services to military and civilian agencies in support of the national defense, including in response to emergency preparedness activities. See Pub. L. No. 81-774, 64 Stat. 798 (1950) (codified, as amended, at 50 U.S.C. §§ 4501 et seq.).

[33] See GAO-18-427 and GAO-04-39.

vaccine manufacturing and distribution activities. However, HHS has not developed a schedule to manage remaining vaccine development, manufacturing, and distribution activities.

Tiberius. The CAG used Tiberius—an integrated information technology database that incorporates information from outside sources, such as vaccine companies and jurisdictions—to help manage and track its COVID-19 vaccine manufacturing, distribution, and administration activities.[34] In particular, according to CAG officials, Tiberius was the principal information system used by jurisdictions to review weekly vaccine allocations. Specifically, Tiberius received a data feed from the electronic system the jurisdictions used to order their vaccines, and then information from that data feed displayed various metrics for each jurisdiction, such as the number of doses available to order and ordered by a jurisdiction.

As part of the transition, HHS officials said they extended a key Tiberius contract for software development through at least July 2022.[35] Additionally, HHS officials told us that the HHS Office of the Chief Information Officer coordinated with officials from the CAG, CDC, and ASPR to transition management of Tiberius to CDC. According to HHS officials, CDC plans to integrate Tiberius into its existing systems, which would allow CDC to continue using the system, as well as determine any long-term plans for using Tiberius after July 2022.

Schedule. HHS has not developed a specific schedule to help manage the remaining COVID-19 vaccine-related responsibilities once the CAG dissolved—such as those related to managing the distribution of vaccine doses for boosters or children, or to address any emerging COVID-19 variants.[36] According to the GAO *Schedule Assessment Guide*, a schedule—as a normal part of project management—assists project managers by providing a road map for systematic project execution, defining when and how long work will occur, and indicating how each activity within a project is related to others, among other benefits.[37] For example, a schedule could include activities for distribution of sufficient vaccine doses across the states and other jurisdictions for boosters, for children, or for addressing variants. As such, a schedule—particularly one that follows best practices such as including all activities, placing them in sequence, assigning resources to them, and establishing their duration— can help managers to identify and mitigate scheduling risks, such as delays. According to the guide, a schedule for a completed project can also be a valuable source of lessons learned—showing what actually happened compared to expectations—when planning similar future projects.

HHS officials told us that the department will no longer use an existing schedule developed by the CAG, as the contract that supported the CAG's schedule has ended.[38] In addition, rather than developing a new schedule, HHS officials told us that the department will instead rely on its project coordination teams to manage the schedules for these activities, by working with the Biomedical Advanced Research and Development Authority (BARDA) and the vaccine

---

[34] According to HHS and DOD officials, the federal government owns the Tiberius software, but licenses the right to use its hosting platform from the private company that established and maintains the platform.

[35] CAG officials estimate that it will cost approximately $32 million per year to maintain and continue to use Tiberius.

[36] Additionally, three COVID-19 vaccines that were part of the CAG remained in development; as of January 2022, the AstraZeneca, Novavax, and Sanofi vaccines were still in development and had not been authorized or licensed for use in the United States.

[37] See GAO-16-89G. Scheduling allows officials to decide between possible sequences of activities, determine the flexibility of the schedule according to available resources, predict the consequences of managerial action or inaction on events, and develop contingency plans to mitigate risks.

[38] In June 2020, the CAG developed a schedule to help manage the alignment of the hundreds of individual tasks needed to support its efforts to develop, manufacture, and distribute the various COVID-19 vaccines. Examples of these tasks include monitoring the timing of clinical trials conducted by vaccine companies; vaccine quality control testing; and the shipment of vaccine doses to specific sites across various jurisdictions for administration.

companies.[39] However, officials have not provided information on how this coordination would result in a reliable schedule that follows best practices.

HHS officials also noted that the information once provided by the CAG's schedule will continue to be made available via the project coordination teams and BARDA officials. However, our separate review of the CAG's schedule indicated that its information was not reliable. Specifically, we found that the CAG's schedule minimally or partially met best practices associated with a "well-constructed" schedule, as defined in the GAO *Schedule Assessment Guide*.[40] In particular, we found a number of missing logical dependencies, which help show how activities that fall behind in the schedule will affect succeeding activities that depend on them, or how these delays would affect the overall project schedule. We also could not identify a valid critical path, and determined the schedule exhibited an unreasonable amount of total float. For more information about the CAG's schedule, including our abridged assessment of it, see appendix III.

Having a schedule that is consistent with identified best practices can help officials have confidence in their ability to manage vaccine development, manufacturing, and distribution efforts. Specifically, developing a schedule that is consistent with best practices could help HHS determine the amount of scheduling flexibility it has, predict the consequences of managerial action or inaction in events, and develop contingency plans to mitigate delays or other risks while completing activities related to vaccines for boosters, for children, or for addressing emerging variants. In addition, developing such a schedule would help HHS to better archive the actual sequence of events for completing its remaining activities, which could be a source of lessons learned to analyze during its planning for any future pandemics.

The CAG Began a Lessons-Learned Review Process, but Its Plans Do Not Include Collecting Information from Stakeholders

The CAG began a joint interagency lessons-learned review process in August 2021 to assess its COVID-19 vaccine development, manufacturing, and distribution efforts, as called for by the April 2021 memorandum. Specifically, the CAG established an interagency workgroup and a review process the CAG would use for collecting lessons learned across each of the nine lines of effort, according to officials. As of September 2021, CAG officials expected they would complete their process of collecting lessons learned no later than December 31, 2021, and that these lessons learned would be available to help guide the transition of CAG responsibilities to HHS. However, we did not receive updated information about the process's completion.

---

[39] According to CAG officials, project coordination teams consisted of federal employees and contractors from HHS and DOD who were responsible for coordinating vaccine development and manufacturing efforts. Additionally, CAG officials told us these teams also served as contact points between the federal government and each of the six vaccine companies that were part of the CAG. Furthermore, CAG officials told us that collectively the project coordination teams fell under the DOD-appointed Director of Vaccines, but each of the six teams were led by HHS officials.

[40] A schedule is well-constructed if all its activities are logically sequenced with the most straightforward logic possible. The best practices of a well-constructed schedule include (1) logical sequencing of all activities—that is, listing the activities in the order in which they are to be logically carried out; (2) confirming that the schedule has a valid critical path—that is, the longest continuous sequence of activities in a schedule and the path that defines the program's earliest completion date or minimum duration; and (3) identifying reasonable total float or slack—the amount of time an activity could be delayed before that delay affects the program's overall estimated finish date.

Officials said they planned to compile the lessons learned collected across all nine lines of effort into a single report, issued no later than March 31, 2022.

We found that the CAG's lessons-learned plan—finalized in September 2021—aligns with some leading practices for conducting lessons-learned reviews that we and others have identified, including collecting and sharing information on any positive and negative experiences.[41] Figure 1 shows these leading practices.

For example, the CAG's lessons-learned plan delineates responsibilities for collecting information on lessons learned by completing after-action reports and exit interviews with CAG officials.[42] It states that prior to departure from the CAG, every official assigned to the CAG should provide input on lessons learned—such as their perspectives on significant challenges and best practices—to their line of effort's point of contact for inclusion in an after-action report.[43] The lessons-learned plan also includes an overview of how CAG officials would transfer or share relevant records with HHS, so that HHS has the necessary information to continue the work.

However, based on our review, the CAG's lessons-learned plan did not meet other leading practices. Specifically, the CAG's planned interagency review process did not include efforts to engage stakeholders in identifying lessons learned. Leading practices emphasize the importance of engaging with key stakeholders—that is, those entities who played significant roles in supporting the CAG's activities. As an example of these leading practices, *The Standard for Program Management*, produced by the Project Management Institute, states that program managers should actively engage key stakeholders throughout the life cycle of a program, which would include lessons-learned processes and evaluation activities, such as completing after-action reviews.[44]

According to CAG officials, the lessons-learned review process is internally focused and does not outline an approach to collect information from key stakeholders outside of the CAG, such as the vaccine companies or other federal agencies that coordinated with the CAG. The six vaccine companies, as well as several HHS and DOD component offices and agencies, were key stakeholders that played significant roles in the CAG's COVID-19 vaccine development, manufacturing, and distribution efforts. As such, they may have valuable contributions to make to the lessons-learned reviews.

CAG officials said their lessons-learned review process was intended to collect information internally from staff assigned to the CAG. Officials added that CAG officials may have chosen

---

[41] See GAO-21-8, GAO-20-104, GAO-19-25, and GAO-12-901. See also Center for Army Lessons Learned, *Establishing a Lessons Learned Program*.

[42] According to the lessons-learned plan, the objective of the after-action reports and associated exit interviews is to provide context to HHS regarding CAG operations and decisions in order to streamline decision-making for efforts to respond to potential future pandemics. The after-action reports will serve as a historic record of accomplishments facilitated by the CAG.

[43] According to CAG officials, the Supply, Production, and Distribution line of effort was subdivided into five separate sections. They said that while one official will continue to serve as the primary point of contact, the official will coordinate with five other individuals who are responsible for completing the after-action reviews for the five subdivided areas under this specific line of effort.

[44] See Project Management Institute, Inc., A Guide to the Project Management Body of Knowledge (PMBOK® Guide), Sixth Edition, 2017. GAO, Disaster Response: HHS Should Address Deficiencies Highlighted by Recent Hurricanes in the U.S. Virgin Islands and Puerto Rico, GAO-19-592 (Washington, D.C.: Sept. 20, 2019). The Project Management Institute is a not-for-profit association that provides global standards for, among other things, project and program management. These standards are utilized worldwide and provide guidance on how to manage various aspects of projects, programs, and portfolios.

to gather information from key stakeholders outside the CAG—at their discretion during the lessons- learned process—but that there was no plan or requirement for them to do so.

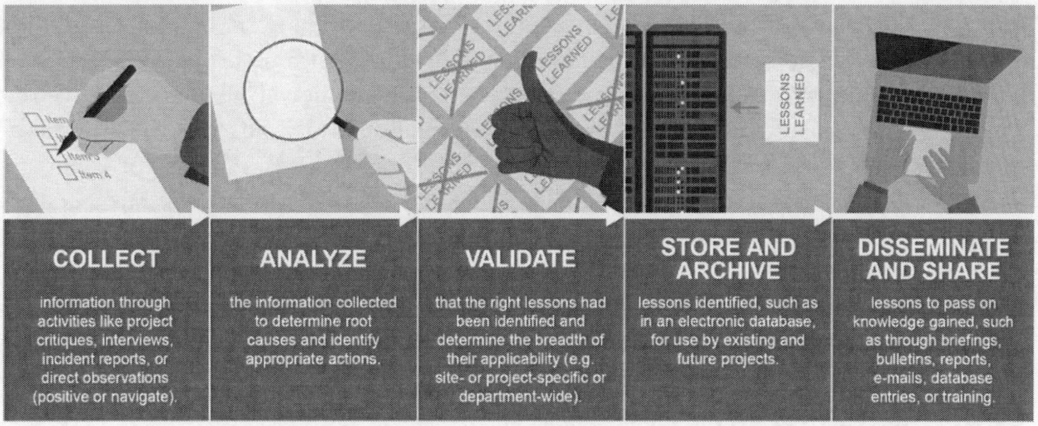

Source: Analysis of prior GAO reports and the Center for Army Lessons Learned report, *Establishing a Lessons learned Program: Observations, Insights, and Lessons*. | GAO-22-104453.

Figure 1. Leading Practices of a Lessons-Learned Review Process.

By expanding the lessons learned review to also obtain and incorporate the perspectives of key external stakeholders, HHS and DOD could better ensure that HHS has the full benefit of capturing perspectives from all of the significant players involved in the CAG's vaccine-related efforts.

Moreover, these perspectives could help provide a more comprehensive understanding of what worked well and of areas for potential improvement to help inform ongoing and any future vaccine development, manufacturing, and distribution efforts.

Preliminary Lessons Learned from the CAG, Federal Agencies, and Vaccine Company Representatives

Based on our review of information from and interviews with CAG officials, federal agency officials, and vaccine company representatives in June 2021 and July 2021, we identified some examples of preliminary lessons learned. The preliminary lessons learned we identified covered several areas, as described below.

Selecting multiple vaccine companies and platforms. According to CAG officials, the CAG's strategy to build a diverse portfolio of vaccine candidates from multiple companies that use different platform technologies worked well.[45] CAG officials highlighted the federal government's strategy to award contracts and OTAs to multiple vaccine companies developing COVID-19 vaccines.

As we have previously reported, the federal government took on financial risk to support or purchase doses of the six vaccine candidates by enabling large-scale manufacturing to start while clinical trials were ongoing, before their safety and effectiveness of the candidates was

---

[45] A vaccine platform is the mechanism used to stimulate an immune response in a recipient.

fully known.[46] We noted that this approach helped to enable distribution of vaccines as soon as possible upon receiving FDA authorization or licensure.

CAG officials noted that including vaccine candidates from different platforms—before knowing whether any would be successful—involved significant costs but helped to allow multiple candidates to receive EUAs within 9 months of establishing the CAG, and to have significant numbers of manufactured doses available for distribution at the time the EUAs were issued. We previously reported that because these platforms use different mechanisms to stimulate an immune response, having a variety of platforms decreases the risk of failure due to safety, effectiveness, or manufacturing factors that may affect some platforms but not others.

Having multiple candidates also increased the chances that one or more candidate would be successful.[47]

Sharing expertise and coordinating across DOD, HHS, and vaccine companies. Officials from the CAG, DOD, HHS, and NIH told us that HHS's expertise in the sciences and DOD's expertise in planning, logistics, programming, and contract management complemented each other, and both were necessary to make the CAG's COVID-19 vaccine development, manufacturing, and distribution efforts successful.

Specifically, according to CAG officials, HHS worked with several vaccine companies as they conducted clinical trials, focusing on the safety and effectiveness of the vaccine candidates throughout the clinical trial process. For example, NIH's National Institute of Allergy and Infectious Diseases made research staff available to several vaccine companies to help collaborate on the companies' clinical trials. NIH staff also helped vaccine companies find sites to conduct clinical trials and solicit enrollees for the trials.

In addition, the CAG DOD team provided operational and logistics expertise, such as delivering personal protective equipment for the clinical trial sites when needed, and installing mobile trailers if additional capacity was required. HHS and DOD's coordination worked well in this instance and both agencies learned from each other, according to CAG officials.

In contrast, representatives from two vaccine companies told us that there were initial coordination challenges in their interactions with the CAG, which improved over time. For example, the representatives said that they sometimes needed to report the same information multiple times to officials from different federal agencies, or to different groups within the same agency. They said that the multiple reporting requirements became time consuming and distracting at times, and led to confusion about who within the government was responsible for making decisions. According to these representatives, coordination and communication with the CAG improved as they continued working with the officials over time.

Using project coordination teams. BARDA officials noted the importance of forming project coordination teams to support vaccine companies' efforts, and including a leader (from BARDA, NIH, or DOD) and a team of program managers and subject matter experts in all

---

[46] See GAO-21-319 and GAO-21-443. Pfizer funded the research and development of its COVID-19 vaccine. The federal government agreed to pay for doses of Pfizer's vaccine upon FDA authorization or licensure and as the doses were delivered. HHS officials stated that this agreement required the government to buy Pfizer vaccine doses upon authorization or licensure, even if other vaccines were found to be more cost effective or efficacious.

[47] See GAO-21-319. It is also possible that a diverse portfolio of vaccine platforms could offer additional benefits over time. Different vaccine platforms may also be more effective in different individuals—for example, older adults or pediatric populations. Further, a diverse portfolio of vaccine platforms may allow for the use of mixed vaccine platform boosters. Scientific studies have shown that mixed boosters might help better address the emergence of SARS-CoV-2 variants and decreasing immunity over time. For example, mixed vaccine platform boosters may help stimulate different parts of the immune system, resulting in better and longer-lasting immune responses, or decrease the risk of adverse events from the original vaccine from developing or happening again.

critical areas of vaccine development and manufacturing. BARDA officials said that in the fall of 2020, project coordination teams would meet daily with each vaccine company to discuss the resources necessary to accelerate vaccine development and to help identify scientific, technical, and strategic risks and any plans for mitigating those risks, among other things. According to CAG officials, the teams continued to conduct meetings 4 times weekly to provide progress updates to the CAG's leadership and other stakeholders about any vaccine-related issues or resource constraints.

Using supply chain managers and the DPA for vaccine manufacturing. CAG officials said that they embedded federal government supply chain managers to work at vaccine manufacturing sites. According to CAG officials, this approach allowed for daily progress updates to its leadership during the fall of 2020, and close coordination between the federal government and manufacturing companies regarding any supply chain issues that could affect manufacturing.

Representatives from two vaccine companies commented on the CAG's efforts to support manufacturing efforts through use of the Defense Production Act (DPA), which has allowed companies to have priority access to necessary materials.[48] Federal agencies used the DPA and other actions more than 100 times to respond to the COVID-19 pandemic and stabilize the medical supply chain through September 2021.[49] Use of the DPA enabled one vaccine company, for example, to have priority access to lipids, bags, and filters to help manufacture its COVID-19 vaccine.

Representatives from one vaccine company said the use of the DPA in limited circumstances could help secure supply-constrained raw materials needed to produce COVID-19 vaccines. However, they added that the company's suppliers have noted that exercising the DPA can create production challenges and disruptions, because it can restrict suppliers' flexibility and ability to maximize capacity.[50]

According to DOD's CAG Continuity Book, use of the DPA requires close coordination of priorities and deliveries to ensure production stability, and is "not a miracle solution." For example, the CAG Continuity Book notes that domestic fill-finish capacity was limited even prior to the COVID-19 pandemic. It states that the need to use existing capacity to address needs during the pandemic meant that less capacity was available for other life-saving medicines. The CAG Continuity Book also emphasizes the importance of expanding manufacturing capacity for future public health emergencies, to ensure sufficient capacity for both routine commercial business and the surge of increased capacity needs due to the emergency.

Contracting for vaccine development and manufacturing. According to CAG officials, constant communication between contracting, legal, and scientific experts was key to obtaining the vaccines. Specifically, DOD's Joint Program Executive Office for Chemical, Biological, Radiological, and Nuclear Defense (JPEO-CBRND) and Army Contracting Command used

---

[48] Contracts with a priority rating under the DPA require a contractor to give preference to these contracts over any other unrated contracts if the contractor cannot meet all required delivery date needs for all contracts. See 50 U.S.C. § 4511.

[49] "Other actions" refers to industrial base expansion projects for medical supplies that have similar goals but were not executed under the DPA Title III authority. See GAO, *COVID-19: Agencies Are Taking Steps to Improve Future Use of Defense Production Act Authorities*. GAO-22-105380. (Washington, D.C.: Dec. 16, 2021).

[50] We previously reported on the unintended consequences that could result from use of the DPA to expedite the receipt of supply-constrained materials for vaccine manufacturing (i.e., creating constrained supplies for other life-saving medicines). See GAO-21-443.

their acquisition workforce expertise and prototype OTA authority—which DOD officials say enabled command officials to negotiate terms and conditions in agreements with five of the six vaccine companies.[51]

In addition, JPEO-CBRND officials said that using a flat organizational structure—with direct contact between acquisition senior leaders and staff—allowed for efficient communication, which enabled quick decision- making when it was necessary. For example, these officials told us that having access to senior leadership on a regular basis, through the leaders' participation in work group meetings and team discussions, helped to reduce the normal acquisition processing times for vaccines by months. Officials added that senior leaders were prepared to review contract documents quickly when they came in for approval, thereby minimizing the contract award time.

CAG officials noted that a challenge they experienced was the initial lack of enough acquisition staff to support the sustained high-volume, high- tempo workload. JPEO-CBRND provided 10-12 employees in direct support of CAG operations, embedded with the project coordination teams, and asked them to work longer hours. According to CAG officials, in approximately May 2021, JPEO-CBRND was authorized to acquire about 75 additional employees and contractors, which helped to relieve the burden on JPEO-CBRND staff.

Communicating COVID-19 vaccine-related activities to the public and vaccine companies. CAG officials told us that the CAG helped to support the federal government's frequent public updates on vaccine development, starting around November 2020. However, the officials noted that the federal government could have better communicated with the public to help people who were unfamiliar with vaccine development understand the inherent unpredictability of the process. Specifically, CAG officials explained that development of biologics, including vaccines, is more unpredictable than other types of drug development and can lead to unforeseen production failures. For example, actual production amounts could be lower than estimated amounts due to the inherent fragility in the process. CAG officials noted that the federal government could work to better communicate expectations for some fluctuation in estimated amounts of available vaccine doses given the nature of vaccine production.

Representatives from one vaccine company noted that ongoing communication with the involved federal agencies allowed them to continuously improve their plans for vaccine rollout. Another vaccine company's representatives stated that the federal agencies provided guidance, feedback, and resources needed through each stage of their clinical trial programs. According to these representatives, direct and frequent communication with federal agencies helped to ensure the vaccine company aligned with safety and effectiveness evaluation practices expected of all federally-funded studies.

---

[51] As we previously reported, OTAs can help agencies contract with entities that have not previously done business with the federal government due to concerns about standard contracting requirements. However, there may be challenges associated with their use, including a risk of reduced accountability and transparency, which we addressed in prior reports. See GAO, *COVID-19 Contracting: Actions Needed to Enhance Transparency and Oversight of Selected Awards*, GAO-21-501 (Washington, D.C.: July 26, 2021) and GAO, *COVID-19 Contracting: Observations on Federal Contracting in Response to the Pandemic*, GAO-20-632 (Washington, D.C.: July 29, 2020).

Conclusion

The accelerated development, manufacturing, and distribution of vaccines has been a critical part of the U.S. response to the COVID-19 pandemic. The federal government has shown it can rapidly and effectively mobilize partnerships to produce safe and effective vaccines to help the nation respond to and recover from the pandemic's catastrophic effects. The CAG partnership between HHS and DOD is an example of a quickly built and effective partnership, as are related agreements between the federal government and private vaccine companies.

As HHS assumes all responsibilities of the CAG, it is vital that the department continues these activities without interruptions. This is especially critical as the pandemic continues well into its second year and the federal government looks to provide greater access to vaccines, such as through the recent availability of boosters and vaccines for children, as well as to prepare for emerging COVID-19 variants and for future pandemics.

HHS and DOD stated that they developed and achieved milestones indicating HHS's readiness to assume the CAG's responsibilities—a critical step to ensuring the successful continuation of the CAG's vaccine work. However, available documentation does not identify most of these milestones, nor does the documentation demonstrate how the milestones were achieved. In addition, while HHS has assessed its workforce's ability to take on tasks that DOD had previously led within the CAG, HHS has yet to address some of the workforce needs that it identified. By developing and implementing a workforce strategy to address HHS's workforce needs, HHS and DOD can mitigate any risks and help ensure that HHS is ready to continue the CAG's work uninterrupted.

Furthermore, HHS has not developed a schedule to help it manage remaining vaccine development, manufacturing, and distribution activities. Developing a schedule that is consistent with best practices would provide a road map for systematic execution of vaccine-related activities, as well as a means by which to help better plan actions, gauge progress, and identify and resolve potential problems. In addition, such a schedule could help HHS better archive the actual sequence of events for completing its remaining activities, which could in turn provide a source of lessons learned for any future pandemics.

Additionally, although HHS and DOD have begun their joint interagency review to help inform HHS's future vaccine activities, the departments do not have plans to gather perspectives from stakeholders outside of the CAG. By also obtaining and incorporating the perspectives of key external stakeholders—such as from vaccine companies or other federal agency officials who worked with the CAG—HHS and DOD have an opportunity to obtain a more comprehensive understanding of what worked well and of areas for potential improvement to inform ongoing and any future vaccine development, manufacturing, and distribution efforts.

Recommendations for Executive Action

We are making a total of five recommendations, including three to the Secretary of Health and Human Services, and two to the Secretary of Defense:

The Secretary of Health and Human Services, in coordination with DOD, should develop and implement workforce strategies to address the workforce needs it identified as part of the CAG's transition to HHS. (Recommendation 1)

The Secretary of Defense, in coordination with HHS, should establish a mechanism—such as through an interagency agreement—to provide support to HHS until it develops and implements workforce strategies to address the workforce needs it identified as part of the CAG's transition to HHS. (Recommendation 2)

The Secretary of Health and Human Services should develop a schedule that is consistent with the best practices established in the GAO Schedule Assessment Guide to manage remaining vaccine-related responsibilities. (Recommendation 3)

The Secretary of Health and Human Services, in coordination with DOD, should expand the CAG's lessons-learned review to also obtain and incorporate input from key external stakeholders, such as vaccine companies and other federal agencies that coordinated with the CAG on its vaccine-related responsibilities. (Recommendation 4)

The Secretary of Defense, in coordination with HHS, should expand the CAG's lessons-learned review to obtain and incorporate input from key external stakeholders, such as vaccine companies and other federal agencies that coordinated with the CAG on its vaccine-related responsibilities. (Recommendation 5)

Agency Comments and Our Evaluation

We provided a draft of this report to HHS and DOD for review and comment. Both departments provided written comments, which are reproduced in appendix IV and V, respectively. HHS also provided technical comments, which we incorporated as appropriate. In written comments from HHS, the department concurred with two recommendations, and did not concur with two other recommendations.

In the draft report, provided to the departments in early December 2021 before the CAG dissolved, we recommended that HHS, in coordination with DOD, should finalize and achieve transition milestones, to help demonstrate HHS's readiness to assume the CAG's responsibilities before DOD formally ended its support. At that time, the CAG had not finalized transition milestones for seven of the nine lines of effort. HHS did not concur with this recommendation because, according to HHS in its comments on our draft report, the department had successfully completed the planned transition of responsibilities to the newly established HHS Coordination Operations and Response Element by its deadline of January 1, 2022. HHS provided memos stating that milestones had been achieved and detailing transition activities. While the memos did not identify or describe such milestones or show how they were achieved, we removed this draft recommendation because the CAG's responsibilities have transferred to HHS. Nonetheless, without a clear understanding of what information the transition was based on—including the specific milestones developed and how those were achieved—we remain concerned that HHS has not demonstrated its readiness to fully assume all responsibilities formerly undertaken by the CAG.

HHS also did not concur with the draft report's second recommendation to complete assessments of its workforce capacity and develop corresponding workforce strategies. In its written comments on our draft report, HHS stated this was because the department completed workforce assessments by January 1, 2022, after we sent the draft report for review. HHS also provided additional documents describing these workforce assessments, and we revised our report to indicate that HHS had completed these assessments. However, as our report indicates, the assessments also identified specific workforce needs, but do not include strategies for addressing those needs. As a result, our report recommends that HHS develop such strategies so that it can mitigate any workforce-related risks and help ensure that it successfully continues its work uninterrupted.

HHS concurred with our recommendation to develop a schedule to manage remaining vaccine-related responsibilities, consistent with best practices. In its written comments, HHS stated that its new office, the HHS Coordination Operations and Response Element, will make assessments regarding the future use of schedules, taking into consideration the best practices established in the GAO Schedule Assessment Guide. HHS also concurred with our recommendation to expand the CAG's lessons-learned review to obtain and incorporate input from key external stakeholders.

In written comments from DOD, the department concurred with the two recommendations directed to it. In the draft report, we recommended that DOD establish a mechanism to formally provide support to HHS until CAG transition milestones are finalized and achieved, and until HHS completes its planned assessments of its workforce capacity and develops corresponding workforce strategies. DOD stated that it concurred with the recommendation, although transition milestones were finalized and achieved by December 31, 2021. As noted above, we also received documentation from HHS that it had finalized milestones and developed workforce assessments. In light of this new information, we modified our recommendation to DOD to provide support to HHS in developing workforce strategies to address the workforce needs it identified as part of the CAG's transition to HHS. DOD also concurred with our recommendation to expand the CAG's lessons-learned review to obtain and incorporate input from key external stakeholders.

Appendix I: Status of U.S. COVID-19 Vaccine Candidates and Related Obligations and Doses

To support the Department of Health and Human Services (HHS)- Department of Defense (DOD) COVID-19 Countermeasures Acceleration Group (CAG) (formerly known as Operation Warp Speed), HHS and DOD awarded contracts and other transaction agreements (OTA) to six vaccine companies and others.[52] We reviewed the related contract documentation and found that these contracts and OTAs were awarded for the development and manufacturing of vaccines, the purchase of vaccine doses, and the acquisition of other critical supplies and services. See table 2 for the status of each of the six vaccine candidates as of January 11, 2022.

[52] The six vaccine companies are AstraZeneca, Janssen, Moderna, Novavax, Pfizer, and Sanofi. Pfizer developed its COVID-19 vaccine in collaboration with BioNTech, and Sanofi is developing its COVID-19 vaccine candidate in collaboration with GSK. Janssen Pharmaceutical Companies are a part of Johnson & Johnson. OTAs are flexible agreements that allow the parties to negotiate terms and conditions without requiring parties to comply with certain federal procurement laws and regulations. See 10 U.S.C. § 2371b.

Table 2. Status of the CAG's six vaccine candidates, as of January 11, 2022

Vaccine company	Findings from phase 3 clinical trials announced	EUA in effect[a]	Biologics license application (BLA) approved[b]
AstraZeneca	•	-	-
Janssen[c]	•	18 and older; booster for 18 and older[d]	-
Moderna	•	18 and older; booster for 18 and older[e]	-
Novavax	•	-	-
Pfizer[f]	•	5-15 years; booster for 12 and older[g]	16 and older[h]
Sanofi[i]	-	-	-

Source: GAO analysis of information provided by vaccine companies, the Food and Drug Administration (FDA), and the Department of Health and Human Services (HHS)-Department of Defense (DOD) COVID-19 Countermeasures Acceleration Group (CAG). | GAO-22-104453.

Note: The CAG was formerly known as Operation Warp Speed. The columns provide information on specific groups for which the vaccines are authorized or licensed.

[a] The Secretary of Health and Human Services may declare that circumstances, prescribed by statute, exist justifying the emergency use of certain medical products, such as vaccines. Once a declaration of an emergency has been made, FDA may temporarily allow use of unlicensed vaccines through an emergency use authorization (EUA), provided certain statutory criteria are met. For FDA to issue an EUA for a vaccine, it must be reasonable to believe that the vaccine may be effective and that the known and potential benefits of the vaccine outweigh the known and potential risks, among other statutory criteria. See 21 U.S.C. § 360bbb-3.

[b] FDA licenses biologics, such as vaccines, through review and approval of BLAs. FDA guidance indicates that licensure is the goal for COVID-19 vaccine candidates, including those that first receive an EUA.

[c] Janssen Pharmaceutical Companies are a part of Johnson & Johnson.

[d] Janssen's one-dose COVID-19 vaccine was first authorized for emergency use on February 27, 2021 for those 18 years of age and older. FDA amended the authorization for Janssen's vaccine on October 20, 2021 to allow a single booster dose to be administered to individuals 18 years and older and who were vaccinated 2 or more months ago.

[e] Moderna's two-dose COVID-19 vaccine was first authorized for emergency use on December 18, 2020 for those 18 years of age and older. FDA has amended the authorization for Moderna's vaccine numerous times, including on August 12, 2021 to allow a third dose to be administered to certain immunocompromised individuals; on October 20, 2021 to allow a single booster dose to be administered 6 months or more after the initial two-dose series to certain groups of individuals; on November 19, 2021 to allow a single booster dose to be administered 6 months or more after the initial two-dose series to individuals ages 18 and older; and on January 7, 2022 to reduce the dosing interval between the initial two-dose series and the booster from 6 months to 5 months.

[f] Pfizer developed its COVID-19 vaccine in collaboration with BioNTech.

[g] Pfizer's two-dose COVID-19 vaccine was first authorized for emergency use on December 11, 2020 for those 16 years of age and older. FDA has amended the authorization for Pfizer's vaccine numerous times, including on May 10, 2021 to include individuals ages 12 to 15; on August 12, 2021 to allow a third dose to be administered to certain immunocompromised individuals; on September 22, 2021 to allow a single booster dose to be administered 6 months or more after the initial two-dose series to certain groups of individuals; on October 29, 2021, FDA amended the authorization again to allow for a lower dose of Pfizer's vaccine to be administered to individuals ages 5 to 11; on November 19, 2021 to allow a single booster dose to be administered 6 months or more after the initial two-dose series to individuals ages 18 and older; and on January 3, 2022 to allow a single booster dose to be administered 5 months or more after the initial two-dose series to individuals 12 and older and to allow a third dose to be administered to certain immunocompromised individuals ages 5 to 11.

[h] On August 23, 2021, FDA licensed Pfizer's COVID-19 vaccine for individuals 16 years and older.

[i] Sanofi is developing its COVID-19 vaccine candidate in collaboration with GSK.

HHS and DOD Vaccine- related Obligations

Our review found that, to support these vaccine candidates, HHS and DOD had obligated at least $29.8 billion as of September 30, 2021, as shown in figure 2.

These obligations were, in part, for contracting to purchase vaccine doses for use in the U.S. As of October 22, 2021, 1.2 billion of these 1.7 billion doses were for vaccines that had been authorized or licensed by the Food and Drug Administration (FDA). (See table 3.)

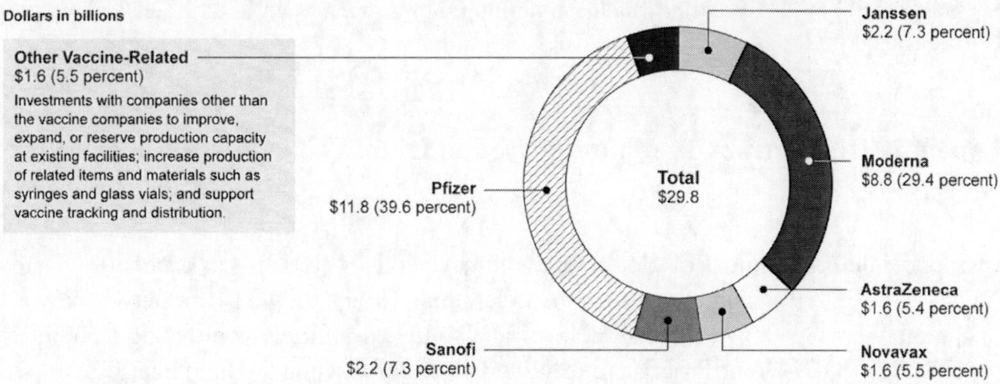

Source: GAO analysis of Federal Procurement Data System – Next Generation data. | GAO-22-104453.

Note: The Department of Health and Human Services (HHS)-Department of Defense (DOD) COVID-19 Countermeasures Acceleration Group (CAG) was formerly known as Operation Warp Speed. We used the HHS Operation Warp Speed website and HHS press releases to determine which contract obligations to include in our analysis. HHS and DOD awarded contracts and other transaction agreements to six vaccine companies and others for the development and manufacturing of vaccines, the purchase of vaccine doses, and the acquisition of other critical supplies and services. HHS announced one award related to distribution for which we could not identify obligations in the Federal Procurement Data System-Next Generation; that award is not included in the chart above.

Figure 2. HHS and DOD Obligations for COVID-19 Vaccine Candidates and Others under the CAG, as of September 30, 2021.

Table 3. Vaccine doses contracted for purchase by the Federal Government for Domestic Use, as of October 22, 2021

Vaccine company	Contracted amount (millions of doses)
AstraZeneca	300
Janssen[a]	100
Moderna	500
Novavax	100[b]
Pfizer[c]	600
Sanofi[d]	100
Total	1,700[e]

Source: GAO analysis of award and other acquisition related documents and information from the Department of Health and Human Services (HHS), the Department of Defense (DOD), Advanced Technology International, and vaccine companies. | GAO-22-104453.

Note: The contracted amount includes base and exercised options. According to officials from the HHS-DOD COVID-19 Countermeasures Acceleration Group (CAG), these doses were intended for domestic use. However, according to these officials, as of September 30, 2021, 122.7 million doses were donated by the federal government for international use.

[a] Janssen Pharmaceutical Companies are a part of Johnson & Johnson.

[b] According to a Novavax representative, the company was also awarded a DOD contract in June 2020 that includes the delivery of 10 million doses. We do not include that amount in this table.

[c] Pfizer developed its COVID-19 vaccine in collaboration with BioNTech.
[d] Sanofi is developing its COVID-19 vaccine candidate in collaboration with GSK.
[e] As of October 22, 2021, 1.2 billion of the 1.7 billion vaccine doses contracted for purchase were authorized or licensed (the Janssen, Moderna, and Pfizer vaccines had received authorization or licensure). COVID-19 vaccine candidates developed by AstraZeneca, Novavax, and Sanofi had not been authorized or licensed as of this date.

Appendix II: Contract Techniques Used to Obtain COVID-19 Vaccines for the U.S.

To support the Department of Health and Human Services (HHS)- Department of Defense (DOD) COVID-19 Countermeasures Acceleration Group (CAG) (formerly known as Operation Warp Speed), DOD and HHS officials utilized multiple contracting techniques.[53] Specifically, DOD's Joint Program Executive Office for Chemical, Biological, Radiological and Nuclear Defense (JPEO-CBRND) and Army Contracting Command leveraged these techniques to obtain vaccine doses from six companies in response to the COVID-19 pandemic.[54] Contracting techniques employed to obtain COVID-19 vaccines included the following:

Broad agency announcements. DOD and HHS used broad agency announcements to solicit vaccine rapid advanced research and development and large scale manufacturing. A broad agency announcement is a notice from the government that requests scientific or research and development proposals from private firms concerning certain areas of interest to the government.[55] Compared to a normal request for proposals, a broad agency announcement does not provide a standard—more specific—statement of work. Rather, it details a problem statement and challenges, and it solicits a solution. Proposals submitted by private firms in response to the announcement may lead to contracts. According to officials from the JPEO-CBRND and Army Contracting Command, vaccine-related broad agency announcements allowed them to obtain input from private companies on how the federal government could meet broad requirements on vaccine development and manufacturing.

Other transaction agreements. DOD awarded prototype other transaction agreements (OTA) to five of the six companies.[56] OTAs are flexible agreements that allow the parties to negotiate terms and conditions without requiring parties to comply with certain federal procurement laws and regulations.[57] This flexibility can help agencies attract and contract with entities that have not previously done business with the federal government due to concerns about standard contracting requirements.[58] For example, OTAs are generally exempt from

[53] We reviewed contract documentation and conducted agency interviews to determine which contract techniques HHS and DOD used.
[54] The six vaccine companies are AstraZeneca, Janssen, Moderna, Novavax, Pfizer, and Sanofi. Pfizer developed its COVID-19 vaccine in collaboration with BioNTech, and Sanofi is developing its COVID-19 vaccine candidate in collaboration with GSK. Janssen Pharmaceutical Companies are a part of Johnson & Johnson.
[55] See Federal Acquisition Regulation (FAR) § 35.016. The Federal Acquisition Regulation (FAR) is the primary regulation for use by all executive agencies in their acquisition of supplies and services with appropriated funds.
[56] The contract with the sixth company was awarded in accordance with the FAR and Defense FAR Supplement.
[57] See 10 U.S.C. § 2371b.
[58] 6See GAO, *COVID-19 Contracting: Observations on Federal Contracting in Response to the Pandemic*, GAO-20-632 (Washington, D.C.: July 29, 2020).

federal procurement laws and regulations, allowing intellectual property rights under each OTA to be tailored to suit the goals of the project.[59]

However, our recent work to review specific aspects of COVID-related OTAs found several challenges associated with their use, including a risk of reduced accountability and transparency.[60] For example, agencies did not accurately reflect all dollars obligated on COVID-19 OTAs in the federal procurement database and, in cases where OTAs were awarded through industry consortia, the agencies did not publicly report which consortium members received the OTA awards because of limitations with the federal procurement database.[61]

Defense Production Act (DPA) awards and priority-rated contracts. DOD and HHS provided priority ratings under the DPA to the contracts with the six vaccine companies to expedite production. The DPA facilitates the supply and timely delivery of products, materials, and services to military and civilian agencies in support of the national defense, including in response to emergency preparedness activities.[62] For example, agencies can require private companies to prioritize fulfilling federal government contracts or orders before fulfilling contracts or orders from other customers. DOD and HHS have also used the DPA to award projects to expand domestic production of health and medical resources. According to officials from the JPEO-CBRND and Army Contracting Command, DPA authorities allowed them to ramp up vaccine production whether they used an OTA or Federal Acquisition Regulation (FAR)- based contract; they believe the DPA use has been instrumental in their ability to quickly obtain vaccine doses.

For other efforts related to securing COVID-19 vaccines, such as increasing manufacturing capacity and obtaining necessary supplies like vials and syringes, DOD used the following contracting techniques:

*Commercial solutions openings***.** The commercial solutions opening pilot program allows DOD to mirror the contracting practices that commercial companies normally use, enabling DOD to solicit company input to design projects, and negotiate payment milestones, intellectual property rights, and other terms and conditions for a desired completion period of within 60 days.[63]

According to officials from the JPEO-CBRND and Army Contracting Command, they leveraged this authority to use commercial solutions openings for the first time during the COVID-19 pandemic to solicit companies for manufacturing facility expansion, including for production of vaccine vials, and to acquire therapeutics. While this authority is set to expire in September 2022, legislation may be enacted to extend the authority.

Technology investment agreements. DOD used technology investment agreements to obtain needed items, such as vials and syringes, as well as for fill-finish work—the process of

---

[59] Under an OTA, the parties can tailor provisions to address concerns about intellectual property and unique government requirements and regulations. The parties are not necessarily bound by FAR-based contract requirements. For example, the Bayh-Dole Act governs intellectual property rights in FAR-based contracts but not in OTAs. 35 U.S.C. §§ 200-212.

[60] See GAO, *COVID-19 Contracting: Actions Needed to Enhance Transparency and Oversight of Selected Awards*, GAO-21-501 (Washington, D.C.: July 26, 2021).

[61] A consortium is comprised of members which can include traditional contractors, nontraditional companies, nonprofit organizations, and academic institutions interested in a specific topic area.

[62] See Pub. L. No. 81-774, 64 Stat. 798 (1950) (codified, as amended, at 50 U.S.C. §§4501 et seq.).

[63] See National Defense Authorization Act for Fiscal Year 2017, Pub. L. No. 114-328, § 879, 130 Stat. 2000, 2312-13 (2016) (codified at 10 U.S.C. § 2303 note). The authority for this pilot program will expire on September 30, 2022.

sealing bulk quantities of vaccines into sterile containers.[64] A technology investment agreement is used to stimulate or support research to foster the best technologies for future defense needs.[65] According to DOD, technology investment agreements are appropriate when research objectives are unlikely to be achieved using other types of contract vehicles.

Appendix III: Abridged Assessment of the Countermeasures Acceleration Group's Schedule

Officials from the Department of Health and Human Services (HHS)- Department of Defense (DOD) COVID-19 Countermeasures Acceleration Group (CAG) (formerly known as Operation Warp Speed) created a schedule to help manage, among other things, tasks needed to support the CAG's efforts to develop, manufacture, and distribute COVID-19 vaccines.[66]

The GAO Schedule Assessment Guide has identified 10 best practices associated with effective schedule estimating, collapsed into four general characteristics that sound schedules should be: well-constructed, comprehensive, credible, and controlled.[67] The best practices of a well- constructed schedule include:

- logical sequencing of all activities—that is, listing the activities in the order in which they are to be logically carried out;
- confirming that the schedule has a valid critical path— that is, the longest continuous sequence of activities in a schedule and the path that defines the program's earliest completion date or minimum duration; and
- identifying reasonable total float or slack—the amount of time an activity could be delayed before that delay affects the program's overall estimated finish date.

Our abridged analysis indicates that as of June 2021, the CAG's schedule partially met one best practice for a well-constructed schedule and minimally met the remaining two, as shown in the table 4 below. For example, we found the schedule was missing a significant number of dependent logical links between related activities. As of June 2021, around 41 percent of remaining incomplete activities in the schedule— including manufacturing potential vaccine booster doses and developing pediatric vaccine doses—were missing a logical link with other activities. According to the GAO Schedule Assessment Guide, unless a schedule identifies all

---

[64] Experts from three pharmaceutical industry groups we interviewed for a previous report said there was a shortage of facilities with capacity to handle fill-finish manufacturing, which could lead to production bottlenecks. See GAO *COVID-19: Federal Efforts Accelerate Vaccine and Therapeutic Development, but More Transparency Needed on Emergency Use Authorizations*, GAO-21-207 (Washington, D.C.: Nov.17, 2020).

[65] See 32 C.F.R. Part 37 (2020).

[66] Schedules typically define when and how long work will occur and how each activity is related to the others. Scheduling allows program management to decide between possible sequences of activities, determine the flexibility of the schedule according to available resources, predict the consequences of managerial action or inaction on events, and develop contingency plans to mitigate risks.

[67] A schedule is *well-constructed* if all its activities are logically sequenced with the most straightforward logic possible. A *comprehensive* schedule includes all activities for both the government and its contractors necessary to accomplish a program's objectives as defined in the program's work breakdown structure. A schedule is *credible* if it is horizontally traceable—that is, it reflects the order of events necessary to achieve aggregated products or outcomes. Finally, a schedule is *controlled* if trained schedulers update it regularly using actual progress and logic—based on information provided by activity owners—to realistically forecast dates for program activities. See GAO, *Schedule Assessment Guide: Best Practices for Project Schedules*, GAO-16-89G (Washington, D.C.: Dec. 22, 2015).

logical dependencies, it will not indicate how activities that fall behind in the schedule will affect succeeding activities that depend on them, or how these delays would affect the overall project schedule.

Table 4. Assessment of the CAG's integrated master schedule, June 2021

GAO Schedule Assessment Guide best practices[a]	Extent incorporated	Description
Sequencing. Schedules should be planned so that important dates can be met. To do this, activities must be logically sequenced and linked—that is, listed in the order in which they are to be carried out and logically linked so that activities that depend on each other can all be completed. The purpose of a logical relationship, or dependency, is to depict the sequence in which activities occur.	◑[b]	Our analysis indicated that the CAG's integrated master schedule missed a significant number of logical links. In some cases, the schedule did not transmit any adjustments for delays in activities deemed necessary to complete other needed activities. For example, the schedule called for a large-scale comparability study for drug substances and products. Though the study was estimated to take 72 days, the schedule showed no effect on expected vaccine completion date if the time frames for this study were extended to as long as 300 days. Without the appropriate predecessor and successor links, the schedule did not indicate how activities that fell behind early in the schedule would have affected later activities that depended on them or the overall project schedule. Additionally, in these instances, the schedule would not have provided confidence to leadership regarding the schedule's dates and indications of key activities that had to be completed.
Critical path. Schedules should identify a critical path—that is, the sequence of activities that determines the program's earliest completion date. The critical path focuses the team's energy and management's attention on the activities that will lead to the project's success.	◔[c]	Our analysis found that the sequence of activities through the schedule did not result in a valid critical path because, among other issues, it was not continuous and was missing logic links to other activities. That is, we could not validate the sequence of critical activities necessary for the CAG to complete a specified goal within its stated timelines, including the vaccine milestones. For example, a critical activity regarding a vaccine company's clinical work did not have a predecessor activity and therefore the schedule did not show what other activities would have needed to be completed before this work have begun. Without a valid critical path, leadership would not have been able to use the schedule to provide realistic timeline estimates, or identify the downstream effects of any changes that occur.
Total float. Schedules should identify reasonable total float—that is, the amount of time a predecessor task can miss its finish date before the delay affects the estimated finish date.	◔[d]	Our analysis identified an unreasonable amount of flexibility in the schedule, so that some activities could have been delayed weeks, months, or years before the schedule would have indicated to leadership an overall delay in milestones. For example, a task which began phase 3 clinical trials for a vaccine candidate could have been delayed 667 days before transferring the delay to the vaccine milestone. Incorrect float estimates may result in an invalid critical path, such that the schedule would not have given reliable indicators of how leadership could have shifted resources to support other critical activities, which could have ultimately delayed completion of those activities.

Source: GAO analysis of the integrated master schedule created by the Department of Health and Human Services (HHS)-Department of Defense (DOD) COVID-19 Countermeasures Acceleration Group (CAG). | GAO-21-104453.

Legend: ● = fully met, ◕ = substantially met, ◑ = partially met, ◔ = minimally met, ○ = not met.

Note: For the best practice assessment described here, we defined the five levels as follows: (1) fully met – CAG officials provided complete evidence that satisfied the entire criterion; (2) substantially met – CAG officials provided evidence that satisfied a large portion of the criterion; (3) partially met – CAG officials provided evidence that satisfied about half of the criterion; (4) minimally met – CAG officials provided evidence that satisfied a small portion of the criterion; and (5) not met – CAG officials provided no evidence that satisfied any of the criterion.

[a] See GAO, *Schedule Assessment Guide: Best Practices for Project Schedules*, GAO-16-89G (Washington, D.C.: Dec. 22, 2015).

[b] We evaluated the schedule against sequencing best practice criterion, such as measuring the number of missing logic links.

[c] We evaluated the schedule against critical path best practice criterion, such as assessing its sequencing and comparing it to the longest path in the schedule.

[d] We evaluated the schedule against total float best practice criterion, such as comparing the average and median values of total float in the schedule and comparing it to the remaining duration of the project schedule.

When we told CAG officials about our analysis, they explained that their schedule was never intended to be fully completed due to time constraints, and because the CAG's work was already underway. For example, CAG officials explained that the limitations in their schedule were due to their work's constricted timeline and the limited amount of information they had regarding certain activities. Specifically, due to the nature of the COVID-19 pandemic, officials said that they had to set overall time frames within the schedule to finish the work as quickly as possible. They also said that they did not consistently have reliable information about the expected duration of some activities conducted by vaccine companies or by different federal agencies, which in turn affected their ability to develop a more specific schedule.

Nonetheless, they said that the schedule—although imperfect—allowed them to better communicate the assumed time frames for activities across the multiple organizations contributing to the CAG's vaccine-related efforts. The integrated master schedule could serve as a critical tool to help HHS officials as they manage remaining vaccine development, manufacturing, and distribution activities following the CAG's dissolution; however the limitations described above could make it less useful for project execution, gauging progress, identifying and resolving potential problems, and promoting accountability.

Appendix IV: Comments from the Department of Health & Human Services

DEPARTMENT OF HEALTH & HUMAN SERVICES

OFFICE OF THE SECRETARY

Assistant Secretary for Legislation
Washington, DC 20201

January 4, 2022

Alyssa M. Hundrup
Director, Health Care
U.S. Government Accountability Office
441 G Street NW
Washington, DC 20548

Dear Ms. Hundrup:

Attached are comments on the U.S. Government Accountability Office's (GAO) report entitled, ***"COVID-19: HHS and DOD Need to Ensure Readiness for Overseeing the Transition of Vaccine Manufacturing and Distribution to HHS"*** (GAO-22-104453).

The Department appreciates the opportunity to review this report prior to publication.

Sincerely,

Melanie Anne Egorin

Melanie Anne Egorin, PhD
Assistant Secretary for Legislation

Attachment

GENERAL COMMENTS FROM THE DEPARTMENT OF HEALTH & HUMAN SERVICES ON THE GOVERNMENT ACCOUNTABILITY OFFICE'S DRAFT REPORT ENTITLED – COVID-19: HHS AND DOD NEED TO ENSURE READINESS FOR OVERSEEING THE TRANSITION OF VACCINE MANUFACTURING AND DISTRIBUTION TO HHS (GAO-22-104453)

The U.S. Department of Health & Human Services (HHS) appreciates the opportunity from the Government Accountability Office (GAO) to review and comment on this draft report.

Recommendation 1
The Secretary of Health and Human Services, in coordination with DOD, should finalize and achieve CAG transition milestones to help demonstrate HHS's readiness to assume the CAG's responsibilities before DOD formally ends its support. **(Recommendation 1)**

HHS Response
HHS non-concurs with this recommendation.

The Department does not concur with this recommendation because HHS has demonstrated readiness to assume the CAG's responsibilities by successfully completing the planned transition of this work to the recently established HHS Coordination Operations and Response Element, or HCORE on January 1, 2022, in accordance with the expiration of the HHS and DOD Memorandum of Understanding (MOU) on December 31, 2021. HCORE institutionalizes the efforts previously led by the CAG within ASPR. It will allow ASPR to build on the progress to date, retain expertise and skills, and continue providing the necessary tools to the American people to respond to the COVID-19 pandemic. HHS has provided the attached memos detailing the remaining workstream transitions, with the exception of the workstreams for Legal and Research and Clinical Trials for Vaccines and Therapeutics, as those were functions already within HHS and, therefore, were not transitioned from DoD. Due to the timing of this GAO engagement and assessment, the draft report was completed ahead of the actual transition timeline. Therefore, the recommendation to finalize and achieve milestones to demonstrate readiness was premature as it was before the timeline established by the MOU to complete the transition.

Recommendation 2
The Secretary of Health and Human Services, in coordination with DoD, should complete assessments of its workforce capacity and develop corresponding workforce strategies demonstrating HHS's readiness to assume the CAG's responsibilities before DoD formally ends its support. **(Recommendation 2)**

HHS Response
HHS non-concurs with this recommendation.

The Department does not concur with this recommendation because HHS has completed workforce assessments in accordance with its planned transition to the recently established HHS Coordination Operations and Response Element, or HCORE on January 1, 2022, prior to the expiration of the HHS and DOD Memorandum of Understanding on December 31, 2021. Organization charts detailing the structure and hiring goals are attached as reference. Due to the

GENERAL COMMENTS FROM THE DEPARTMENT OF HEALTH & HUMAN SERVICES ON THE GOVERNMENT ACCOUNTABILITY OFFICE'S DRAFT REPORT ENTITLED — COVID-19: HHS AND DOD NEED TO ENSURE READINESS FOR OVERSEEING THE TRANSITION OF VACCINE MANUFACTURING AND DISTRIBUTION TO HHS (GAO-22-104453)

timing of this GAO engagement and assessment, the draft report was completed ahead of the actual transition timeline. Therefore, the recommendation to complete the workforce planning was premature.

Recommendation 4
The Secretary of Health and Human Services should develop a schedule that is consistent with the best practices established in the GAO Schedule Assessment Guide to manage remaining vaccine-related responsibilities. **(Recommendation 4)**

HHS Response
HHS concurs with this recommendation.

Now that the transition has completed, HCORE will make assessments regarding the future use of schedules and will take into consideration the best practices established in the GAO Schedule Assessment Guide.

Recommendation 5
The Secretary of Health and Human Services, in coordination with DoD, should expand the CAG's lessons-learned review to also obtain and incorporate input from key external stakeholders, such as vaccine companies and other federal agencies who coordinated with the CAG on its vaccine-related responsibilities. **(Recommendation 5)**

HHS Response
HHS concurs with this recommendation.

Appendix V: Comments from the Department of Defense

OFFICE OF THE ASSISTANT SECRETARY OF DEFENSE

1200 DEFENSE PENTAGON
WASHINGTON, DC 20301-1200

HEALTH AFFAIRS

Ms. Alyssa Hundrup
Director, Health Care
U.S. Government Accountability Office
441 G Street, Northwest
Washington, DC 20548

Dear Ms. Hundrup,

This is the Department of Defense response to the Government Accountability Office (GAO) Draft Report, GAO-22-104453, "COVID-19: HHS and DOD Need to Ensure Readiness for Overseeing the Transition of Vaccine Manufacturing and Distribution to HHS," dated December 6, 2021 (GAO Code 104453).

The Department acknowledges receipt.

My point of contact and the primary action officer for this issue is COL Michael Berecz who may be reached at (703) 681-8463 or michael.j.berecz.mil@mail.mil.

Sincerely,

SMITH.DAVID.J.1085480975 Digitally signed by SMITH.DAVID.J.1085480975 Date: 2022.01.07 13:42:00 -05'00'

David J. Smith, M.D.
Performing the Duties of the Assistant Secretary of Defense for Health Affairs

GAO DRAFT REPORT DATED DECEMBER 6, 2021
GAO-22-104453 (GAO CODE 104453)

"COVID-19: HHS AND DOD NEED TO ENSURE READINESS FOR OVERSEEING THE TRANSITION OF VACCINE MANUFACTURING AND DISTRIBUTION TO HHS"

DEPARTMENT OF DEFENSE COMMENTS
TO THE GAO RECOMMENDATION

The Secretary of Health and Human Services, in coordination with DOD, should finalize and achieve CAG transition milestones to help demonstrate HHS's readiness to assume the CAG's responsibilities before DOD formally ends its support. (Recommendation 1)

HHS answered this recommendation.

The Secretary of Health and Human Services, in coordination with DOD, should complete assessments of its workforce capacity and develop corresponding workforce strategies demonstrating HHS's readiness to assume the CAG's responsibilities before DOD formally ends its support. (Recommendation 2)

HHS answered this recommendation.

The Secretary of Defense, in coordination with HHS, should establish a mechanism—such as through an interagency agreement—to formally provide support to HHS until CAG transition milestones are finalized and achieved, and until HHS completes its planned assessments of its workforce capacity and develops corresponding workforce strategies. (Recommendation 3)

DoD concurs with this recommendation, although the transition milestones were finalized and achieved prior to the expiration of the Memorandum of Understanding on December 31, 2021.

The Secretary of Health and Human Services should develop a schedule that is consistent with the best practices established in the GAO Schedule Assessment Guide to manage remaining vaccine-related responsibilities. (Recommendation 4)

HHS answered this recommendation.

The Secretary of Health and Human Services, in coordination with DOD, should expand the CAG's lessons-learned review to also obtain and incorporate input from key external stakeholders, such as vaccine companies and other federal agencies who coordinated with the CAG on its vaccine-related responsibilities. (Recommendation 5)

HHS answered this recommendation.

2

The Secretary of Defense, in coordination with HHS, should expand the CAG's lessons-learned review to obtain and incorporate input from key external stakeholders, such as vaccine companies and other federal agencies who coordinated with the CAG on its vaccine-related responsibilities. (Recommendation 6)

DoD concurs with this recommendation.

Chapter 11

COVID-19 Vaccination: Selected U.S. Data Sources*

Ada S. Cornell and Angela Napili

The sources below can help congressional staff track the progress of the U.S. Coronavirus Disease 2019 (COVID-19) vaccination campaign at the national, state, and local levels.

Sources were selected for having commonly cited and frequently requested data. This list is not intended to be comprehensive. Because different resources use different methodologies, readers should check websites' notes and caveats, and use caution when comparing data.

About Vaccine Data

In the COVID-19 vaccine program, doses are first *allocated* and made available to states and other jurisdictions for ordering. Once ordered, doses are *delivered* (distributed) to appropriate state and jurisdictional sites. States then allocate and deliver doses to health departments, health care systems, pharmacies, and multi-county entities, which can further re-allocate to local clinical sites. Providers then *administer* doses to patients and report administration data to jurisdictions and CDC. (See CDC's How COVID-19 Vaccines Get to You and About COVID-19 Vaccine Delivered and Administration Data.) Federal health care programs (e.g., Veterans Health Administration) manage vaccine data through a similar process.

Comirnaty (the Pfizer-BioNTech COVID-19 vaccine) is approved as a two-dose vaccine for ages 16+. Comirnaty is also authorized for uses that fall outside the scope of its approval—that is, as a two-dose regimen in individuals aged 5-15 (with a lower dose authorized for children 5-11), as a third dose for certain immunocompromised individuals aged 12+, and as a single booster dose to be given at least six months after the primary series in individuals aged 18.

Vaccines manufactured by Moderna (a two-dose vaccine) and J&J/Janssen (a single-dose vaccine) are currently authorized for emergency use for ages 18+. The Moderna vaccine is also authorized as a third dose for certain immunocompromised individuals 18+ and as a single booster dose (half dose) to be given at least six months after the primary series in individuals

* This is an edited, reformatted and augmented version of Congressional Research Service Publication No. IN11595, updated December 7, 2021.

In: COVID-19 Vaccines
Editor: John Schroder
ISBN: 979-8-88697-150-7

18+. FDA has also authorized a single J&J/Janssen booster dose to be given at least two months after a first dose. Any of the available vaccines can be used as a "mix and match" booster dose in eligible individuals.

CDC Sources

CDC provides data on doses and people vaccinated. Some aggregated national data are available for federal entities (Bureau of Prisons, Department of Defense, Indian Health Service, and Veterans Health Administration; see "Data Table"). CDC also tracks rates of COVID-19 cases, deaths, and hospitalizations by vaccination status. CDC continues to study vaccine effectiveness in real-world conditions.

CDC compiles links to state dashboards, which may also track local data.

Non-CDC Sources

Non-CDC sources provide different visualizations and analyses of CDC data and incorporate data from various jurisdiction-specific sources:

- Bloomberg
- Covid Act Now (and Harvard analysis with congressional district estimates as of September 2021)
- Johns Hopkins University & Medicine (JHU)
- Kaiser Family Foundation (KFF)
- *New York Times* (*NYT*) (subscription required)
- *Washington Post (WP)*

Centers for Medicare & Medicaid Services (CMS) posts nursing home-reported data. The Health Resources & Services Administration (HRSA) posts data on the Health Centers Vaccination Program.

Vaccination Data Sources

Table 1. Vaccination Data

Measure	National	State	Local
Doses delivered			
Number	CDC *NYT*	CDC *NYT*	—
Per capita	—	CDC	—
By vaccine type (J&J/Janssen, Moderna, Comirnaty/Pfizer-BioNTech)	CDC	CDC (download Data Table)	—

Doses administered			
Number	CDC (also trend) Bloomberg JHU NYT	CDC (also trend) Bloomberg JHU NYT	Harvard (congressional district)[a]
Per capita	CDC (download Data Table) Bloomberg	CDC Bloomberg	—
Per day (daily count and 7-day average, trend)	CDC[b] Bloomberg KFF[c] NYT WP	CDC[b] Bloomberg KFFc NYT WP	—
By vaccine type	CDC NYT (trend)	CDC (download Data Table)	—
Percentage of delivered doses that have been administered	Bloomberg ("Supply used") NYT ("Doses used")	Bloomberg ("Supply used") NYT ("Doses used")	—
People vaccinated			
People who received ≥1 dose (number)	CDC (also trend)[b]	CDC (also trend)[b]	CDC (county) CDC (CBSA)[d] Harvard (congressional district)[a]
People who received ≥1 dose (percentage)	CDC Bloomberg Covid Act Now NYT (also trend)	CDC Bloomberg Covid Act Nowe NYT (also trend)	CDC (county) CDC (CBSA)[d] Covid Act Now (county, metro area)[e] Harvard (congressional district)[a]
People fully vaccinated[f] (number)	CDC (also trend)[b] JHU (see "People fully vaccinated") WP	CDC (also trend)[b] JHU WP	CDC (county) CDC (CBSA)[d] Harvard (congressional district)[a]
People fully vaccinated[f] (percentage)	CDC Bloomberg JHU NYT WP	CDC Bloomberg Covid Act Nowe JHU NYT WP	CDC (county, also case rates and testing positivity map) CDC (CBSA)[d] Covid Act Now (county, metro area)[e] Harvard (congressional district)[a] NYT (county) WP (county)
People fully vaccinated[f] by vaccine type	CDC	CDC (download Data Table)	—
People who received additional (including booster) doses	CDC[g] (also trend) Bloomberg WP	CDCg (download Data Table) Bloomberg WP	—

Table 1. (Continued)

Demographics[h]	CDC (race/ethnicity, sex, age; also trends) CDC (aged 65+) CDC (trends by age, alongside cases) CDC (disability status and age, race/ethnicity) CDC (pregnant people by race/ethnicity, trend) CDC (urban/rural, trend) KFF (race/ethnicity) NYT (age) WP (race/ethnicity, age trends) HRSA (race/ethnicity, health centers program)	CDC (aged 65+) CDC (urban/rural, trend) Bloomberg (race/ethnicity) KFF (race/ethnicity) NYT (age) HRSA (race/ethnicity, health centers program)	CDC (age, county and CBSA)[d] CDC (aged 65+, county) CDC (social vulnerability, urban/rural, county) NYT (aged 65+, county)
Nursing homes			
Percent of residents and staff vaccinated	CDC (trend) CMS	CDC (trend) CMS	CMS (facility-level data in "Search for a nursing home") Medicare.gov (facility-level data; search for a nursing home)

Source: CRS based on sources as of December 1, 2021.

Notes: Some sources report similar data, but with different visualizations and analysis.

[a] Data were last updated September 2021 but may be of historical interest.

[b] See also 7-day average trend alongside cases or deaths, see "View (right axis)."

[c] Click "Vaccines": "Daily."

[d] Scroll to Excel spreadsheets under "Attachments." Metropolitan and Micropolitan Statistical Areas are collectively known as Core-Based Statistical Areas (CBSAs).

[e] Search state, city, or county, then scroll to "% Vaccinated" for trend.

[f] As defined in these data sources, "fully vaccinated" people have received the second dose of a two-dose vaccine or one dose of a single-shot vaccine (CDC).

[g] Includes number, percentage, and by vaccine type.

[h] Not all states report demographics on vaccine recipients.

Chapter 12

Occupational Safety and Health Administration (OSHA): COVID-19 Emergency Temporary Standards (ETS) on Health Care Employment and Vaccinations and Testing for Large Employers*

Scott D. Szymendera

Summary

On June 21, 2021, the Occupational Safety and Health Administration (OSHA) promulgated an Emergency Temporary Standard (ETS) for the prevention of the transmission of SARS-CoV-2, the virus that causes COVID-19 in health care employment settings. On December 27, 2021, OSHA announced that it was withdrawing all provisions of this ETS, with the exception of certain COVID-19 reporting requirements.

On November 5, 2021, OSHA promulgated a separate ETS that requires employers with 100 or more employees to require that all employees either be fully vaccinated against COVID-19 by January 4, 2022, or test negative for COVID-19 weekly in order to work onsite. After earlier actions by the U.S. Courts of Appeals for the Fifth and Sixth Circuits, on January 13, 2022, the U.S. Supreme Court granted a stay of the OSHA COVID-19 vaccination and testing ETS pending additional judicial review by the U.S. Court of Appeals for the Sixth Circuit. On January 25, 2022, OSHA announced that it was withdrawing all provisions of this ETS. The ETS will continue to serve as a proposed permanent standard subject to normal rulemaking.

The Occupational Safety and Health Act of 1970 (OSH Act) gives OSHA the ability to promulgate an ETS that would remain in effect for up to six months without going through the normal review and comment process of rulemaking. OSHA, however, has rarely used this authority prior to the COVID-19 pandemic—not since the courts struck down its ETS on asbestos in 1983.

All employers are required to comply with the general duty clause of the OSH Act as well as existing OSHA standards on respiratory protection and recordkeeping that may apply to the current COVID-19 pandemic. Pursuant to guidance issued by OSHA

* This is an edited, reformatted and augmented version of Congressional Research Service Publication No. R46288, updated January 26, 2022.

In: COVID-19 Vaccines
Editor: John Schroder
ISBN: 979-8-88697-150-7

on May 22, 2021, employers are not required to record or report any injuries or illnesses caused by the COVID-19 vaccine. This guidance supersedes earlier OSHA guidance that had required employers to record and report adverse reactions to the vaccine if vaccination was a condition of employment.

The California Division of Occupational Safety and Health (Cal/OSHA), which operates California's state occupational safety and health plan, has had an aerosol transmissible disease (ATD) standard since 2009. This standard includes, among other provisions, the requirement that employers provide covered employees with respirators, rather than surgical masks, when these workers interact with ATDs, such as known or suspected COVID-19 cases. In addition, according to the Cal/OSHA ATD standard, certain procedures require the use of powered air purifying respirators (PAPR). Cal/OSHA has also promulgated an ETS to specifically address COVID-19 exposure in the workplace. The agency that operates the state occupational safety health plan in Michigan (MIOSHA) has promulgated an ETS, which was later rescinded and replaced with the OSHA COVID-19 ETS for health care employers, to specifically address COVID-19 in workplaces. In January 2021, the Virginia state plan (VOSH) promulgated a permanent standard to supersede its ETS, and in May 2021, the Oregon state plan (Oregon OSHA) replaced its ETS with a permanent standard.

Occupational Safety and Health Administration Standards

Section 6 of the Occupational Safety and Health Act of 1970 (OSH Act) grants the Occupational Safety and Health Administration (OSHA) of the Department of Labor the authority to promulgate, modify, or revoke occupational safety and health standards that apply to private sector employers, the United States Postal Service, and the federal government as an employer.[1] In addition, Section 5(a)(1) of the OSH Act, commonly referred to as the general duty clause, requires that all employers under OSHA's jurisdiction provide workplaces free of "recognized hazards that are causing or are likely to cause death or serious physical harm" to their employees.[2] OSHA has the authority to enforce employer compliance with its standards and with the general duty clause through the issuance of abatement orders, citations, and civil monetary penalties. The OSH Act does not cover state or local government agencies or units. Thus, certain entities that may be affected by Coronavirus Disease 2019 (COVID-19), such as state and local government hospitals, local fire departments and emergency medical services, state prisons and county jails, and public schools, are not covered by the OSH Act or subject to OSHA regulation or enforcement.

State Plans

Section 18 of the OSH Act authorizes states to establish their own occupational safety and health plans and preempt standards established and enforced by OSHA.[3] OSHA must approve

[1] 29 U.S.C. §655. The provisions of the Occupational Safety and Health Act of 1970 (OSH Act) are extended to the legislative branch as an employer by the Congressional Accountability Act (P.L. 104-1).

[2] 29 U.S.C. §654(a)(1).

[3] 29 U.S.C. §667.

state plans if they are "at least as effective" as OSHA's standards and enforcement.[4] If a state adopts a state plan, it must also cover state and local government entities, such as public schools, not covered by OSHA. Currently, 21 states and Puerto Rico have state plans that cover all employers, and 5 states and the U.S. Virgin Islands have state plans that cover only state and local government employers not covered by the OSH Act.[5] In the remaining states, state and local government employers are not covered by OSHA standards or enforcement. State plans may incorporate OSHA standards by reference, or states may adopt their own standards that are at least as effective as OSHA's standards. State plans do not have jurisdiction over federal agencies and generally do not cover maritime workers and private sector workers at military bases or other federal facilities.

Promulgation of OSHA Standards

OSHA may promulgate occupational safety and health standards on its own initiative or in response to petitions submitted to the agency by various government agencies, the public, or employer and employee groups.[6] OSHA is not required, however, to respond to a petition for a standard or to promulgate a standard in response to a petition. OSHA may also consult with one of the two statutory standing advisory committees—the National Advisory Committee on Occupational Safety and Health (NACOSH) or the Advisory Committee on Construction Safety and Health (ACCSH)—or an ad-hoc advisory committee for assistance in developing a standard.[7]

Notice and Comment

OSHA's rulemaking process for the promulgation of standards is largely governed by the provisions of the Administrative Procedure Act (APA) and Section 6(b) of the OSH Act.[8] Under the APA informal rulemaking process, federal agencies, including OSHA, are required to provide notice of proposed rules through the publication of a Notice of Proposed Rulemaking in the *Federal Register* and to provide the public a period of time to comment on the proposed rules.

Section 7(b) of the OSH Act mirrors the APA in that it requires notice and comment in the rulemaking process.[9] After publishing a proposed standard, the public must be given a period of at least 30 days to provide comments. In addition, any person may submit written objections to the proposed standard and may request a public hearing on the standard.

---

[4] For additional information on Occupational Safety and Health Administration (OSHA) state plans, see CRS Report R43969, *OSHA State Plans: In Brief, with Examples from California and Arizona.*

[5] Information on specific state plans is available from the OSHA website at https://www.osha.gov/stateplans.

[6] Per Section 6(b)(1) of the OSH Act [29 §655(b)(1)], a petition may be submitted by "an interested person, a representative of any organization of employers or employees, a nationally recognized standards-producing organization, the Secretary of Health and Human Services (HHS), the National Institute for Occupational Safety and Health, or a state or political subdivision."

[7] The National Advisory Committee on Occupational Safety and Health (NACOSH) was established by Section 7(a) of the OSH Act [29 U.S.C. §656(a)]. The Advisory Committee on Construction Safety and Health (ACCSH) was established by Section 107 of the Contract Work Hours and Safety Act (P.L. 87-581). Section 7(b) of the OSH Act provides OSHA the authority to establish additional advisory committees.

[8] The Administrative Procedure Act (APA) is codified at 5 U.S.C. §§500-596. For detailed information on federal agency rulemaking and the APA, see CRS Report RL32240, *The Federal Rulemaking Process: An Overview.*

[9] 29 U.S.C. §655(b).

Statement of Reasons

Section 6(e) of the OSH Act requires OSHA to publish in the *Federal Register* a statement of the reasons the agency is taking action whenever it promulgates a standard, conducts other rulemaking, or takes certain additional actions, including issuing an order, compromising on a penalty amount, or settling an issued penalty.[10]

Other Relevant Laws and Executive Order 12866

In addition to the APA and OSH Act, other federal laws that generally apply to OSHA rulemaking include the Paperwork Reduction Act,[11] Regulatory Flexibility Act,[12] Congressional Review Act,[13] Information Quality Act,[14] and Small Business Regulatory Enforcement Fairness Act (SBREFA).[1515] Also, Executive Order 12866, issued by President Clinton in 1993, requires agencies to submit certain regulatory actions to the Office of Management and Budget (OMB) and Office of Information and Regulatory Affairs (OIRA) for review before promulgation.[16]

OSHA Rulemaking Time Line

OSHA rulemaking for new standards has historically been a relatively time-consuming process. In 2012, at the request of Congress, the Government Accountability Office (GAO) reviewed 59 significant OSHA standards promulgated between 1981 (after the enactments of the Paperwork Reduction Act and Regulatory Flexibility Act) and 2010.[17] For these standards, OSHA's average time between beginning formal consideration of the standard—either through publishing a Request for Information or Advance Notice of Proposed Rulemaking in the *Federal Register* or placing the rulemaking on its semiannual regulatory agenda—and promulgation of the standard was 93 months (7 years, 9 months). Once the Notice of Proposed Rulemaking was published for these 59 standards, the average time until promulgation of the standard was 39 months (3 years, 3 months).

In 2012, OSHA's Directorate of Standards and Guidance published a flowchart of the OSHA rulemaking process on the agency's website.[18] This flowchart includes estimated duration ranges for a variety of rulemaking actions, beginning with pre-rule activities—such as developing the idea for the standard and meeting with stakeholders—and ending with promulgation of the standard. The flowchart also includes an estimated duration range for post-promulgation activities, such as judicial review. The estimated time from the start of preliminary rulemaking to the promulgation of a standard ranges from 52 months (4 years, 4 months) to 138 months (11 years, 6 months). After a Notice of Proposed Rulemaking is published in the *Federal Register*, the estimated length of time until the standard is promulgated ranges from 26 months (2 years, 2 months) to 63 months (5 years, 3 months). *Table 1* provides

---

[10] 29 U.S.C. §655(e).

[11] 44 U.S.C. §§3501-3520.

[12] 5 U.S.C. §§601-612.

[13] 5 U.S.C. §§801-808.

[14] 44 U.S.C. §3516 note.

[15] 5 U.S.C. §601 note. For information on these additional laws that apply to OSHA rulemaking, see U.S. Government Accountability Office (GAO), *Workplace Safety and Health: Multiple Challenges Lengthen OSHA's Standard Setting*, GAO-12-330, April 2012, Appendix II, at https://www.gao.gov/products/GAO-12-330 (hereinafter cited as GAO-12- 330, *Workplace Safety and Health*).

[16] Executive Order 12866, "Regulatory Planning and Review," 58 *Federal Register* 51735, October 4, 1993.

[17] GAO-12-330, *Workplace Safety and Health.*

[18] OSHA, Directorate of Standards and Guidance, *The OSHA Rulemaking Process*, October 15, 2012.

OSHA's estimated time lines for six major pre-rulemaking and rulemaking activities leading to the promulgation of a standard.

Table 1. OSHA rulemaking process: estimated durations of activities

Stage	Activities	Estimated Duration
1	Preliminary rulemaking activities	12-36 months
2	Developing the proposed rule	12-36 months
3	Publishing the Notice of Proposed Rulemaking (NPRM)	2-3 months
4	Developing and analyzing the rulemaking record, including public comments and hearings	6-24 months
5	Developing the final rule, including Office of Information and Regulatory Affairs (OIRA) submission	18-36 months
6	Publishing the final rule (promulgating the new standard)	2-3 months
Total estimated duration		52-138 months
Estimated duration from NPRM to final rule		26-63 months

Source: Congressional Research Service (CRS) with data from Occupational Safety and Health Administration (OSHA), Directorate of Standards and Guidance, The OSHA Rulemaking Process, October 15, 2012.

Judicial Review

Both the APA and the OSH Act provide for judicial review of OSHA standards. Section 7(f) of the OSH Act provides that any person who is "adversely affected" by a standard may file, within 60 days of its promulgation, a petition challenging the standard with the U.S. Court of Appeals for the circuit in which the person lives or maintains his or her principal place of business.[19] A petition for judicial review does not automatically stay the implementation or enforcement of the standard. However, the court may order such a stay. OSHA estimates that post-promulgation activities, including judicial review, can take between four and 12 months after the standard is promulgated.[20]

Emergency Temporary Standards

Section 6(c) of the OSH Act provides the authority for OSHA to issue an Emergency Temporary Standard (ETS) without having to go through the normal rulemaking process. OSHA may promulgate an ETS without supplying any notice or opportunity for public comment or public hearings. An ETS is immediately effective upon publication in the Federal Register. Upon promulgation of an ETS, OSHA is required to begin the full rulemaking process for a permanent standard with the ETS serving as the proposed standard for this rulemaking. An ETS is valid until superseded by a permanent standard, which OSHA must promulgate within six months of publishing the ETS in the Federal Register.[21] An ETS must include a statement of reasons for the action in the same manner as required for a permanent standard.

---

[19] 29 U.S.C. §655(f).

[20] OSHA, Directorate of Standards and Guidance, *The OSHA Rulemaking Process*, October 15, 2012.

[21] 29 U.S.C. §655(c)(2). The statute is not clear on what happens if OSHA is unable to promulgate a permanent standard within six months. For additional information see the section "ETS Duration" later in this report.

State plans are required to adopt or adhere to an ETS, although the OSH Act is not clear on how quickly a state plan must come into compliance with an ETS.

ETS Requirements

Section 6(c)(1) of the OSH Act requires that both of the following determinations be made in order for OSHA to promulgate an ETS:

- that employees are exposed to grave danger from exposure to substances or
- agents determined to be toxic or physically harmful or from new hazards, and
- that such emergency standard is necessary to protect employees from such danger.

Grave Danger Determination

The term *grave danger*, used in the first mandatory determination for an ETS, is not defined in statute or regulation. The legislative history demonstrates the intent of Congress that the ETS process "not be utilized to circumvent the regular standard-setting process," but the history is unclear as to how Congress intended the term grave danger to be defined.[22]

In addition, although the federal courts have ruled on challenges to previous ETS promulgations, the courts have provided no clear guidance as to what constitutes a grave danger. In 1984, the U.S. Court of Appeals for the Fifth Circuit in *Asbestos Info. Ass'n v. OSHA* issued a stay and invalidated OSHA's November 1983 ETS lowering the permissible exposure limit for asbestos in the workplace.[23] In its decision, the court stated that "gravity of danger is a policy decision committed to OSHA, not to the courts."[24] The court, however, ultimately rejected the ETS, in part on the grounds that OSHA did not provide sufficient support for its claim that 80 workers would ultimately die because of exposures to asbestos during the six-month life of the ETS.

Necessity Determination

In addition to addressing a grave danger to employees, an ETS must also be *necessary* to protect employees from that danger. In *Asbestos Info. Ass'n*, the court invalidated the asbestos ETS for the additional reason that OSHA had not demonstrated the necessity of the ETS. The court cited, among other factors, the duplication between the respirator requirements of the ETS and OSHA's existing standards requiring respirator use. The court dismissed OSHA's argument that the ETS was necessary because the agency felt that the existing respiratory standards were "unenforceable absent actual monitoring to show that ambient asbestos particles are so far above the permissible limit that respirators are necessary to bring employees' exposure within the PEL of 2.0 f/cc."[25] The court determined that "fear of a successful judicial challenge to enforcement of OSHA's permanent standard regarding respirator use hardly justifies resort to the most dramatic weapon in OSHA's enforcement arsenal."[26]

---

[22] U.S. Congress, Senate Labor and Public Welfare, Subcommittee on Labor, *Legislative History of the Occupational Safety and Health Act of 1970 (*S. 2193, *P.L. 91-596)*, committee print, prepared by Subcommittee on Labor, 91st Cong., 1 sess., June 1971, 52-531 (Washington: GPO, 1971), p. 1218.

[23] 727 F.2d at 415, 425-427 (5th Cir. 1984).

[24] 727 F.2d at 427 (5th Cir. 1984).

[25] 727 F.2d at 427 (5th Cir. 1984). The ETS mandated a permissible exposure limit (PEL) for asbestos of two asbestos fibers per cubic centimeter of air (2.0 f/cc).

[26] 727 F.2d at 427 (5th Cir. 1984).

In 2006, the agency considered a petition from the United Food and Commercial Workers (UFCW) and International Brotherhood of Teamsters (IBT) for an ETS on diacetyl, a compound then commonly used as an artificial butter flavoring in microwave popcorn and a flavoring in other food and beverage products. The UFCW and IBT petitioned OSHA for the ETS after the National Institute for Occupational Safety and Health (NIOSH) and other researchers found that airborne exposure to diacetyl was linked to the lung disease *bronchiolitis obliterans*, now commonly referred to as "popcorn lung."[27] According to GAO's 2012 report on OSHA's standard-setting processes, OSHA informed GAO that although the agency may have been able to issue an ETS based on the grave danger posed by diacetyl, the actions taken by the food and beverage industries, including reducing or removing diacetyl from products, made it less likely that the necessity requirement could be met.[28]

ETS Duration

Section 6(c)(2) of the OSH Act provides that an ETS is effective until superseded by a permanent standard promulgated pursuant to the normal rulemaking provisions of the OSH Act. Section 6(c)(3) of the OSH Act requires OSHA to promulgate a permanent standard within six months of promulgating the ETS. As shown earlier in this chapter, six months is well outside of historical and currently expected time frames for developing and promulgating a standard under the notice and comment provisions of the APA and OSH Act, as well as under other relevant federal laws and executive orders. This dichotomy between the statutory mandate to promulgate a standard and the time lines that, based on historical precedent, other provisions in the OSH Act might realistically require for such promulgation raises the question of whether or not OSHA could extend an ETS's duration without going through the normal rulemaking process. The statute and legislative history do not clearly address this question.

OSHA has used its ETS authority sparingly in its history. As shown in *Table A-1*, in the 11 times OSHA has issued an ETS, the courts have fully vacated or stayed the ETS in four cases and partially vacated the ETS in one case.[29] In five of the seven ETSs that were not challenged, were fully or partially upheld by the courts, or are still active, OSHA issued a permanent standard either within the six months required by the statute or within several months of the six-month period and always within one year of the promulgation of the ETS.[30] Each of these five cases, however, occurred before 1980, after which a combination of additional federal laws and court decisions added additional procedural requirements to the OSHA rulemaking process. OSHA did not attempt to extend the ETS's expiration date in any of these cases.

Although the courts have not ruled directly on an attempt by OSHA to solely extend the life of an ETS, in 1974, the U.S. Court Appeals for the Fifth Circuit held in *Florida Peach Growers Ass'n v. United States Department of Labor* that OSHA was within its authority to

---

[27] See, for example, Centers for Disease Control and Prevention (CDC): National Institute for Occupational Safety and Health (NIOSH), *NIOSH Alert: Preventing Lung Disease in Workers who Use or Make Flavorings*, DHHS (NIOSH) publication no. 2004-110, December 2003, at https://www.cdc.gov/niosh/docs/2004-110/.

[28] GAO-12-330, *Workplace Safety and Health.*

[29] Mark A. Rothstein, "Substantive and Procedural Obstacles to OSHA Rulemaking: Reproductive Hazards as an Example," *Boston College Environmental Affairs Law Review*, vol. 12, no. 4 (August 1985), p. 673.

[30] For example, OSHA promulgated the Acrylonitrile (vinyl cyanide) ETS on January 17, 1978, and the permanent standard on October 3, 1978, with an effective date of November 2, 1978. The preamble to the permanent standard published in the *Federal Register* does not include information on the status of the ETS during the time between its expiration and the promulgation of the permanent standard. OSHA, "Occupational Exposure to Acrylonitrile (Vinyl Cyanide)," 43 *Federal Register* 45762, October 3, 1978.

amend an ETS without going through the normal rulemaking process.[31] The court stated that "it is inconceivable that Congress, having granted the Secretary the authority to react quickly in fast-breaking emergency situations, intended to limit his ability to react to developments subsequent to his initial response."[32] The court also recognized the difficulty OSHA may have in promulgating a standard within six months due to the notice and comment requirements of the OSH Act, stating that in the case of OSHA seeking to amend an ETS to expand its focus, "adherence to subsection (b) procedures would not be in the best interest of employees, whom the Act is designed to protect. Such lengthy procedures could all too easily consume all of the temporary standard's six months life."[33]

OSHA COVID-19 ETS for Health Care Employers— Withdrawn

On June 21, 2021, OSHA promulgated an ETS for the prevention of COVID-19 in health care employment.[34] The ETS required a covered employer to create a COVID-19 plan, included provisions for the prevention of COVID-19 in the workplace, required new recordkeeping in COVID-19 cases, and (in certain circumstances) permitted employers to forgo the medical evaluation and fit-testing requirements of the OSHA respiratory protection standard. The ETS became effective with its publication in the *Federal Register*, with covered employers required to comply with all provisions of the ETS—with the exceptions of the physical distancing, building ventilation, training, and mini-respiratory-protection provisions—by July 6, 2021. Covered employers were required to comply with the physical distancing, building ventilation, training, and mini-respiratory-protection provisions by July 21, 2021.

On December 27, 2021, OSHA announced that it was withdrawing all provisions of the ETS for health care employers, with the exceptions of certain recordkeeping requirements.[35] In the withdrawal announcement, OSHA cited the fact that six months had elapsed since the promulgation of the ETS and that the agency was not able to promulgate a permanent standard during this six-month period.

Recordkeeping and Reporting[36]

Under the recordkeeping and reporting provisions of the ETS, which remain in force, health care employers with more than 10 employees must take the following actions:

---

[31] 489 F.2d. 120 (5th Cir. 1974).

[32] 489 F.2d. at 127 (5th Cir. 1974).

[33] 489 F.2d. at 127 (5th Cir. 1974).

[34] OSHA, "Occupational Exposure to COVID-19; Emergency Temporary Standard," 86 *Federal Register* 32376, June21, 2021.

[35] OSHA, *Statement on the Status of the OSHA COVID-19 Healthcare ETS*, December 27, 2021, at https://www.osha.gov/coronavirus/ets. In its withdrawal announcement, OSHA states that the recordkeeping and reporting requirements are authorized by Section 8 of the OSH Act (29 U.S.C. §657) and thus are not subject to the six- month time limit of the ETS.

[36] For additional information on OSHA's COVID-19 recordkeeping and reporting requirements for employers not covered by the ETS, see the section "COVID-19 Recordkeeping" later in this report.

- Establish and maintain a log of COVID-19 cases among employees, regardless of whether or not they are connected to workplace exposures;[37]
- Provide, by the end of the next business day upon request, the individual COVID-19 log entry of an employee to that employee and any person who has the written consent of the employee;[38]
- Provide, by the end of the next business day upon request, a version of the COVID-19 log with personally identifiable information of employees removed to any employees or their personal or authorized representatives;[39]
- Provide, by the end of the next business day, all COVID-19 records to OSHA;[40]
- Report to OSHA any work-related COVID-19 fatality within eight hours of learning of the fatality;[41] and
- Report to OSHA any work-related COVID-19 inpatient hospitalization within 24 hours of learning of the hospitalization.[42]

OSHA ETS on COVID-19 Vaccination and Testing—Withdrawn

On November 5, 2021, OSHA promulgated an ETS on COVID-19 vaccination and testing for all large employers.[43] This ETS required that all employers with 100 or more employees develop written policies requiring that employees be fully vaccinated against COVID-19. As an alternative, employers could develop written policies that allow employees to choose to either be fully vaccinated against COVID-19 or provide proof of weekly negative COVID-19 tests and wear face coverings while in the workplace. Employers would not be required to pay for COVID- 19 tests or pay for or provide face coverings. Employers were to develop vaccination and testing plans within 30 days of the publication of the ETS (December 5, 2021) and enforce the requirements for testing of unvaccinated employees within 60 days (January 4, 2022).[44]

While the *Federal Register* announcement did not specify a specific duration for the COVID-19 ETS, per the OSH Act, an ETS is effective until replaced by a permanent standard within six months. The publication of the COVID-19 ETS in the *Federal Register* also included a request for comments on the ETS and on whether the ETS should become a permanent standard. In the preamble to the ETS, OSHA provided that all state plans must adopt the ETS within 30 days of its publication and notify OSHA within 15 days of the actions they plan to take to adopt the ETS.

---

[37] 29 C.F.R. §502(q)(2)(ii).
[38] 29 C.F.R. §502(q)(3)(ii).
[39] 29 C.F.R. §502(q)(3)(iii).
[40] 29 C.F.R. §502(q)(3)(iv).
[41] 29 C.F.R. §502(r)(1)(i).
[42] 29 C.F.R. §502(r)(1)(ii).
[43] OSHA, "COVID-19 Vaccination and Testing; Emergency Temporary Standard," 86 *Federal Register* 61402, November 5, 2021.
[44] After the U.S. Court of Appeals for the Sixth Circuit dissolved the stay on the ETS, OSHA announced that it would not issue citations for noncompliance with any provision of the ETS until January 10, 2022, and for noncompliance with the testing requirements until February 9, 2022, provided employers are making good faith efforts to comply with the ETS (OSHA, "Litigation Update," December 17, 2022, at https://www.osha.gov/coronavirus/ets2#litigation).

Petitions for Judicial Review and Withdrawal by OSHA

Petitions for judicial review of the COVID-19 vaccination and testing ETS were filed by 27 states and numerous employers in the U.S. Courts of Appeals for the First, Fourth, Fifth, Sixth, Seventh, Eighth, Ninth, Eleventh, and District of Columbia Circuits.[45] In addition, labor unions and employee groups filed petitions for judicial review in the Second, Third, Fourth, Ninth, Tenth, and District of Columbia Circuits.

On November 6, 2021, the U.S. Court of Appeals for the Fifth Circuit ordered that the COVID-19 vaccination and ETS be stayed pending judicial review. This stay was reaffirmed by the court on November 12, 2021, and applied nationally.[46]

On November 16, 2021, the United States Judicial Panel on Multidistrict Litigation consolidated the petitions for judicial review of the COVID-19 vaccination and testing ETS and randomly assigned these consolidated cases to the U.S. Court of Appeals for the Sixth Circuit.[47] On December 17, 2021, the court dissolved the stay.

On December 17, 2021, numerous states and other petitioners requested that the U.S. Supreme Court review the ETS by filing an application for a stay of the ETS and an alternative petition for writ of certiorari before judgment. On January 13, 2022, U.S. Supreme Court granted a stay pending additional judicial review by the U.S. Court of Appeals for the Sixth Circuit.[48]

On January 25, 2022, OSHA announced that it was withdrawing the COVID-19 vaccination and testing ETS but that the ETS would continue to serve as a proposed permanent standard subject to the normal rulemaking process.[49]

Other OSHA Standards Related to COVID-19

While the COVID-19 ETS applies only to health care employers, all employers are required to comply with other OSHA standards that, while not specific to COVID-19, may cover situations related to the prevention of COVID-19 transmission in the workplace. OSHA may enforce the general duty clause in the absence of a standard if it can be determined that an employer has failed to provide a worksite free of "recognized hazards" that are "causing or are likely to cause death or serious physical harm" to workers.[50] In addition, OSHA's standards for the use of PPE

---

[45] The states of Louisiana, Mississippi, South Carolina, Texas and Utah (Fifth Circuit); Idaho, Kansas, Kentucky, Ohio, Oklahoma, Tennessee, and West Virginia (Sixth Circuit); Indiana (Seventh Circuit); Alaska, Arizona, Arkansas, Iowa, Missouri, Montana, Nebraska, New Hampshire, North Dakota, South Dakota, and Wyoming (Eighth Circuit); and Alabama, Florida, and Georgia (Eleventh Circuit) were plaintiffs in these cases.

[46] For additional information on judicial review of the OSHA COVID-19 vaccination and testing ETS, see CRS Legal Sidebar LSB10658, *Fifth Circuit Stays OSHA Vaccination and Testing Standard.*

[47] In Re: Occupational Safety and Health Administration, Interim Final Rule: COVID-19 Vaccination and Testing; Emergency Temporary Standard, 86 Fed. Reg. 61402, Issued on November 4, 2021, MCP No. 165 (J.P.M.L. November 16, 2021).

[48] National Federation of Independent Business, et al. v. Department of Labor, Occupational Safety and Health Administration, et al. and Ohio, et al. v. Department of Labor, Occupational Safety and Health Administration, et al. Nos. 21A244 and 21A247 (U.S. January 13, 2022).

[49] OSHA, *Statement on the Status of the COVID-19 Vaccination and Testing ETS*, January 25, 2022, at https://www.osha.gov/coronavirus/ets2.

[50] 29 U.S.C. §654(a)(1).

may apply in cases in which workers require eye, face, hand, or respiratory protection against COVID-19 exposure.[51]

OSHA Respiratory Protection Standard

National Institute for Occupational Safety and Health Certification

The OSHA respiratory protection standard requires the use of respirators certified by NIOSH in cases in which engineering controls, such as ventilation or enclosure of hazards, are insufficient to protect workers from breathing contaminated air.[52] Surgical masks, procedure masks, and dust masks are not considered respirators. NIOSH certifies respirators pursuant to federal regulations.[53] For nonpowered respirators, such as filtering face piece respirators commonly used in health care and construction, NIOSH classifies respirators based on their efficiency at filtering airborne particles and their ability to protect against oil particles. Under the NIOSH classification system, the letter (N, R, or P) indicates the level of oil protection as follows: N—no oil protection; R—oil resistant; and P—oil proof. The number following the letter indicates the efficiency rating of the respirator as follows: 95—filters 95% of airborne particles; 97—filters 97% of airborne particles; and 100—filters 99.7% of airborne particles. Thus an N95 respirator, the most common type, is one that does not protect against oil particles and filters out 95% of airborne particles. An R or P respirator can be used in place of an N respirator.

A respirator that is past its manufacturer-designated shelf life is no longer considered to be certified by NIOSH. However, in response to potential shortages in respirators, NIOSH has tested and approved certain models of respirators for certified use beyond their manufacturer-designated shelf lives.[54]

Respirators designed for certain medical and surgical uses are subject to both certification by NIOSH (for oil protection and efficiency) and regulation by the FDA as medical devices. In general, respirators with exhalation valves cannot be used in surgical and certain medical settings because, although the presence of an exhalation valve does not affect the respirator's protection afforded the user, it may allow unfiltered air from the user into a sterile field. On March 2, 2020, FDA issued an EUA to approve for use in medical settings certain NIOSH-certified respirators not previously regulated by FDA.[55]

Medical Evaluation and Fit Testing

The OSHA respiratory protection standard requires that the employer provide a medical evaluation to the employee to determine if the employee is physiologically able to use a respirator. This medical evaluation must be completed before any fit testing. For respirators designed to fit tightly against the face, the specific type and model of respirator that an employee is to use must be fit tested in accordance with the procedures provided in Appendix

[51] 29 C.F.R. §§1910.133, 1910.134, and 1910.138.

[52] 29 C.F.R. §1910.134.

[53] 42 C.F.R. Part 84.

[54] NIOSH, Release of Stockpiled Filtering Facepiece Respirators Beyond the Manufacturer-Designated Shelf Life: Considerations for the COVID-19 Response, February 28, 2020, at https://www.cdc.gov/coronavirus/2019-ncov/release-stockpiled-N95.html.

[55] Letter from RADM Denise M. Hinton, chief scientist, FDA, to Robert R. Redfield, Director, CDC, March 2, 2020, at https://www.fda.gov/media/135763/download.

A of the OSHA respiratory protection standard to ensure there is a complete seal around the respirator when worn.[56] Once an employee has been fit tested for a respirator, he or she is required to be fit tested annually or whenever the model of respirator, but not the actual respirator itself, is changed. Each time an individual uses a respirator, he or she is required to perform a check ofthe seal of the respirator to his or her face in accordance with the procedures provided in Appendix B of the standard.[57] On March 14, 2020, OSHA issued guidance permitting employers tosuspend annual fit testing of respirators for employees that have already been fit tested on the same model respirator.

Temporary OSHA Enforcement Guidance on the Respiratory Protection Standard

In response to shortages of respirators and other PPE during the national response to the COVID- 19 pandemic, OSHA has issued five sets of temporary enforcement guidance to permit the following exceptions to the respiratory protection standard:

1. employers may suspend annual fit testing of respirators for employees that have already been fit tested on the same model respirator;[58]
2. employers may permit the use of expired respirators and the extended use or reuse of respirators, provided the respirator maintains its structural integrity and is not damaged, soiled, or contaminated (e.g., with blood, oil, or paint);[59]
3. employers may permit the use of respirators not certified by NIOSH, but approved under standards used by the following countries or jurisdictions, in accordance with the protection equivalency tables provided in Appendices A and B of the enforcement guidance document:

   - Australia,
   - Brazil,
   - European Union,
   - Japan,
   - Mexico,
   - People's Republic of China, and
   - Republic of Korea.[60]

---

[56] 29 C.F.R. §1910.134 Appendix A. PAPRs that do not require a seal to the user's face do not need to be fit tested.

[57] 29 C.F.R. §1910.134 Appendix B.

[58] OSHA, *Temporary Enforcement Guidance—Health Care Respiratory Protection Annual Fit-Testing for N95 Filtering Facepieces During the COVID-19 Outbreak*, March 14, 2020, at https://www.osha.gov/memos/2020-03-14/ temporary-enforcement-guidance-healthcare-respiratory-protection-annual-fit; and OSHA *Expanded Temporary Enforcement Guidance on Respiratory Protection Fit-Testing for N95 Filtering Facepieces in All Industries During the Coronavirus Disease 2019 (COVID-19) Pandemic*, April 8, 2020, at https://www.osha.gov/memos/2020-04-08/expanded-temporary-enforcement-guidance-respiratory-protection-fit-testing-n95.

[59] OSHA, *Enforcement Guidance for Respiratory Protection and the N95 Shortage Due to the Coronavirus Disease 2019 (COVID-19) Pandemic*, April 3, 2020, at https://www.osha.gov/memos/2020-04-03/enforcement-guidance-respiratory-protection-and-n95-shortage-due-coronavirus. Under this guidance, employers are required to address in their written respiratory protection plans when respirators are contaminated and not available for use or reuse.

[60] OSHA, *Enforcement Guidance for Use of Respiratory Protection Equipment Certified under Standards of Other Countries or Jurisdictions During the Coronavirus Disease 2019 (COVID-19) Pandemic*, April 3, 2020, at https://www.osha.gov/memos/2020-04-03/enforcement-guidance-use-respiratory-protection-equipment-certified-under.

4. employers may permit the re-use of respirators decontaminated in accordance with CDC decontamination guidance;[61] and
5. employers may permit the use of NIOSH-approved tight-fitting PAPRs in place of respirators when respirator fit testing is not feasible due to supply issues.[62]

COVID-19 Recordkeeping

Sections 8(c) and 24(a) of the OSH Act require employers to maintain records of occupational injuries and illnesses in accordance with OSHA regulations.[63] OSHA's reporting and recordkeeping regulations require that employers with 10 or more employees must keep records of work-related injuries and illnesses that result in lost work time for employees or that require medical care beyond first aid.[64] Employers must also report to OSHA, within eight hours, any workplace fatality and, within 24 hours, any injury or illness that results in in-patient hospitalization, amputation, or loss of an eye. Employers in certain industries determined by OSHA to have lower occupational safety and health hazards are listed in the regulations as being exempt from the recordkeeping requirements but not the requirement to report to OSHA serious injuries, illnesses, and deaths.[65] Offices of physicians, dentists, other health practitioners and outpatient medical clinics are included in the industries that are exempt from the recordkeeping requirements.

OSHA regulations require the employer to determine if an employee's injury or illness is related to his or her work and thus subject to the recordkeeping requirements.[66] The regulations provide a presumption that an injury or illness that occurs in the workplace is work-related and recordable unless one of the exemptions provided in the regulations applies.[67] One of the listed exemptions is "The illness is the common cold or flu (Note: contagious diseases such as tuberculosis, brucellosis, hepatitis A, or plague are considered work-related if the employee is infected at work)."[68]

Because of the nature of COVID-19 transmission, which can occur outside of work as well as in the workplace, it can be difficult to determine the exact source of any person's COVID-19 transmission. Absent any specific guidance, this may make it difficult for employers to determine if an employee's COVID-19 is subject to the recordkeeping requirements.

---

[61] OSHA, Enforcement Guidance on Decontamination of Filtering Facepiece Respirators in Healthcare During the Coronavirus Disease 2019 (COVID-19) Pandemic, April 24, 2021, at https://www.osha.gov/memos/2020-04-24/enforcement-guidance-decontamination-filtering-facepiece-respirators-healthcare; and CDC, Implementing Filtering Facepiece Respirator (FFR) Reuse, Including Reuse after Decontamination, When There Are Known Shortages of N95 Respirators, October 19, 2021, at https://www.cdc.gov/coronavirus/2019-ncov/hcp/ppe-strategy/decontamination- reuse-respirators.html.

[62] OSHA, Temporary Enforcement Guidance—Tight-Fitting Powered Air Purifying Respirators (PAPRs) Used During the Coronavirus Disease 2019 (COVID-19) Pandemic, October 2, 2021, at https://www.osha.gov/memos/2020-10-02/temporary-enforcement-guidance-tight-fitting-powered-air-purifying-respirators.

[63] 29 U.S.C. §§657(c) and 673(a).

[64] OSHA's reporting and recordkeeping regulations are at Title 29, Part 1904, of the Code of Federal Regulations.

[65] The list of exempted industries is at Title 29, Subpart B, Appendix A, of the Code of Federal Regulations. States with state occupational safety and health plans may require employers in these exempted industries to comply with the recordkeeping requirements.

[66] 29 C.F.R. §1904.5.

[67] 29 C.F.R. §1905.5(a).

[68] 29 C.F.R. §1904.5(b)(2)(viii).

Initial OSHA Recordkeeping Guidance

On April 10, 2020, OSHA issued enforcement guidance on how cases of COVID-19 should be treated under the recordkeeping requirements.[69] This guidance stated that COVID-19 cases were recordable if they were work-related.

Under this guidance, employers in the following industry groups were to fully comply with the recordkeeping regulations, including the requirement to determine if COVID-19 cases were work-related:

- health care;
- emergency response, including firefighting, emergency medical services, and law enforcement; and
- correctional institutions.

For all other employers, OSHA required employers to determine if COVID-19 cases were work- related and subject to the recordkeeping requirements only if both of the following two conditions were met:

1. There was objective evidence that a COVID-19 case may have been work-related. This could have included, for example, a number of cases developing among workers who worked closely together without an alternative explanation.
2. The evidence of work-relatedness was reasonably available to the employer. For purposes of this guidance, examples of reasonably available evidence included information given to the employer by employees, as well as information that an employer learned regarding its employees' health and safety in the ordinary course of managing its business and employees.

Updated OSHA Recordkeeping Guidance

OSHA issued new guidance, effective May 26, 2020, on recordkeeping of COVID-19 cases.[70] This new guidance rescinds the previous guidance issued by OSHA on April 10, 2020. Under this new guidance, all employers, regardless of type of industry or employment, are subject to the recordkeeping and reporting regulations for work-related cases of COVID-19. To determine if an employer has made a reasonable determination that a case of COVID-19 was work-related, OSHA says it will consider the following factors:

- the reasonableness of the employer's investigation of the COVID-19 case and its transmission to the employee,
- the evidence that is available to the employer, and
- the evidence that COVID-19 was contracted at work.

---

[69] OSHA, *Enforcement Guidance for Recording Cases of Coronavirus Disease 2019 (COVID-19)*, April 10, 2020, at https://www.osha.gov/memos/2020-04-10/enforcement-guidance-recording-cases-coronavirus-disease-2019-covid-19.

[70] OSHA, *Revised Enforcement Guidance for Recording Cases of Coronavirus Disease 2019 (COVID-19)*, May 19, 2020, at https://www.osha.gov/memos/2020-05-19/revised-enforcement-guidance-recording-cases-corona virus-disease-2019-covid-19.

The guidance provides examples of evidence that can be used to demonstrate that a COVID-19 case was or was not work-related, such as if an employee had frequent close contact with members of the public in an area with ongoing community transmission of COVID-19.

Injuries and Illnesses Caused by the COVID-19 Vaccine Are Not Subject to Recording and Reporting Requirements

OSHA guidance, issued in the form of questions and answers on the OSHA COVID-19 Frequently Asked Questions webpage on May 22, 2021, provides that the agency will not require any employers to record or report any injuries or illness resulting from the COVID-19 vaccine even if vaccination is a condition of employment. This guidance is to remain in effect through May 2022.[71]

Whistleblower Protections

Section 11(c) of the OSH Act prohibits any person from retaliating or discriminating against any employee who exercises certain rights provided by the OSH Act.[72] Commonly referred to as the whistleblower protection provision, this provision protects any employee who takes any of the following actions:

- files a complaint with OSHA related to a violation of the OSHAct;
- causes an OSHA proceeding, such as an investigation, to be instituted;
- testifies or is about to testify in any OSHA proceeding; and
- exercises on his or her own behalf, or on behalf of others, any otherrights afforded by the OSH Act.[73]

Other rights afforded by the OSH Act that are covered by the whistleblower protection provision include the right to inform the employer about unsafe work conditions; the right to access material safety data sheets or other information required to be made available by the employer; and the right to report a work-related injury, illness, or death to OSHA.[74] In limited cases, the employee has the right to refuse to work if conditions reasonably present a risk of serious injury or death and there is not sufficient time to eliminate the danger through other means.[75]

---

[71] OSHA, *COVID-19: Frequently Asked Questions*, at https://www.osha.gov/coronavirus/faqs#vaccine. This guidance supersedes previous guidance, issued on April 21, 2021, that required employers to record and report injuries and illnesses from the COVID-19 vaccine if the employers required the vaccine as a condition of employment.

[72] 29 U.S.C. §660(c). OSHA also enforces whistleblower provisions in 22 other federal statutes. Information on statutes with whistleblower provisions enforced by OSHA is at OSHA, *Whistleblower Statutes Summary Chart*, October 17, 2009, at https://www.whistleblowers.gov/sites/wb/files/2019-12/WB-Statute-Summary-Chart-10.8-Final.pdf.

[73] 29 C.F.R. §1977.3. Public sector employees, except employees of the U.S. Postal Service, are not protected by the whistleblower provision but may be covered by whistleblower provisions in other federal and state statutes.

[74] For additional information on other rights covered by the whistleblower protection provision, see OSHA, January 9, 2019, *Investigator's Desk Aid to the Occupational Safety and Health Act (OSH Act) Whistleblower Protection Provision*, pp. 5-7, at https://www.osha.gov/sites/default/files/11cDeskAid.pdf.

[75] 29 C.F.R. §1977.12(b)(2).

In the 116th Congress, the COVID-19 Every Worker Protection Act of 2020 (H.R. 6559/S. 3677) would have required OSHA to promulgate an ETS and required the ETS and permanent standard promulgated pursuant to the legislation to expand the protections for whistleblowers. The following additional activities taken by employees would have granted them protection from retaliation and discrimination from employers and agents of employers:

- reporting to the employer; a local, state, or federal agency; or the media or on a social media platform the following:
  - a violation of the ETS or permanent standard promulgated pursuant to the legislation,
  - a violation of the infectious disease control plan required by the ETS or permanent standard, or
  - a good-faith concern about an infectious disease hazard in the workplace;
- seeking assistance from the employer or a local, state, or federal agency with such a report; and
- using personally supplied PPE with a higher level of protection than offered by the employer.

State Occupational Safety and Health Standards

States have the authority to establish their own occupational safety and health plans and preempt standards established and enforced by OSHA.[76] OSHA must approve state plans if they are "at least as effective" as OSHA's standards and enforcement. If a state adopts a state plan, it must also cover state and local government entities, such as public schools, not covered by OSHA.

State plans may incorporate OSHA standards by reference, or states may adopt their own standards that are at least as effective as OSHA's standards. If a state has a standard that is stricter than an OSHA standard, the state standard would apply.

Two states, California and Michigan, have issued temporary standards under their state plans that directly address COVID-19 exposure, with Michigan's temporary standards rescinded and replaced by the OSHA COVID-19 ETS for health care employers. In addition, Oregon and Virginia have issued permanent COVID-19 standards, and California has had a permanent state standard covering aerosol transmission of diseases since 2009. *Table A-2* in the Appendix to this report provides a summary of these state standards.

California: Cal/OSHA Aerosol Transmissible Disease Standard

The California Division of Occupational Safety and Health (Cal/OSHA), under its state plan, promulgated its aerosol transmissible disease (ATD) standard in 2009.[77] The ATD standard

---

[76] 29 U.S.C. §667.

[77] *Aerosol Transmissible Diseases*, Cal. Code Regs. tit. 8, §5199, available at https://www.dir.ca.gov/title8/5199.html. The California state plan covers all state and local government agencies and all private sector workers in the state, with the exception of maritime workers; workers on military bases and in national parks, monuments, memorials,

covers most health care workers (including emergency medical services and police transport or detention of infected persons) and laboratory workers, as well as workers in correctional facilities, homeless shelters, and drug treatment programs. Under the ATD standard, SARS-CoV-2, the virus that causes COVID-19, is classified as a disease or pathogen requiring airborne isolation. This classification subjects the virus to stricter control standards than diseases requiring only droplet precautions, such as seasonal influenza.[78] The key requirements of the ATD standard include

- written ATD exposure control plan and procedures;
- training of all employees on COVID-19 exposure, use of PPE, and procedures if exposed to COVID-19;
- engineering and work practice controls to control COVID-19 exposure, including the use of airborne isolation rooms;
- provision of medical services to exposed employees, including post-exposure evaluation of employees and treatment and vaccines, if available;
- the removal, without penalty to the employees, of exposed employees,
- specific requirements for laboratory workers, and
- PPE requirements.

Cal/OSHA Aerosol Transmissible Disease PPE Requirements

The Cal/OSHA ATD standard requires that employers provide employees PPE, including gloves, gowns or coveralls, eye protection, and respirators certified by NIOSH at least at the N95 level whenever workers

- enter or work in an airborne isolation room or area with a case or suspected case;
- are present during procedures or services on a case or suspected case;
- repair, replace, or maintain air systems or equipment that may contain pathogens;
- decontaminate an area that is or was occupied by a case or suspected case;
- are present during aerosol generating procedures on cadavers of cases or suspected cases;
- transport a case or suspected case within a facility or within a vehicle when the patient is not masked; or
- are working with a viable virus in the laboratory.

In addition, a PAPR with a high-efficiency particulate air (HEPA) filter must be used whenever a worker performs a high-hazard procedure on a known or suspected COVID-19 case.[79] High- hazard procedures are those in which "the potential for being exposed to aerosol transmissible pathogens is increased due to the reasonably anticipated generation of aerosolized

---

and recreation areas; workers on federally recognized Native American reservations and trust lands; and U.S. Postal Service contractors.

[78] Cal. Code Regs. tit. 8, §5199 Appendix A.

[79] A PAPR uses a mechanical device to draw in room air and filter it before expelling that air over the user's face. In general, PAPRs do not require a tight seal to the user's face and do not need to be fit tested.

pathogens"— they include intubation, airway suction, and caring for patients on positive pressure ventilation.[80] Emergency medical services (EMS) workers may use N100, R100, or P100 respirators in place of PAPRs.

Cal/OSHA COVID-19 ETS

On November 19, 2020, the California Occupational Safety and Health Standards Board approved an ETS to specifically address COVID-19 exposure in the workplace.[81] This ETS became effective on November 30, 2020. The Cal/OSHA ETS applies to all covered employers in the state, including state and local government entities, and provides for broader protections than the Cal/OSHA ATD standard. The Cal/OSHA ETS includes specific provisions that apply to employer-provided housing and transportation. On June 17, 2021, the California Occupational Safety and Health Standards Board voted to amend the Cal/OSHA ETS to permit fully vaccinated employees to work indoors without facemasks or face coverings and all employees, regardless of vaccination status, to work outdoors without facemasks or face coverings. The amended Cal/OSHA ETS expired on January 14, 2022, but was extended with some revisions through April 14, 2022.

Michigan: MIOSHA COVID-19 Emergency Rules

On October 14, 2020, the director of the Michigan Department of Labor and Economic Opportunity, which operates Michigan's state occupational safety and health plan (MIOSHA), promulgated emergency rules, with a duration of six months, to address workplace exposure to COVID-19. On April 10, 2021, the MIOSHA emergency rules were extended for an additional six months through October 14, 2021. These rules were amended, effective May 24, 2021, based on updated CDC guidance, and the amended rules were to remain in effect through October 14, 2021.[82] On June 22, 2021, the Michigan Department of Labor and Economic Opportunity rescinded the MIOSHA COVID-19 emergency rules and replaced them with the OSHA COVID- 19 ETS for health care employers. After OSHA's withdrawal of the COVID-19 ETS for health care employers, this ETS is no longer in force in Michigan.

Oregon: Oregon OSHA COVID-19 Permanent Administrative Rules

On November 6, 2020, the Oregon Department of Consumer and Business Services, which operates Oregon's state plan (Oregon OSHA), adopted temporary administrative rules to specifically address COVID-19 exposures in the workplace. These rules were set to expire on

---

[80] Cal. Code Regs. tit. 8, §5199(b).

[81] *COVID-19 Prevention*, Cal. Code Regs. tit. 8, §§3205-3205.4, available at https://www.dir.ca.gov/ dosh/coronavirus/ETS.html.

[82] *Emergency Rules: Coronavirus 2019 (COVID-19)*, available at https://www.michigan.gov//documents/leo/Final_MIOSHA_Rules_705164_7.pdf. The Michigan state plan covers all state and local government agencies and all private sector workers in the state, with the exception of maritime workers, U.S. Postal Service contractors, workers at businesses owned or operated by tribal members at Indian reservations, and aircraft cabin crew members.

May 4, 2021. On May 4, 2021, permanent administrative rules became effective.[83] These permanent rules will remain in effect until repealed or revised by Oregon OSHA. Since the promulgation of the permanent administrative rules, Oregon has adopted multiple temporary amendments to the rules, some of which were incorporated into permanent amendments to the administrative rules on December 21, 2021.

Virginia: VOSH COVID-19 Permanent Standard

On July 15, 2020, the Virginia Safety and Health Codes Board adopted an ETS to specifically protect employees from exposure to SARS-CoV-2, the virus that causes COVID-19.[84] On January 12, 2021, the Virginia Safety and Health Codes Board voted to promulgate a permanent COVID- 19 standard that supersedes the ETS.[85]

This ETS, promulgated under Virginia's state occupational safety and health plan (VOSH), was the first state standard to specifically address COVID-19 in the workplace.[86] As an ETS, the VOSH standard was to expire within six months of its effective date, upon expiration of the governor's state of emergency, when superseded by a permanent standard, or when repealed by the Virginia Safety and Health Codes Board, whichever came first. The VOSH permanent standard applies to all state and local government agencies and all covered private sector employees in the state and does not contain additional requirements for any specific industries.

Among the concerns raised by groups opposed to the VOSH permanent standard was that, because the standard is permanent, employers would be required to comply with the COVID-19 prevention requirements even after the COVID-19 pandemic has ended.[87] While the standard is permanent, a provision in the standard requires that within 14 days of expiration of the governor's COVID-19 state of emergency and the commissioner of health's COVID-19 declaration of public emergency, the Virginia Safety and Health Codes Board must meet to determine if there is a continued need for the standard.

---

[83] *Addressing COVID-19 Workplace Risks*, Or. Admin. R. 437-001-0744, available at https://osha.oregon.gov/OSHARules/div1/437-001-0744.pdf. The Oregon state plan covers all state and local government agencies and all private sector workers in the state, with the exception of maritime workers, private sector establishments within the boundaries of Indian reservations and federal military reservations, employment at Crater Lake National Park and the U.S. Department of Energy Albany Research Center, U.S. Postal Service contractors, and aircraft cabin crew members during flight operations.

[84] *Infectious Disease Prevention: SARS-CoV-2 Virus That Causes COVID-19*, 16 Va. Admin. Code §25-220, available at https://www.doli.virginia.gov/wp-content/uploads/2020/07/RIS-filed-RTD-Final-ETS-7.24.2020.pdf. This ETS was effective upon publication in a Richmond, VA, newspaper during the week of July 27, 2020.

[85] *Infectious Disease Prevention of the SARS-CoV-2 Virus That Causes COVID-19*, 16 Va. Admin. Code §25-220, available at http://www.doli.virginia.gov/wp-content/uploads/2021/01/Final-Standard-for-Infectious-Disease-Prevention-of-COVID-19-16VAC25-220-1.15.2021.pdf. This permanent standard is effective on January 27, 2021.

[86] The Virginia state plan covers all state and local government agencies and all private sector workers in the state, with the exception of maritime workers, U.S. Postal Service contractors, workers at military bases or other federal enclaves in which the federal government has civil jurisdiction, workers at the U.S. Department of Energy's Southeastern Power Administration Kerr-Philpott System, and aircraft cabin crew members.

[87] See, for example, letter from Hobey Bauhan, President, Virginia Poultry Federation, to Princy Doss, Director of Policy, Planning and Public Information, and Jay Withrow, Director, Division of Legal Support, Virginia Department of Labor and Industry, January 7, 2021.

Appendix.

Table A-1. OSHA Emergency Temporary Standards (ETS)

Year	Subject of ETS	*Federal Register* Citation of ETS	Result of Judicial Review	Judicial Review Case Citation
1971	Asbestos	36 *Federal Register* 23207 (December 7, 1971)	Not challenged	—
1973	Organophosphor--ous pesticides	38 *Federal Register* 10715 (May 1, 1973); amended by 38 *Federal Register* 17214 (June 29, 1973)	Vacated	*Florida Peach Growers Ass'n v. United States Department of Labor,* 489 F.2d 120 (5th Cir. 1974)
1973	Fourteen carcinogens	38 *Federal Register* 10929 (May 3, 1973)	Twelve upheld, two vacated	*Dry Color Mfrs. Ass'n v. Department of Labor,* 486 F.2d 98 (3d Cir. 1973)
1974	Vinyl chloride	39 *Federal Register* 12342 (April 5, 1974)	Not challenged	—
1976	Diving operations	41 *Federal Register* 24271 (June 15, 1976)	Stayed	*Taylor Diving & Salvage Co. v. Department of Labor*, 537 F.2d 819 (5th Cir. 1976)
1977	Benzene	42 *Federal Register* 22515 (May 3, 1977)	Stayed	*Industrial Union Dep't v. Bingham*, 570 F.2d 965 (D.C. Cir. 1977)
1977	1,2 Dibromo-3-chloropropane (DBCP)	42 *Federal Register* 45535 (September 9, 1977)	Not challenged	—
1978	Acrylonitrile (vinyl cyanide)	43 *Federal Register* 2585 (January 17, 1978)	Stay denied	*Vistron v. OSHA*, 6 OSHC 1483 (6th Cir. 1978)
1983	Asbestos	48 *Federal Register* 51086 (November 4, 1983)	Stayed	*Asbestos Info. Ass'n v. OSHA*, 727 F.2d 415 (5th Cir. 1984)
2021	COVID-19 for health care employers	86 *Federal Register* 32376 (June 21, 2021)	Petitions for review filed on June 24, 2021. ETS withdrawn by OSHA on December 27, 2021.	*United Food and Commercial Workers and American Federation of Labor and Congress of Industrial Organizations v. OSHA, et al.*, Docket No. 21-1143 (D.C. Cir. June 24, 2021)
2021	COVID-19 vaccination and testing	86 Federal Register 61402 (November 5, 2021)	Stay ordered by U.S. Court of Appeals for the Fifth Circuit on November 6, 2021, and reaffirmed on November 12, 2021. Stay dissolved by U.S. Court of Appeals for Sixth Circuit on December 17, 2021. Stay ordered by U.S. Supreme Court on January 13, 2022.ETS withdrawn by OSHA on January 25, 2022.	*Numerous petitions for judicial review consolidated as National Federation of Independent Business, et al. v. Department of Labor, Occupational Safety and Health Administration, et al., (Docket No. 21A244), and Ohio, et al. v. Department of Labor, Occupational Safety and Health Administration, et al. (Docket No. 21A247), before the U.S. Supreme Court.*

Source: CRS with data from Mark A. Rothstein, "Substantive and Procedural Obstacles to OSHA Rulemaking: Reproductive Hazards as an Example," Boston College Environmental Affairs Law Review, vol. 12, no. 4 (August 1985), p. 673.

[a] For additional information on judicial review of the OSHA COVID-19 vaccination and testing ETS, see CRS Legal Sidebar LSB10658, Fifth Circuit Stays OSHA Vaccination and Testing Standard.

Table A-2. State occupational safety and health standards that apply to COVID-19

State	Standard	Covered Employers	Issued	Expires
California (Cal/OSHA)	Aerosol Transmissible Disease (ATD)[a]	Health care, laboratories, corrections facilities, homeless shelters, and drug treatment centers	July 6, 2009	Permanent
	COVD-19 Prevention[b]	All employers	November 30, 2020 June 17, 2021 (amended) January 5, 2022 (amended)	April 14, 2022
Michigan (MIOSHA)	Emergency Rules: Coronavirus 2019 (COVID-19)[c]	All employers, with additional rules for specific industries	October 14, 2020, April 10, 2021 (extended) May 24, 2021 (amended)	Rescinded on June 22, 2021, and replaced with OSHA COVID-19 ETS for health care employers, which expired with OSHA's
				withdrawal of the ETS.
Oregon (Oregon OSHA)	Addressing COVID-19 Workplace Risks[d]	All employers, with additional rules for specific industries	November 6, 2020 (ETS), reissued December 11, 2020 May 4, 2021 (permanent standard) December 21, 2021 (amended)	Permanent[e]
Virginia (VOSH)	Infectious Disease Prevention: SARS-CoV-2 Virus that Causes COVID-19[f]	All employers	July 27, 2020 (ETS), January 12, 2021 (permanent standard)	Permanent[g]

Source: Congressional Research Service (CRS).

[a] Available at https://www.dir.ca.gov/title8/5199.html.

[b] Available at https://www.dir.ca.gov/dosh/coronavirus/ETS.html.

[c] Available at https://www.michigan.gov//documents/leo/Final_MIOSHA_Rules_705164_7.pdf.

[d] Available at https://osha.oregon.gov/OSHARules/div1/437-001-0744.pdf.

[e] Oregon OSHA is required to consult with state agencies and other stakeholders to determine when the permanent rules can be amended or repealed, with the first of these consultations to occur no later than July 2021. After the first consultations, ongoing consultations are required every two months until the rules are repealed.

[f] Available at http://www.doli.virginia.gov/wp-content/uploads/2021/01/Final-Standard-for-Infectious-Disease- Prevention-of-COVID-19-16VAC25-220-1.15.2021.pdf.

[g] Within 14 days of expiration of the governor's COVID-19 state of emergency and the commissioner of health's COVID-19 declaration of public emergency, the Virginia Safety and Health Codes Board must meet to determine if there is a continued need for the standard.

Chapter 13

State and Federal Authority to Mandate COVID-19 Vaccination*

Wen W. Shen

Summary

The Coronavirus Disease 2019 (COVID-19) vaccines licensed or authorized by the U.S. Food and Drug Administration (FDA) are a critical tool to reduce the spread and severity of COVID-19. FDA initially authorized the vaccines, between December 2020 and February 2021, under Section 564 of the Federal Food, Drug, and Cosmetic Act (FD&C Act), a regulatory pathway that allows certain medical products to be made available in the market prior to full FDA approval under specified circumstances, including during a public health emergency. In August 2021, FDA licensed the first COVID- 19 vaccine, Pfizer's Comirnaty, for the prevention of COVID-19 in individuals 16 years of age and older, after determining that the vaccine, for the licensed use, meets the standards for safety, purity, and potency (i.e., effectiveness) under the Public Health Service Act.

Given the data supporting the safety and efficacy of the licensed and authorized COVID-19 vaccines, many public health experts view promoting high COVID-19 vaccination rates—along with continued engagement in community mitigation activities that prevent transmission, such as mask wearing in certain settings—as key components of the United States' pandemic response.

One available legal tool for increasing vaccination rates is for governments to require vaccination. In 2021, various state, local, and federal governmental entities instituted COVID-19 vaccination requirements to address the pandemic, particularly as the Delta variant—a highly contagious strain of SARS-CoV-2 (the virus that causes COVID-19)—spread in the United States. Under the United States' federalist system, states and the federal government share regulatory authority over public health matters, with states traditionally exercising the bulk of the authority in this area pursuant to their general police power. That power authorizes states, within constitutional limits, to enact laws "to provide for the public health, safety, and morals" of the states' inhabitants. In contrast to this general power, the federal government's powers are confined to those enumerated in the Constitution.

* This is an edited, reformatted and augmented version of Congressional Research Service Publication No. R46745, dated January 18, 2022.

In: COVID-19 Vaccines
Editor: John Schroder
ISBN: 979-8-88697-150-7

This chapter provides an overview of state and federal authority to mandate vaccination. The first part of the chapter provides background on state and local authority to mandate vaccination under the states' general police power. It discusses the Supreme Court's long-standing recognition of state and local authority to mandate vaccination as an exercise of their police power, and modern courts' analyses of more recent challenges to state vaccination mandates based on the First Amendment's Free Exercise Clause. The chapter then analyzes the Supreme Court's evolving free exercise jurisprudence and the questions it raises regarding whether and when governments must provide for or grant religious exemptions to vaccination requirements. It then looks at how courts have addressed challenges to COVID-19 vaccination requirements imposed by states and state entities.

The second part of the chapter provides an overview of federal authority to mandate vaccination. It discusses several sources of existing federal statutory authority that could serve, or have been invoked, as the basis for federal COVID-19 vaccination mandates. It then provides an overview of four employment-based civilian mandates issued by the executive branch to date directed at (1) federal executive agency civilian employees; (2) federal contractors for executive departments, agencies, and offices; (3) most Medicare- and Medicaid-certified providers and suppliers; and (4) employers with 100 or more employees. The chapter then discusses the state of litigation challenging these mandates. This part also reviews the extent of Congress's constitutional authority under the Constitution's Spending and Commerce Clauses to mandate vaccination.

The chapter concludes with a brief discussion of a legal issue specific to COVID-19 vaccination mandates, particularly before FDA's licensure of Comirnaty. Namely, it reviews how courts have addressed some litigants' argument that the Emergency Use Authorization status of COVID-19 vaccines preclude entities from mandating COVID-19 vaccination.

The Coronavirus Disease 2019 (COVID-19) vaccines licensed or authorized by the U.S. Food and Drug Administration (FDA) are a critical tool to reduce the spread and severity of COVID-19.[1] Until August 2021, all COVID-19 vaccines were authorized under Section 564 of the Federal Food, Drug, and Cosmetic Act (FD&C Act),[2] a regulatory pathway that allows certain medical products to be made available in the market prior to FDA approval under specified circumstances, including during public health emergencies.[3] FDA issued the Emergency Use Authorizations (EUAs) under Section 564 after determining that the COVID-

[1] *See, e.g., Vaccines Prevented Up to 140,000 COVID-19 Deaths in U.S.*, NAT'L INST. HEALTH, NIH RESEARCH MATTERS (Aug. 24, 2021), https://www.nih.gov/news-events/nih-research-matters/vaccines-prevented-140000-covid- 19-deaths-us; Eric C. Schneider et al., *How Many COVID-19 Hospitalizations and Deaths Can Be Averted if States Immediately Accelerate Their Vaccination Efforts?*, COMMONWEALTH FUND BLOG (Oct. 5, 2021), https://www.commonwealthfund.org/blog/2021/how-many-covid-19-hospitalizations-deaths-averted-states-accelerate- vaccination.

[2] FDA authorized three COVID-19 vaccines under Emergency Use Authorizations between December 2020 and February 2021. *See FDA Takes Key Action in Fight Against COVID-19 by Issuing Emergency Use Authorization for First COVID-19 Vaccine*, U.S. FOOD & DRUG ADMIN. (Dec. 11, 2020), https://www.fda.gov/news-events/press-announcements/fda-takes-key-action-fight-against-covid-19-issuing-emergency-use-authori zation-first-covid-19; *FDA Takes Additional Action in Fight Against COVID-19 by Issuing Emergency Use Authorization for First COVID-19 Vaccine*, U.S. FOOD & DRUG ADMIN. (Dec. 18, 2020), https://www.fda.gov/news-events/press-announcements/fda-takes-additional-action-fight-against-covid-19-issuing-emergency-use-authorization-second-covid; *FDA Issues Emergency Use Authorization for Third COVID-19 Vaccine*, U.S. FOOD & DRUG ADMIN, (Feb. 27, 2021), https://www.fda.gov/news-events/press-announcements/fda-issues-emergency-use-authorization-third-covid-19- vaccine [hereinafter, and collectively, FDA EUA Press Releases].

[3] *See* 21 U.S.C. § 360bbb-3. *See also* CRS In Focus IF10745, *Emergency Use Authorization and FDA's Related Authorities*, by Agata Bodie.

19 vaccines met the applicable statutory standards and the Agency's specific safety and efficacy standards.[4] Among other information, data supporting the EUA requests show that the vaccines are effective at preventing symptomatic COVID-19 in vaccinated individuals.[5] Since receiving the EUAs, each COVID-19 vaccine manufacturer, building on the clinical trial safety and effectiveness data previously submitted to FDA in support of their EUA requests, has submitted or is in the process of submitting a biologics license application (BLA) to obtain full approval of the vaccines for specified uses.[6] In August 2021, FDA licensed the first COVID-19 vaccine, Pfizer's Comirnaty, for the prevention of COVID-19 in individuals 16 years of age and older, after determining that the vaccine, for the licensed use, meets the standards for safety, purity, and potency (i.e., effectiveness) under the Public Health Service Act (PHSA).[7]

Given the data supporting the safety and efficacy of the licensed and authorized COVID-19 vaccines, many public health experts view promoting high COVID-19 vaccination rates—along with continued engagement in community mitigation activities that prevent transmission, such as mask wearing in certain settings—as key components of the United States' pandemic response.[8] One available legal tool for increasing vaccination rates is for governmental entities to require vaccination.[9] During 2021, various state, local, and federal governmental entities instituted COVID-19 vaccination requirements to address the pandemic, particularly as the Delta variant—a highly contagious strain of SARS-CoV-2 (the virus that causes COVID-19)—

---

[4] FDA EUA Press Releases, *supra* note 2. *See also* CRS Report R46399, *Legal Issues in COVID-19 Vaccine Development and Deployment*, by Kevin J. Hickey, Wen W. Shen, and Erin H. Ward, at 12–14.

[5] FDA EUA Press Releases, *supra* note 2. At the time of the COVID-19 vaccines' authorization, data supporting their EUA requests showed that the vaccines were between 67%–95% effective at preventing symptomatic COVID-19. *See id.*

[6] See FDA Approves First COVID-19 Vaccine, U.S. FOOD & DRUG ADMIN. (Aug. 23, 2021), https://www.fda.gov/news- events/press-announcements/fda-approves-first-covid-19-vaccine [hereinafter FDA Comirnaty Press Release]; Moderna Completes Submission of Biologics License Application to the U.S. Food and Drug Administration for Its COVID-19 Vaccine, MODERNA (Aug. 25, 2021), https://investors.modernatx.com/news-releases/news-release-details/moderna-completes-submission-biologics-license-application-us; Johnson & Johnson Single-Shot COVID-19 Vaccinations to Resume in the U.S. for All Adults Aged 18 and Older Following CDC and FDA Decision, JOHNSON & JOHNSON (Apr. 23, 2021), https://www.jnj.com/ johnson-johnson-single-shot-covid-19-vaccinations-to-resume-in-the-u-s-for-all-adults-aged-18-and-older-following-cdc-and-fda-decision.

[7] See FDA Comirnaty Press Release, supra note 6. See also 42 U.S.C. § 262(a)(2)(C). For more information about FDA's approval of Comirnaty, see CRS Report R46913, FDA Approval of the Pfizer-BioNTech COVID-19 Vaccine: Frequently Asked Questions, by Kevin J. Hickey, Erin H. Ward, and Agata Bodie.

[8] See, e.g., COVID-19: Prevent Getting Sick, CTRS FOR DISEASE CONTROL & PREVENTION (Apr. 27, 2021), https://www.cdc.gov/coronavirus/2019-ncov/prevent-getting-sick/index.html; Stacy Wood & Kevin Schulman, Beyond Politics—Promoting Covid-19 Vaccination in the United States, NEW ENG. J. MED. (Feb. 18, 2021), https://www.nejm.org/doi/full/10.1056/NEJMms2033790; Mary Van Beusekom, Experts Propose Steps to Promote, Distribute COVID Vaccine, CIDRAP NEWS (Dec. 15, 2020), https://www.cidrap.umn.edu/news-perspective/2020/12/ experts-propose-steps-promote-distribute-covid-vaccine; Gypsyamber D'Souza & David Dowdy, Rethinking Herd Immunity and the COVID-19 Response End Game, JOHNS HOPKINS (Sept. 13, 2021), https://publichealth.jhu.edu/2021/what-is-herd-immunity-and-how-can-we-achieve-it-with-covid-19.

[9] While it is beyond the scope of this report, there are also a range of public policy and other legal tools available (such as education, accessibility, and outreach efforts) to increase vaccine uptake short of a mandate. See Kevin G. Volpp et al., Behaviorally Informed Strategies for a National COVID-19 Vaccine Promotion Program, JAMA (Dec. 14, 2020), https://jamanetwork.com/journals/jama/fullarticle/2774381; Matt Motta et al., Encouraging COVID-19 Vaccine Uptake Through Effective Health Communication, FRONTIER IN POL. SCI. (Jan. 28, 2021), https://www.frontiersin.org/articles/ 10.3389/fpos.2021.630133/full. See also Dorit Rubinstein Reiss & Lois A. Weithorn, Responding to the Childhood Vaccination Crisis: Legal Frameworks and Tools in the Context of Parental Vaccine Refusal, 63 BUFF. L. REV. 881, 958–79 (2015) (describing a continuum of legal tools to increase vaccination rates).

spread in the United States.[10] For instance, some states imposed COVID-19 vaccination requirements on certain state employees and/or health care workers;[11] many state entities, such as public universities, likewise imposed vaccination requirements on their staff and students.[12] Several cities issued ordinances or orders that require certain indoor business establishments to verify their patrons' proof of vaccination before permitting entry.[13] The federal government issued several employment- or workforce-based mandates that either directly require certain employees to receive COVID-19 vaccinations or direct certain employers to impose a vaccination or vaccination-and-testing requirement on their employees or staff.[14] With the exception of a few state health care worker vaccination requirements that provide only for medical exemptions, the governmental vaccination mandates issued to date generally provide exceptions from the vaccination requirements based on a disability, medical condition, or sincerely held religious belief.[15]

Under the United States' federalist system, states and the federal government share regulatory authority over public health matters, with states traditionally exercising the bulk of the authority in this area pursuant to their general police power.[16] This power authorizes states, within constitutional limits, to enact laws "to provide for the public health, safety, and morals" of the states' inhabitants.[17] In contrast to this general power, the federal government's powers are confined to those enumerated in the Constitution.[18]

---

[10] Delta Variant: What We Know About the Science, CTRS. FOR DISEASE CONTROL & PREVENTION (Aug. 26, 2021), https://www.cdc.gov/coronavirus/2019-ncov/variants/delta-variant.html. As of December 20, 2021, a new variant of SARS-CoV-2 first detected in the United States in late November 2021—the Omicron variant—has overtaken Delta to become the dominant strain for new COVID-19 infections in the United States. See COVID Data Tracker, CTRS. FOR DISEASE CONTROL & PREVENTION, https://covid.cdc.gov/covid-data-tracker/#variant-proportions (last accessed Dec. 21, 2021).

[11] *See, e.g.*, N.M. DEP'T OF HEALTH, AMENDED PUBLIC HEALTH EMERGENCY ORDER REQUIRING ALL SCHOOL WORKERS COMPLY WITH CERTAIN HEALTH REQUIREMENTS AND REQUIRING CONGREGATE CARE FACILITY WORKERS, HOSPITAL WORKERS, AND EMPLOYEES OF THE OFFICE OF THE GOVERNOR BE FULLY VACCINATED (Sept. 15, 2021), https://www.nmhealth.org/publication/view/rules/6875/; OFF. OF THE GOVERNOR, COMMONWEALTH OF MASS., IMPLEMENTING A REQUIREMENT FOR COVID-19 VACCINATION FOR THE COMMONWEALTH'S EXECUTIVE DEPARTMENT EMPLOYEES (Aug. 19, 2021), https://www.mass.gov/doc/august-19-2021-executive-department-employee-vaccination- order/download; Code Me. R. tit. 10-144, ch. 264, § 2 (2021) (emergency regulation issued by Maine's Department of Health and Human Services adding COVID-19 vaccination to the list of required vaccinations for most health care workers); 10 N.Y.C.R.R. § 2.61 (emergency regulation issued by the New York Department of Health requiring COVID-19 vaccination for certain health care workers).

[12] *See* Elissa Nadworny, *Full FDA Approval Triggers More Universities to Require the COVID-19 Vaccine*, NPR (Sept. 1, 2021), https://www.npr.org/2021/09/01/1031385629/full-fda-approval-triggers-more-universities-to-require- the-covid-19-vaccine.

[13] *See, e.g.*, 10 L.A. Municipal Code § 200.122 (2021), https://clkrep.lacity.org/onlinedocs/2021/21-0878_ord_187219_ 11-08-21.pdf; CITY OF N.Y., EMERGENCY EXECUTIVE ORDER NO. 228, § 4 (Aug. 25, 2021), https://www1.nyc.gov/assets/home/downloads/pdf/executive-orders/2021/eeo-228.pdf.

[14] *See infra* "Executive Branch Authority to Mandate Vaccination."

[15] *See infra* "State COVID-19 Vaccination Mandates and Related Litigation" and "Executive Branch Authority to Mandate Vaccination." In addition to governmental entities, private entities—especially private employers—have also opted to institute vaccination requirements in response to the pandemic. For more information about legal constraints on vaccination requirements imposed by private employers, see CRS Legal Sidebar LSB10573, *COVID-19 Vaccination Requirements: Potential Constraints on Employer Mandates Under Federal Law*, by April J. Anderson and Victoria L. Killion.

[16] *See* Elizabeth Y. McCuskey, *Body of Preemption: Health Law Traditions and the Presumption Against Preemption*, 89 TEMPLE L. REV. 95, 113–20 (2016).

[17] Barnes v. Glen Theatre, Inc., 501 U.S. 560, 569 (1991).

[18] *See* CRS Report R45323, *Federalism-Based Limitations on Congressional Power: An Overview*, coordinated by Andrew Nolan and Kevin M. Lewis, at 1.

This chapter provides an overview of state and federal authority to mandate vaccination. The first part of the chapter provides background on state and local authority to mandate vaccination under the states' general police power. It discusses the Supreme Court's long-standing recognition of state and local authority to mandate vaccination as an exercise of their police power, and modern courts' analyses of more recent challenges to state vaccination mandates based on the First Amendment's Free Exercise Clause. It then analyzes the Supreme Court's evolving Free Exercise Clause jurisprudence and the questions it raises regarding whether and when governments must provide for or grant religious exemptions to vaccination requirements.[19] It then takes a look at how courts have addressed challenges to COVID-19-vaccination requirements imposed by state and state entities to date.[20]

The second part of the chapter provides an overview of federal authority to mandate vaccination. It begins by discussing several sources of existing federal statutory authority that could serve, or have been invoked, as the basis for federal COVID-19 vaccination mandates. It then provides an overview of four employment-based civilian mandates issued by the executive branch to date directed at (1) federal executive agency civilian employees; (2) federal contractors for executive departments, agencies, and offices; (3) most Medicare- and Medicaid-certified providers and suppliers; and (4) employers with 100 or more employees. The chapter then analyzes the litigation challenging these mandates,[21] before reviewing the extent of Congress's constitutional authority under the Spending and Commerce Clauses to potentially mandate vaccination.[22]

The chapter concludes with a brief discussion of a legal issue specific to COVID-19 vaccination mandates, particularly before FDA's licensure of Comirnaty. Namely, it looks at how courts have addressed some litigants' argument that the EUA status of COVID-19 vaccines precludes entities from mandating COVID-19 vaccination.[23]

State and Local Authority to Mandate Vaccination

Legal Background

State and local vaccination requirements—as government actions—are subject to constitutional constraints, including those that protect individual rights.[24] For instance, the government is prohibited by the Bill of Rights from infringing the free exercise of religion or violating due process of law.[25] For more than a century, however, the Supreme Court has recognized few rights- based constraints on states' ability to mandate vaccination, holding instead that the states' general police power to promote public health and safety encompasses authority to mandate vaccination.[26]

---

[19] *See infra* "Legal Background."

[20] *See infra* "State COVID-19 Vaccination Mandates and Related Litigation."

[21] *See infra* "Executive Branch Authority to Mandate Vaccination."

[22] *See infra* "Congress's Constitutional Authority to Mandate Vaccination."

[23] *See infra* "Emergency Use Authorization and Vaccination Mandates."

[24] *See* U.S. CONST. art. XIV, cl. 1, § 1; Edmonson v. Leesville Concrete Co., 500 U.S. 614, 619 (1991) ("The Constitution's protections of individual liberty and equal protection apply in general only to action by the government.").

[25] *See* U.S. CONST. amends. I & XIV.

[26] *See* Jacobson v. Massachusetts, 197 U.S. 11, 39 (1905).

In the early part of the 20th century, the Supreme Court twice considered constitutional challenges to state vaccination mandates.[27] Each time, the Court rejected the challenges to the mandates and recognized such laws as falling squarely within the states' police power.[28] In 1905, the Supreme Court in *Jacobson v. Massachusetts* upheld a state law that gave municipal boards of health the authority to require the vaccination of persons over the age of 21 against smallpox, determining the vaccination program had a "real [and] substantial relation to the protection of the public health and safety."[29] In doing so, the Court rejected an argument that such a program violated a liberty interest that, under more modern jurisprudence, the plaintiff might have asserted as a substantive due process right.[30]

Less than two decades later, in *Zucht v. King*, parents of a child who was excluded from school due to her unvaccinated status challenged the local ordinance requiring vaccination for schoolchildren, arguing that the ordinance violated the Fourteenth Amendment's Equal Protection and Due Process Clauses.[31] Relying on *Jacobson*, the Supreme Court rejected the constitutional challenges, concluding "it is within the police power of a State to provide for compulsory vaccination" and that the ordinance bestowed "only that broad discretion required for the protection of the public health."[32]

Based on the Supreme Court's recognition of this authority, states and localities have enacted vaccination mandates for certain populations and circumstances. All 50 states and the District of Columbia, for instance, currently have laws requiring all students enrolled in both public and private schools to receive specified vaccines as a condition of school entry.[33] With respect to adults, states—to the extent they have mandated vaccination—have typically limited the mandates to health care workers, who are required to be vaccinated against certain vaccine-preventable diseases as a condition of their employment.[34] These vaccination requirements are generally subject to certain exemptions, which vary from state to state.[35] While most vaccination mandates generally provide for some degree of medical exemption (i.e., when individuals have a contraindication to a vaccine that makes receipt of the vaccine harmful or unsafe),[36] many mandates also include exemptions for those whose religious beliefs counsel against immunization.[37] In the case of student vaccination mandates, several states also provide

---

[27] *Id.*; Zucht v. King, 260 U.S. 174 (1922).

[28] *Jacobson*, 197 U.S. at 39; *Zucht*, 260 U.S. at 175–77.

[29] *Jacobson*, 197 U.S. at 31.

[30] *See* Reiss & Weithorn, *supra* note 9, at 897–98.

[31] *Zucht*, 260 U.S. at 175–77.

[32] *Id.* at 176–77.

[33] *States with Religious and Philosophical Exemptions From School Immunization Requirements*, NAT'L CONF. OF STATE LEGISLATURES (NCSL) (Nov. 22, 2021), https://www.ncsl.org/research/health/school-immuni zation-exemption- state-laws.aspx.

[34] *See* Brian Dean Abramson, *Vaccine Law in the Health Care Workplace*, 12 J. HEALTH & LIFE SCI. L. 22, 24–27 (2019) (describing different approaches states have taken to impose vaccination requirements on health care workers: some states require health care workers to receive annual flu vaccines; several others require hospitals or other health care facilities to ensure their employees have been vaccinated against certain vaccine-preventable diseases, including hepatitis B, rubella, and mumps; and still others require hospital employees to provide proof of immunization against certain vaccine-preventable diseases).

[35] *See id.* at 28–31 (describing scope of medical and religious exemptions for vaccination mandates for health care workers); NCSL, *supra* note 33 (describing exemptions for student vaccination mandates).

[36] *See, e.g.*, N.Y. Pub. Health Law § 2164(8) (providing a medical exemption from school vaccination requirements if a licensed physician "certifies that such immunization may be detrimental to a child's health").

[37] Abramson, *supra* note 34, at 28–31; NCSL, *supra* note 33.

a broader philosophical exemption for those who object to immunizations because of personal, moral, or other beliefs.[38]

These state and local vaccination mandates have withstood more recent legal challenges.[39] While the Supreme Court's constitutional jurisprudence has evolved substantially since *Jacobson* and *Zucht*,[40] modern courts have continued to rely on these cases to reject due process and equal protection claims against vaccination mandates, giving considerable deference to the states' use of their police power to require immunizations to protect public health.[41]

Prior to the COVID-19 pandemic, courts have also generally upheld state vaccination requirements that do not provide for a religious exemption. While most states' school vaccination requirements provide for religious exemptions, several states—some in response to concerns over outbreaks of vaccine-preventable diseases and/or declining vaccination rates—have eliminated those exemptions to permit only medical exemptions.[42]

In the modern era, these mandates without religious exemptions have been subject to several legal challenges, in which plaintiffs have argued the applicable mandate violated their rights under the First Amendment's Free Exercise Clause.[43] Courts generally rejected these claims and concluded that a state is not constitutionally required to provide for a religious exemption.[44] The courts reasoned that, under *Employment Division v. Smith* and its progeny, the vaccination mandates at issue were neutral, generally applicable laws—i.e., laws that do not single out religion or selectively burden religiously motivated conduct.[45] As such, the

---

[38] NCSL, *supra* note 33.

[39] *See, e.g.*, Phillips v. City of New York, 775 F.3d 538, 542–44 (2d Cir. 2015); Workman v. Mingo Cty. Bd. of Edu. 419 F. App'x 348 (4th Cir. 2011); Whitlow v. California, 203 F. Supp. 3d 1079, 1085–89 (S.D. Cal. 2016); Boone v. Boozman, 217 F. Supp. 2d 938, 952–57 (E.D. Ark. 2002). Prior to the COVID-19 pandemic, challenges against state vaccination mandates have primarily occurred in the context of student vaccination requirements. However, in 2009, following the emergence of a new strain of type A influenza (H1N1), New York State issued a regulation that made vaccination against seasonal and H1N1 influenza a condition of employment for health care workers who have direct contact with patients or who may expose patients to disease. This directive drew several legal challenges from local health care workers who argued that the regulation violated the Fourteenth Amendment's Due Process Clause, the First Amendment's Free Exercise Clause, and the right to "freedom of contract" guaranteed by the Fifth and Fourteenth Amendments. *See* Alexander M. Stewart, *Mandatory Vaccination of Health Care Workers*, NEW ENG. J. OF MED. (Nov. 19, 2009), https://www.nejm.org/ doi/full/10.1056/nejmp0910151. The litigation, however, was mooted in its early stages after the governor suspended the regulation due to a vaccine shortage. *See* Joe Nocera, *When New York Mandated Vaccinations, Nurses Sued*, BLOOMBERG BUSINESSWEEK (Mar. 23, 2020), https://www. bloombergcom/news/articles/ 2020-03-23/can-states-mandate-vaccinations-for-health-care-workers.

[40] Commentators have observed, for instance, that the Supreme Court decided *Jacobson* and *Zucht* before the advent of tiered scrutiny, which may subject regulations that infringe upon certain fundamental liberty interests to heightened scrutiny. Reiss & Weithorn, *supra* note 9, at 896–97. A regulation survives the most heightened level of scrutiny only if it is narrowly tailored to serve a compelling government interest. *See* Reno v. Flores, 507 U.S. 292, 301–02 (1993).

[41] *See, e.g.*, *Phillips*, 775 F.3d at 543; *Workman*, 419 F. App'x at 352–54; *Whitlow*, 203 F. Supp. 3d at 1085–87.

[42] *See* James Colgrove & Abigail Lowin, *A Tale of Two States: Mississippi, West Virginia, And Exemptions to Compulsory School Vaccination Laws*, HEALTH AFFS. (Feb. 2016), https://www.healthaffairs.org/ doi/10.1377/hlthaff.2015.1172. From 1979 to 2016, Mississippi and West Virginia were the only two states that did not offer nonmedical exemptions. Since 2016, four additional states—California, New York, Maine, and Connecticut—have eliminated nonmedical exemptions. *See* NCSL, *supra* note 33.

[43] *See, e.g.*, *Phillips*, 775 F.3d at 543; *Workman*, 419 F. App'x at 352–54; *Whitlow*, 203 F. Supp. 3d at 1085–87; *Boone*, 217 F. Supp. 2d at 952–55.

[44] *See, e.g.*, *Phillips*, 775 F.3d at 543; *Workman*, 419 F. App'x at 352–54; *Whitlow*, 203 F. Supp. 3d at 1085–87; *Boone*, 217 F. Supp. 2d at 952–55. The alleged violation of the Free Exercise Clause was not a claim available to the plaintiffs in *Jacobson* or *Zucht* because at that time, the Supreme Court had not yet held that the First Amendment applied to the states. *See Phillips*, 775 F.3d at 543.

[45] *See, e.g.*, *Phillips*, 775 F.3d at 543; *Workman*, 419 F. App'x at 352–54; *Whitlow*, 203 F. Supp. 3d at 1085–87; *Boone*, 217 F. Supp. 2d at 952–55.

vaccination mandates, in these courts' view, were not subject to heightened scrutiny under *Smith*.[46] Applying rational-basis review, a lenient standard under which courts generally uphold laws that reasonably further legitimate government interests, courts have held that "the right to free exercise of religion . . . [is] subordinated to society's interest in protecting against the spread of disease."[47]

In 2021, however, the Supreme Court issued two decisions that potentially weaken these precedents involving free exercise challenges to vaccination mandates. In *Tandon v. Newsom*, the Court ruled that a law is not neutral and generally applicable if it treats "*any* comparable secular activity more favorably than religious exercise."[48] "[W]hether two activities are comparable for purposes of the Free Exercise Clause," the Court explained, depends on "the asserted government interest that justifies the regulation at issue."[49] Applying this standard, the Court concluded that the state regulations at issue in *Tandon*, which limited religious gatherings in response to the COVID-19 pandemic, treated some comparable secular activities—such as getting haircuts and retail shopping—more favorably without showing that these secular activities posed a lower risk of transmission of COVID-19.[50] Thus, the Court applied heightened scrutiny and granted a preliminary injunction, staying enforcement of the state regulations during pendency of the litigation.[51]

A few months after the *Tandon* ruling, the Supreme Court, in *Fulton v. City of Philadelphia*, considered whether a city's contract provision prohibiting sexual orientation discrimination by contractors violated a religious foster care agency's free exercise rights.[52] The contract provision at issue generally prohibited providers from rejecting a child or family for services based on their sexual orientation unless a specified city official, at his "sole discretion," granted an exception.[53] Even though the City had never granted an exception under the provision, the Court held that this exemption system meant that the nondiscrimination policy was not generally applicable under *Smith*.[54] This system, in the Court's view, "incorporate[d] a system of individual exemptions" that invited the government "to decide which reasons for not complying with the policy are worthy of solicitude."[55] Because a law lacks general applicability "if it prohibits religious conduct while permitting secular conduct

---

[46] *See, e.g.*, *Phillips*, 775 F.3d at 543; *Workman*, 419 F. App'x at 352–54; *Whitlow*, 203 F. Supp. 3d at 1085–87; *Boone*, 217 F. Supp. 2d at 952–55.

[47] *Boone*, 217 F. Supp. 2d at 954; *see also Phillips*, 775 F.3d at 543; *Workman*, 419 F. App'x at 352–54; *Whitlow*, 203 F. Supp. 3d at 1085–87. In cases where a vaccination mandate includes a religious exemption, plaintiffs have also filed suit to challenge their unsuccessful invocation of the exemption. In these cases, courts, applying the relevant state law, typically considered whether the plaintiffs' objections to vaccination are based on a sincerely held religious belief. *See, e.g.*, N.M. v. Hebrew Acad. Long Beach, 155 F. Supp. 3d 247, 257–58 (E.D.N.Y. 2016) (finding that plaintiff failed to establish her objections to vaccination were religious in nature); *In re* Christine M., 157 Misc. 2d 4, 21 (N.Y. 1992) (finding that plaintiff's objections to vaccination were based on plaintiff's personal and medical, rather than religious, beliefs); Lewis v. Sobol, 710 F. Supp. 506, 516 (S.D.N.Y. 1989) (finding that plaintiffs' objections to vaccination stemmed from their religious beliefs, which entailed "views of spiritual perfection" that they apply in their dietary and medical practices).

[48] 141 S. Ct. 1294, 1296 (2021) (per curiam) (alteration in original). The Supreme Court's *Tandon* ruling was issued on the Court's non-merits docket. For more information about the potential differences in the precedential value of the Court's non-merits versus merits decisions, see *infra* note 110.

[49] *Tandon*, 141 S. Ct. at 1296.

[50] *Id.* at 1297.

[51] *Id.* at 1297–98.

[52] 141 S. Ct. 1868

[53] *Id.* at 1878.

[54] *Id.*

[55] *Id.* at 1879.

that undermines the government's asserted interest in a similar way," the Court held that the City "may not refuse to extend that exemption system to cases of religious hardship without compelling reason."[56] The Court concluded that the City failed to offer any compelling reason for "why it has a particular interest in denying an exception to [the plaintiff foster care agency] while making them available to others."[57]

Together, *Fulton* and *Tandon* could suggest that where a governmental requirement provides a secular exemption from the requirement (but no religious exemption), and the exemption system is to some extent discretionary, the requirement may not be neutral and generally applicable for purposes of the Free Exercise Clause.[58] This interpretation would mean that a governmental requirement with only a secular exemption—assuming that the secular exemption is comparable to a hypothetical religious exemption as measured against the asserted government interest underlying the requirement—may be subject to heightened scrutiny.[59]

For state vaccination requirements—which typically provide, at a minimum, medical exemptions to those with contraindications—*Fulton* and *Tandon* thus raise a number of questions that potentially unsettle the law concerning vaccination requirements and religious freedom. These questions include whether a vaccination requirement that provides only for a medical exemption—a secular exemption—is not neutral and generally applicable; whether that analysis depends on the extent to which the medical exemption process is discretionary; and whether medical and religious exemptions—as measured against the relevant underlying government interest for vaccination requirements—are comparable exemptions in the context of this analysis. To the extent a vaccination requirement that provides only a medical exemption would be subject to heightened scrutiny, *Fulton* and *Tandon* also leave unanswered whether there are certain circumstances under which the requirement would survive such scrutiny.

While courts have historically upheld state vaccination requirements generally, more recent developments in the Supreme Court's free exercise jurisprudence raise questions regarding whether, when, and under what circumstances states must provide or grant religious exemptions to a vaccination requirement.

State COVID-19 Vaccination Mandates and Related Litigation

In 2021, various state and local entities instituted COVID-19 vaccination requirements to address the pandemic, particularly as the Delta variant began to cause surges in COVID-19 cases across the country. Many public universities, for instance, imposed vaccination requirements on their students and staff as a condition of in-person attendance and employment.[60] A few cities required certain indoor business establishments in their jurisdictions to verify their patrons' proof of vaccination before permitting their entry.[61] To date, only a few states have imposed statewide vaccination requirements, and these requirements are generally limited to health care workers.[62] At least one state—California—

[56] *Id.* at 1877–78 (internal alterations and quotations omitted) (quoting Emp. Div., Dep't of Hum. Res. of Or. v. Smith, 494 U.S. 872, 884 (1990)).
[57] *Id.*
[58] *See id.* at 1878–79; Tandon v. Newsom, 141 S. Ct. 1294, 1297–98 (2021) (per curiam).
[59] *See Fulton*, 141 S. Ct. at 1878–79; *Tandon*, 141 S. Ct. at 1297–98.
[60] *See supra* note 12 and accompanying text.
[61] *See supra* note 13 and accompanying text.
[62] *See supra* note 11 and accompanying text.

announced in 2021 plans to add COVID-19 vaccination to the list of required student vaccinations. The requirement is expected to be phased-in by grade span in 2022, applying to grades 7 through 12 starting on July 1, 2022.[63] With the exception of several state health care worker mandates (as well as California's expected student vaccination requirements) that provide only for a medical exemption,[64] most of these state and local vaccination requirements provide for both medical and religious exemptions.

Many of these state COVID-19 vaccination requirements have drawn legal challenges. To date, consistent with the discussion in the preceding section, courts have generally upheld these requirements, particularly if the requirements provide for both medical and religious exemptions.[65] Some of the common claims raised in these challenges include, for instance, an alleged violation of the plaintiffs' substantive due process rights to bodily integrity or right to refuse unwanted medical treatment, or an alleged violation of their equal protection rights. Courts have generally rejected these claims, relying on *Jacobson* to conclude that a fundamental right or a suspect class is not implicated by the vaccination mandates, which reasonably further a legitimate government interest under rational-basis review.[66]

The principal area of legal uncertainty as to state vaccination requirements, as explained in the preceding section, is whether and when state vaccination requirements must provide for religious exemptions, and the circumstances under which such exemptions may be granted or denied. On this issue, the federal courts of appeals have reached arguably conflicting results.

In *Dahl v. Board of Trustees of Western Michigan University*, the district court preliminarily enjoined (i.e., temporarily suspended) a state university's policy requiring student-athletes to be vaccinated in order to participate in team activities.[67] The university's policy—which applied only to student-athletes and not the student body at large—provided that "[m]edical or religious exemptions and accommodations will be considered on an individual basis."[68] Several student- athletes who were denied religious exemptions and barred from participation sued to challenge the policy, alleging, among other claims, that the policy violated their free exercise rights.[69] In considering the university's motion to lift the preliminary

---

[63] *California Becomes First State in Nation to Announce COVID-19 Vaccine Requirements for Schools*, OFF. OF GOVERNOR (Oct. 1, 2021), https://www.gov.ca.gov/2021/10/01/california-becomes-first-state-in-nation-to-announce- covid-19-vaccine-requirements-for-schools/.

[64] As noted *supra* in note 42, California eliminated, in 2016, nonmedical exemptions for its student vaccination requirements generally.

[65] *See, e.g.*, Klaassen v. Trustees of Ind. Univ., 7 F.4th 592 (7th Cir. 2021) (affirming district court's denial of a motion to enjoin a state university's policy requiring COVID-19 vaccination as a condition of in-person attendance); Norris v. Stanley, No. 1:21-CV-756, 2021 WL 4738827, at *4 (W.D. Mich. Oct. 8, 2021) (denying plaintiff's motion to enjoin a state university policy requiring employees to receive COVID-19 vaccination); Kheriaty v. Regents of the Univ. of Cal., No. 8:21-cv-01367, 2021 WL 4714664 (C.D. Cal. Sept. 29, 2021) (similar); Dixon v. De Blasio, No. 21-cv-5090, 2021 WL 5740187, at *14 (E.D.N.Y. Oct. 12, 2021) (denying plaintiffs' motion to enjoin several mayoral executive orders that require certain business entities to prevent individuals who have not received a COVID-19 vaccine from remaining in certain indoor facilities); Valdez v. Grisham, No. 21-cv-783, 2021 WL 4145746, at *4–5 (D.N.M. Sept. 13, 2021) (denying plaintiffs' motion to enjoin state public health orders that require all hospital workers and state fair exhibitors to be vaccinated against COVID-19).

[66] *See, e.g., Klaasen*, 7 F.4th at 592–94; *Norris*, 2021 WL 4738827, at *2-4; *Dixon*, 2021 WL 5740187, at *4–6, *8–9; *Valdez*, 2021 WL 4145746, at *5–9. In addition to these claims, another common claim raised by plaintiffs challenging COVID-19 vaccination requirements—particularly before FDA fully approved a COVID-19 vaccine—is a claim asserting that the vaccination requirements in question violate the EUA provision of the FD&C Act. *See infra* "Emergency Use Authorization and Vaccination Mandates" for additional discussion.

[67] 2021 WL 3891620, at *3 (W.D. Mich. Aug. 31, 2021).

[68] Dahl v. Bd. of Tr. of W. Mich. Univ., 15 F.4th 728, 730 (6th Cir. 2021) (per curiam).

[69] *See id.*

injunction, the U.S. Court of Appeals for the Sixth Circuit (Sixth Circuit) concluded that the university's discretionary exemption process provided a "mechanism for individualized exemptions" under *Fulton* that rendered the policy *not* generally applicable, subjecting it to heightened scrutiny.[70] Applying heightened scrutiny, the Sixth Circuit concluded that the student-athletes were likely to succeed on their free exercise claim because while the university had a compelling interest "in fighting COVID-19," the policy was not narrowly tailored to achieve that.[71] The court reasoned that nonathlete students were not required to be vaccinated, undermining the university's stated interest in prohibiting conduct that created health risks.[72] The court also drew comparisons to other university policies that allowed exemptions, suggesting the university's vaccination policy might have been unnecessarily "severe."[73]

In *Does v. Mills*, the U.S. Court of Appeals for the First Circuit (First Circuit) considered Maine's August 2021 emergency regulation that added COVID-19 vaccination to the list of required vaccinations that employees of licensed health care facilities must receive.[74] The state legislature in 2019 eliminated all nonmedical exemptions to the state's health care worker and student vaccination requirements, citing declining vaccination rates and the need to protect those who are immunocompromised and reliant on others' vaccinations for protection.[75] In issuing the August 2021 regulation, the Maine Department of Health and Human Services and Maine's Center for Disease Control determined that the rule was necessary because the highly contagious Delta variant had caused a 300% increase in COVID-19 cases between June and July 2021; health care facilities are uniquely susceptible to outbreaks of infectious diseases like COVID-19; such outbreaks hamper the state's ability to care for its residents suffering from both COVID-19 and other conditions; the size of Maine's health care workforce is limited; alternatives to vaccination (such as regular testing or reliance on personal protective equipment) would not be as effective; and no health care facility types at the time—despite the states' various efforts at promoting voluntary vaccination—had achieved vaccination rates above 90%, which the state public health agency determined was the minimum rate required to prevent community transmission of the Delta variant.[76] Several then-unvaccinated health care workers sued to challenge the regulation, alleging, among other claims, that the COVID-19 vaccination requirement violates their free exercise rights because it lacks a religious exemption.[77]

In affirming the district court's denial of a preliminary injunction, the First Circuit concluded that the plaintiffs were not likely to succeed on their free exercise claim. In the court's view, Maine's vaccination requirement was a neutral and generally applicable law that (1) did not "single[] out religious objections . . . because of their religious nature" and (2) "applie[d] equally across the board" without requiring the state government "to exercise

---

[70] *Id.* at 733–34.
[71] *Id.* at 734–35.
[72] *Id.*
[73] *Id.* On November 18, 2021, the parties in *Dahl* voluntarily dismissed the appeal after entering into a consent decree, wherein the university agreed not to prevent plaintiffs from participating in team activities because of their unvaccinated status. Under the consent decree, the university may require unvaccinated plaintiffs to submit to COVID- 19 testing weekly or more frequently, and may also require them to wear face coverings during team activities. *See* Dahl v. Bd. of Tr. of W. Mich. Univ., Consent Decree ¶ 2, ECF No. 46, Nov. 16, 2021 (M.D. Mich.). Accordingly, no final decision on the merits is expected in this case.
[74] 16 F.4th 20, 28 (2021).
[75] *Id.* at 24–25. The amended exemptions became effective in 2020. *See id.*
[76] *See id.* at 27–28.
[77] *Id.* at 28.

discretion in evaluating individual requests for exemptions."[78] According to the First Circuit, the availability of a general medical exemption to employees who provide a written statement from specified licensed medical professionals that the vaccination is medically inadvisable did not render the vaccination requirement not generally applicable. Unlike the exemption system at issue in *Fulton*, the medical exemption, in the court's view, was "a single objective exemption" that did not call for discretionary evaluation, nor did it permit "secular conduct that undermines the government's asserted interests in a similar way" as would a religious exemption.[79] Instead, according to the court, exempting only those whose health would be endangered by vaccination *reinforced* the state's underlying interests in protecting the health and safety of its residents, including that of the health care workforce and those who are most vulnerable because they cannot be vaccinated for medical reasons.[80] Because the medical exemption is meaningfully different from a religious exemption—the availability of which would *undermine* the relevant state interests—the court concluded that Maine's vaccination requirement was generally applicable and subject to rational- basis review, which it "easily satisfie[d]."[81]

Even though the court did not need to reach this issue, the First Circuit further concluded that even if heightened scrutiny applied, the vaccination requirement would likely survive such scrutiny. According to the court, the state has a compelling interest in both stemming the spread of COVID-19 and in denying an exception to plaintiffs, who provide health care services, because exemptions from the requirement for non-health-related reasons threaten "the most vulnerable Mainers."[82] The vaccination requirement, according to the court, was also sufficiently narrowly tailored to achieve those interests, given that (1) Maine considered alternatives such as testing, masking, and social distancing, but found them to be inadequate in meeting the state's goals particularly in the face of the spread of the Delta variant; (2) Maine "demonstrated that it ha[d] tried many alternatives to get its healthcare workers vaccinated short of a mandate" but such efforts failed to achieve the at least 90% vaccination rate necessary to halt community transmission; and (3) the requirement was not underinclusive—in that it applies to all except those who have a medical contraindication—or overinclusive—in that it was limited to "the narrow sphere of healthcare workers . . . who regularly enter healthcare facilities."[83]

In *We the Patriots USA, Inc. v. Hochul*, the U.S. Court of Appeals for the Second Circuit (Second Circuit) considered an emergency rule adopted by the New York Department of Health, 10 N.Y.C.R.R. § 2.61, that directed specified health care facilities in the state to require certain employees to receive COVID-19 vaccines.[84] Like the Maine emergency regulation, New York's vaccination requirement provided only a medical exemption, which applied "only until such immunization is found no longer to be detrimental to [the employees'] health and must be supported by a certification from a licensed physician or nurse practitioner issued in accordance with generally accepted medical standards, including recommendations of the Advisory Committee on Immunization Practices."[85] Several health care workers sued to

---

[78] *Id.* at 30.
[79] *Id.* at 30–31.
[80] *Id.*
[81] *Id.* at 31–32.
[82] *Id.* at 32.
[83] *Id.* at 32–33.
[84] 17 F.4th 266, 274 (2d Cir. 2021) (per curiam).
[85] *Id.* at 275.

challenge New York's rule, asserting, among other claims, that it violated the Free Exercise Clause.[86]

The Second Circuit concluded that the plaintiffs did not demonstrate a likelihood of success on their free exercise claim at the preliminary injunction phase.[87] Like the First Circuit, the Second Circuit concluded that the plaintiffs did not meet their burden to show that New York's rule—by providing a medical but not a religious exemption—was not a neutral, generally applicable law under *Smith*, or that the rule did not satisfy rational-basis review.[88] Similar to the First Circuit, the Second Circuit found that the medical and religious exemptions were not "comparable" exemptions relative to the asserted government interests—which included protecting the health of health care employees to reduce staffing shortages that can compromise patient safety—because a medical exemption furthered those interests while a religious exemption would undermine them.[89] Also similar to the First Circuit, the Second Circuit found that § 2.61's medical exemption did not create a system of individualized exemptions under *Fulton* because the rule "provide[d] for an objectively defined category of people to whom the vaccine requirement does not apply"— i.e., those who present the appropriate certification from a specified medical professional in accordance with generally accepted medical standards.[90] Because the plaintiffs, in the court's view, did not demonstrate that § 2.61 is not neutral or generally applicable, the court applied rational-basis review. An emergency rule that requires health care employees to be vaccinated in the face of an especially contagious variant of the virus that has claimed the lives of more than 750,000 in the United States and some 55,000 in New York, the court reasoned, "easily m[et] that standard."[91]

In sum, *Dahl* on one hand, and *Does* and *We the Patriots* on the other hand, highlight some of the unsettled questions raised by *Fulton* and *Tandon* as they apply to vaccination requirements and the circumstances under which states may be constitutionally required to provide for or grant religious exemptions. Whereas *Dahl* suggests that the availability of a medical exemption may render a vaccination requirement not generally applicable and thus subject to heightened scrutiny, for instance, *Does* and *We the Patriots* indicate that, at least in the health care employment context, a vaccination requirement providing for only a medical exemption is a generally applicable requirement subject to rational-basis review.

The Supreme Court has so far rejected applications to stay the Maine and New York emergency rules at issue in *Does* and *We the Patriots*, allowing for their implementation.[92] The plaintiffs in *Does* filed a petition for certiorari, and the Court, if it grants the petition, may provide further clarification on these open questions.

---

[86] *Id.* at 273.
[87] *Id.*
[88] *Id.*
[89] *Id.* at 285.
[90] *Id.* at 289.
[91] *Id.* at 290.
[92] *See* Dr. A v. Hochul, 142 S. Ct. 552 (2021); Does v. Mills, 142 S. Ct. 17 (2021). Justices Neil Gorsuch, Clarence Thomas, and Samuel Alito dissented from the application denial in both cases. Among other determinations, the dissent concluded that the vaccination requirements at issue were not generally applicable, including because the medical exemption process was "individualized" and because both medical and religious exemptions are comparable exemptions as measured against the states' asserted interest in infectious disease control and protecting the states' health care infrastructure. *See Does*, 142 S. Ct. at 19–20; *Dr. A*, 142 S. Ct. at 556–57.

Federal Authority to Mandate Vaccination

Like state vaccination requirements, federal vaccination requirements are government actions subject to constitutional constraints.[93] In addition to constitutional constraints based on individual rights—which apply in broadly similar ways to both state and federal vaccination mandates— federal vaccination requirements must fall within the powers granted to the federal government in the Constitution.[94] Federal requirements imposed by the executive branch are also subject to statutory constraints. Such requirements generally must rely on the federal government's existing statutory authorities.[95] Depending on the circumstances, the requirements may also be subject to statutory requirements under the Administrative Procedure Act (APA), the Religious Freedom Restoration Act of 1993 (RFRA),[96] or other context-specific statutory limits.[97]

This part begins by discussing the executive branch's authority to mandate vaccination, including the asserted statutory authority for the non-military federal COVID-19 vaccination mandates issued to date, and the state of the litigation challenging these mandates. This part then reviews the extent of Congress's constitutional authority under the Constitution's Spending and Commerce Clauses to mandate vaccination.

Executive Branch Authority to Mandate Vaccination

Prior to the COVID-19 pandemic, federal vaccination requirements were primarily limited to the immigration,[98] military,[99] and certain federal health care employment contexts.[100] Certain

---

[93] *See, e.g.*, Pub. Util. Comm'n of D.C. v. Pollak, 343 U.S. 451, 461 (1952).

[94] *See* Nolan & Lewis, *supra* note 18, at 1.

[95] *See, e.g.*, City of Arlington v. Fed. Commc'ns Comm'n, 569 U.S. 290, (2013) (stating that agencies' "power to act and how they are to act is authoritatively prescribed by Congress" and thus a question concerning agencies' statutory authority "is always whether the agency has gone beyond what Congress has permitted it to do").

[96] The APA generally establishes the procedures that federal agencies use for rulemaking and adjudication, and the procedures for how courts may review those agency actions. RFRA generally imposes a heightened standard of review for federal government actions that substantially burden a person's religious exercise and creates a private right of action to those so burdened to assert that violation as a claim or defense and obtain appropriate relief against the government. For more information about the APA, see CRS In Focus IF10003, *An Overview of Federal Regulations and the Rulemaking Process*, by Maeve P. Carey; and CRS Legal Sidebar LSB10558, *Judicial Review Under the Administrative Procedure Act (APA)*, by Jonathan M. Gaffney. For more information about RFRA, see CRS In Focus IF11490, *The Religious Freedom Restoration Act: A Primer*, by Whitney K. Novak.

[97] In the military context, for instance, additional waiver requirements under 10 U.S.C. § 1107a may apply to the administration of medical products subject to EUAs to servicemembers.

[98] Under 8 U.S.C. § 1182(a)(1)(A), for instance, immigrants seeking permanent residence in the United States must present documentation showing they have been vaccinated against certain specified vaccine-preventable diseases.

[99] The Department of Defense's Immunization Program, for instance, requires all health care personnel working in the Department's medical treatment facilities, as well as all active duty and selected reserve personnel, to receive annual seasonal influenza vaccines or to obtain a medical or administrative exemption. DEP'T OF DEFENSE INSTRUCTION 6205.02 § 1.2b (July 23, 2019), https://www.esd.whs.mil/Portals/54/Documents/DD/ issuances/ dodi/620502p.pdf?ve r=2019-07-23-085404-617. For more information about the military's vaccination requirements, see CRS In Focus IF11816, *Defense Health Primer: Military Vaccinations*, by Bryce H. P. Mendez.

[100] The Indian Health Service, for instance, has required proof of immunization for measles and rubella as a condition of employment for all health care personnel since 1991. The agency added seasonal influenza vaccine as a mandatory vaccination for all health care personnel in 2015. *See* SGM 21-04, Memorandum from Elizabeth A. Fowler, Acting Director of Indian Health Serv. to all agency employees, *available at* https://www.ihs.gov/ sites/ihm/themes/responsive2017/display_objects/documents/sgm/2021/covid-19-immunizations-require ment.pdf.

existing statutory authorities, however, could potentially encompass the authority to mandate vaccination in specified contexts.

Earlier in the COVID-19 pandemic, and even before the pandemic, some commentators believed that one likely source of authority for federal public health orders—including those related to vaccination requirements—may be Section 361(a) of the PHSA.[101] This provision, codified at 42U.S.C. § 264(a), grants the Secretary of HHS the authority—delegated in part to the Centers for Disease Control and Prevention (CDC)[102]—to make and enforce regulations necessary "to prevent the introduction, transmission, or spread of communicable diseases from foreign countries into the States or possessions, or from one State or possession into any other State or possession."[103] Following this text, Section 361(a) states that "[f]or purposes of carrying and enforcing such regulations," the Agency "may provide for such inspection, fumigation, disinfection, sanitation, pest extermination, destruction of animals or articles found to be so infected or contaminated as to be sources of dangerous infection to human beings, and other measures, as in [its] judgment may be necessary."[104] Based on this statutory text, some have argued that a broad construction of CDC's Section 361(a) authority may permit CDC to issue regulations requiring vaccination in circumstances that would prevent the foreign or interstate transmission of COVID-19.[105]

Before the COVID-19 vaccines became available under EUAs during the Trump Administration, the CDC invoked PHSA Section 361 to issue a nationwide eviction moratorium in September 2020. CDC based the moratorium on its findings that evictions threatened to increase the spread of COVID-19 as they would force people to live in new shared housing or congregate settings.[106] Numerous legal challenges to the eviction moratorium followed. By June 2021, the U.S. Court of Appeals for the District of Columbia Circuit (D.C. Circuit) and the Sixth Circuit—in the context of reviewing procedural motions to stay or lift the stay of the district courts' preliminary injunction orders[107]—had reached different conclusions as to the CDC's statutory authority to issue the order. The D.C. Circuit, adopting a broad construction of Section 361, concluded that "the CDC's eviction moratorium f[ell] within the plain text of 42 U.S.C. § 264(a)."[108] The Sixth Circuit, in contrast, characterized the enumerated measures under Section 361(a) as "property interest restrictions" and concluded that the eviction moratorium was "radically unlike" such restrictions and thus "f[ell] outside the scope of the statute."[109]

---

[101] *See, e.g.*, Lindsay F. Wiley, *CDC's Boundary-Pushing Eviction Freeze*, AM. CONST. SOC'Y (Sept. 3, 2020), https://www.acslaw.org/expertforum/cdcs-boundary-pushing-eviction-freeze/(prior to the availability of COVID-19 vaccines, noting that "[t]he most likely source of authority for federal executive action to mandate and support social distancing and face covering is Section 361(a) of the Public Health Service Act"); Christopher T. Robertson, *Vaccines and Airline Travel: A Federal Role to Protect the Public Health*, 42 AM. J.L. & MED. 543, 566 (2016) (suggesting CDC has authority under Section 361 "to require vaccinations as a condition of airline travel").

[102] *See Legal Authorities for Isolation and Quarantine*, CTRS. FOR DISEASE CONTROL & PREVENTION (Feb. 24, 2020), https://www.cdc.gov/quarantine/aboutlawsregulationsquarantineisolation.html.

[103] 42 U.S.C. § 264(a).

[104] *Id.* § 264(a).

[105] *See* Robertson, *supra* note 101, at 566.

[106] 85 Fed. Reg. 55,292, 55,296 (Sept. 4, 2020).

[107] As discussed *infra* in note 110 in more detail, these orders were issued on the courts' non-merits dockets without full briefing or oral argument from the parties; thus, their precedential value beyond the cases in which they were issued is uncertain.

[108] Ala. Ass'n of Realtors v. U.S. Dep't of Health & Human Servs., No. 21-5093, 2021 WL 2221646, at *1 (D.C. Cir. June 2, 2021).

[109] Tiger Lily, LLC v. U.S. Dep't of Hous. & Urb. Dev., 992 F.3d 518, 521, 524 (6th Cir. 2021).

The eviction moratorium litigation introduced much legal uncertainty over the scope of CDC's authority under PHSA Section 361(a), including the agency's authority to issue regulations relating to public health measures, such as vaccination, that arguably bear more directly on infectious disease control than eviction moratoria. Uncertainty as to the reach of Section 361(a) deepened after August 2021, when the Supreme Court—in the context of granting a procedural motion to lift a stay of the eviction moratorium in *Alabama Ass'n of Realtors v. Department of Health and Human Services*—concluded that the plaintiffs challenging the eviction moratorium were likely to succeed on their statutory claim.[110] Characterizing the enumerated measures under Section 361(a) as measures "directly relate[d] to preventing the interstate spread of disease by identifying, isolating, and destroying the disease itself," the Court concluded that the eviction moratorium "relate[d] to interstate infection far more indirectly" and the sheer scope of CDC's claimed authority counseled against the government's interpretation. The government has since voluntarily dismissed its appeal, and a final decision on the merits is not expected in the case. In short, while the eviction moratorium litigation indicates that the CDC's authority under Section 361(a) does not extend to issuing eviction moratoriums, it leaves unresolved the precise scope of the agency authority under the provision to take other measures to prevent the spread of communicable diseases.

To address the spread of the Delta variant in 2021, the President and several executive agencies— including the Centers for Medicare and Medicaid Services (CMS) and the Occupational Safety and Health Administration (OSHA)—ultimately invoked several other statutory authorities to issue several employment- or workforce-based COVID-19 vaccination mandates for civilians.

These vaccination requirements include those that apply to (1) federal executive agency civilian employees (federal employee mandate);[111] (2) federal contractors for executive departments, agencies, and offices (federal contractor mandate);[112] (3) most Medicare- and Medicaid-certified providers and suppliers (CMS's Medicare/Medicaid provider mandate);[113] and (4) employers with 100 or more employees (OSHA's large-employer vaccination and testing mandate).[114] Subject to accommodations required by federal law for medical disabilities and religious beliefs, these employment-based mandates either directly require certain employees to receive COVID-19 vaccinations or direct certain employers to impose a vaccination or vaccination-and-testing requirement on their employees or staff.[115] (See *Table 1* for a summary of these mandates.)

---

[110] 141 S. Ct. 2485, 2488–89 (2021) (per curiam). This order was issued on the Supreme Court's non-merits or motions docket—sometimes informally called the Court's "shadow docket"—without full briefing and oral argument. Unlike the Court's majority merits decisions, which are generally issued after considering both briefs and oral arguments from the parties as well as input from non-parties known as *amici curiae*, the precedential value of a non-merits orders beyond the case in which it was issued is more uncertain, and lower courts have not traditionally treated such orders as binding. For more discussion about the Supreme Court's non-merits orders, see CRS Legal Sidebar LSB10637, *The "Shadow Docket:" The Supreme Court's Non-Merits Orders*, by Joanna R. Lampe.

[111] Exec. Order No. 14,043 of Sept. 9, 2021, 86 Fed. Reg. 50,989 (Sept. 14, 2021).

[112] Exec. Order No. 14,042 of Sept. 9, 2021, 86 Fed. Reg. 50,985 (Sept. 14, 2021).

[113] 86 Fed. Reg. 61,555 (Nov. 5, 2021).

[114] 86 Fed. Reg. 61,402 (Nov. 5, 2021). In addition to these mandates, the Secretary of Defense mandated COVID-19 vaccination for servicemembers. For more information about the military's COVID-19 vaccination mandate, see CRS Insight IN11764, *The Military's COVID-19 Vaccination Mandate*, by Bryce H. P. Mendez.

[115] For more information about reasonable accommodations employers may need to provide—including providing exceptions from the vaccination requirement to employees who do not get vaccinated because of a disability or a sincerely held religious belief—see Anderson & Killion, *supra* note 15.

Federal Employee Mandate

Executive Order 14,043, issued on September 9, 2021, instructs each executive agency to implement a program to require COVID-19 vaccination for all federal employees, subject to exceptions required by law, including those based on a disability, medical condition, or a sincerely held religious belief.[116] The federal employee mandate directs the Safer Federal Workforce Task Force (Task Force) to issue guidance on this requirement's implementation.[117] The mandate is based on the President's statutory authority under 5 U.S.C. §§ 3301, 3302, and 7301.[118] These provisions grant the President general authority to prescribe rules and/or regulations for executive branch employees.[119]

Under the Task Force's guidance, federal employees must have been fully vaccinated (i.e., two weeks after completing either a one-dose vaccine or a two-dose vaccine series) or have obtained an exception by November 22, 2021.[120] The vaccination requirement applies to employees who are under maximum telework or remote-work arrangements.[121] Employees who refuse to be vaccinated or provide proof of vaccination, and have neither an exception nor an exception request under consideration, are subject to disciplinary measures, up to and including removal or termination.[122] Under the guidance, any removal or termination would be preceded by a brief period of education and counseling and a suspension period of generally up to 14 days.[123]

Several federal employees and at least one employee union have sued to challenge the federal employee mandate.[124] These suits raise a variety of claims, including some claims common to challenges to state vaccination requirements.[125] As discussed above, courts have generally rejected these claims.[126]

Plaintiffs have also asserted several claims specific to the federal employee mandate, based on certain generally applicable statutory requirements under the RFRA and APA. One set of claims, for instance, challenged the agencies' alleged denial of religious exemption requests as violating RFRA and the First Amendment's Free Exercise Clause.[127] In a November 2021

---

[116] 86 Fed. Reg. 50,989, 50,990 (Sept. 14, 2021).

[117] *Id.*

[118] *Id.* at 50,989.

[119] *See* 5 U.S.C. §§ 3301 (authorizing the President to "prescribe such regulations for the admission of individuals into the civil service in the executive branch as will best promote the efficiency of that service" and to "ascertain the fitness of applicants as to . . . health"), 3302 (authorizing the President to "prescribe rules governing the competitive service"), 7301 (authorizing the President to "prescribe regulations for the conduct of employees in the executive branch").

[120] *See FAQs – Vaccinations: Vaccination Requirement for Federal Employees*, SAFER FEDERAL WORKFORCE TASK FORCE, https://www.saferfederalworkforce.gov/faq/vaccinations/ (last accessed Dec. 7, 2021).

[121] *See id.* ("Employees who are on maximum telework or working remotely are not excused from this requirement, including because employees working offsite may interact with the public as part of their duties and agencies may need to recall employees who are on maximum telework or working remotely").

[122] *See FAQs – Vaccinations: Enforcement of Vaccination Requirement for Employees*, SAFER FEDERAL WORKFORCE TASK FORCE, https://www.saferfederalworkforce.gov/faq/vaccinations/ (last accessed Dec. 7, 2021).

[123] *See id.*

[124] *See, e.g.*, Brnovich v. Biden, No. 2:21-cv-01568, Second Amended Complaint, ECF No. 70 (D. Ariz. filed Nov. 19, 2021) [hereinafter Brnovich Second Amended Complaint]; Church v. Biden, No. 1:21-cv02815, Complaint, ECF No. 1 (D.D.C. filed Oct. 24, 2021); Am. Fed. of Gov't Emp. v. Biden, No. 1:21-cv-23828, Complaint, ECF No. 1 (D. Fla. filed Oct. 30, 2021).

[125] *See, e.g.*, Brnovich Second Amended Complaint, *supra* note 124, ¶¶ 47, 55–57.

[126] *See supra* note 66 and accompanying text.

[127] *See* Order Denying Emergency Application for Temporary Restraining Order and Mot. for Preliminary Injunction, ECF No. 17, Church v. Biden, No. 1:21-cv02815 (D.D.C. Nov. 8, 2021).

decision, however, the district court considering these claims rejected them as unripe—or too early—for review, given that each plaintiff had a pending request for exemption and had not suffered any adverse employment consequence.[128] Another claim, raised by an employee union, challenges the manner by which the mandate was implemented. According to the plaintiffs, the vaccination requirement was implemented without undergoing the notice-and-comment rulemaking procedures required by the APA.[129] The district court in December 2021 dismissed the case for lack of standing, concluding, among other determinations, that the plaintiff failed to allege that any of its members had suffered an injury-in-fact because it was "speculative as to whether [they] would be disciplined for failure to become vaccinated because, for example, they may choose to become vaccinated or receive an exemption."[130]

Federal Contractor Mandate

Executive Order 14,042, also issued on September 9, 2021, directs federal executive departments and agencies to include in certain contracts a clause requiring compliance with the Task Force's workplace safety guidance.[131] The Task Force guidance, issued on September 24, 2021, requires federal contractors and subcontractors with a covered contract to conform to several workplace safety protocols, including COVID-19 vaccination of covered contractor-employees, subject to exceptions required by law.[132] Covered contractor-employees include those working on or in connection with a covered contract or working at a covered contractor workplace.[133] Covered contractor-employees working remotely are subject to the vaccination requirements.[134]

Consistent with the executive order, the federal contractor mandate sets forth a phase-in period for the new clause to be added to federal contracts.[135] Generally, new contracts awarded on or after November 14, 2021, must include the new clause, while contracts awarded prior to October 15, 2021, would incorporate the new clause only at the point at which the government renews the contract or exercises an option.[136] By January 18, 2022, covered contractors must ensure that their covered employees are fully vaccinated by the first day of performance of a new contract or when there is a renewal, extension, or exercised option on an existing contract.[137] The Task Force guidance instructs that "significant actions, such as termination of

---

[128] *See id.* at 1.

[129] *See* Mot. for Preliminary Injunction at 9–10, ECF No. 19, Am. Fed. of Gov't Emp. v. Biden, No. 1:21-cv-23828 (S.D. Fla. filed Nov. 12, 2021).

[130] *See* Order Dismissing Case for Lack of Subject Matter Jurisdiction, ECF No. 33, Am. Fed. of Gov't Emp. v. Biden, No. 1:21-cv-23828 (S.D. Fla. Dec. 22, 2021).

[131] Exec. Order No. 14,042 of Sept. 9, 2021, 86 Fed. Reg. 50,985, 50,985 (Sept. 14, 2021).

[132] SAFER FEDERAL WORKFORCE TASK FORCE, COVID-19 WORKPLACE SAFETY: GUIDANCE FOR FEDERAL CONTRACTORS AND SUBCONTRACTORS (updated Nov. 10, 2021), https://www.saferfederalworkforce.gov/downloads/Guidance%20for%20Federal%20Contractors_Safer%20Federal%20Workforce%20Task%20Force_20211110.pdf [hereinafter TASK FORCE FEDERAL CONTRACTOR GUIDANCE].

[133] *Id.* at 3.

[134] *See FAQs – Federal Contractors: Workplaces*, SAFER FEDERAL WORKFORCE TASK FORCE, https://www.saferfederalworkforce.gov/faq/contractors/ (last accessed Dec. 7, 2021).

[135] *See FAQs – Federal Contractors: Scope and Applicability of Task Force Guidance for Federal Contractors*, SAFER FEDERAL WORKFORCE TASK FORCE, https://www.saferfederalworkforce.gov/faq/contractors/ (last accessed Dec. 7, 2021).

[136] *See id.*

[137] TASK FORCE FEDERAL CONTRACTOR GUIDANCE, *supra* note 132, at 5.

the contract," should be taken if a contractor does not take steps to comply with the requirements.[138]

The Federal Contractor executive order is based on the President's authorities under 3 U.S.C.§ 301 and the Federal Property and Administrative Services Act (Procurement Act), including 40U.S.C. § 121.[139] The Procurement Act empowers the President to "prescribe policies and directives that the President considers necessary to carry out" the Act if they are consistent with the Act,[140] the purpose of which is to provide "an economical and efficient system" for, among other objectives, federal procurement.[141] The Federal Contractor executive order states that it was issued to promote this purpose "by ensuring that the parties that contract with the Federal Government provide adequate COVID-19 safeguards to their workers" performing on or in connection with a covered contract.[142] The President determined that the safeguards would "decrease worker absence, reduce labor costs, and improve the efficiency of contractors and subcontractors at sites where they are performing work for the Federal Government."[143]

The executive order, pursuant to 3 U.S.C. § 301, tasked the Director of the Office of Management and Budget (OMB) with determining whether the Task Force's guidance "will promote economy and efficiency in Federal contracting."[144] In accordance with this delegation, the OMB Director made an affirmative determination in a *Federal Register* notice published on the same date of the Task Force guidance's release.[145] The executive order also directs the Federal Acquisition Regulatory Council to make corresponding amendments to the Federal Acquisition Regulation, and to issue guidance to federal agencies on how to comply with the federal contractor mandate in the interim.[146] The Council issued the guidance on September 30, 2021.[147]

More than 20 states, on behalf of their state agencies and political subdivisions that may have a covered contract subject to the federal contractor mandate, have filed at least four separate suits in different district courts to challenge the mandate.[148] Plaintiffs in each case filed a motion for preliminary injunction seeking to enjoin the mandate while the litigation is pending. In November 2021, one district court—in *Kentucky v. Biden*, a challenge filed by Kentucky, Ohio, and Tennessee—granted the states' motion and enjoined the mandate in those three states while the litigation is pending.[149] In December 2021, another district court—in

[138] *See FAQs – Federal Contractors: Compliance*, SAFER FEDERAL WORKFORCE TASK FORCE, https://www.saferfederalworkforce.gov/faq/contractors/ (last accessed Dec. 7, 2021). For more information about the Federal Contractor EO's requirements, see CRS Insight IN11803, *Executive Order 14042 Requirements for COVID-19 Vaccination of Federal Contractors*, coordinated by Heidi M. Peters.

[139] *See* 86 Fed. Reg. 50,985, 50,985 (Sept. 14, 2021).

[140] 40 U.S.C. § 121(a).

[141] *Id.* § 101.

[142] 86 Fed. Reg. 50,985, 50,985 (Sept. 14, 2021).

[143] *Id.*

[144] *Id.* at 50,985–50,986.

[145] *See* 86 Fed. Reg. 53,691 (Sept. 24, 2021).

[146] 86 Fed. Reg. 50,985, 50,986 (Sept. 14, 2021).

[147] Memorandum from the Fed. Acquisition Regul. Council to Chief Acquisition Officers, Senior Procurement Executives, Defense Acquisition Regulations Council, Civilian Agency Acquisition Council (Sept. 30, 2021), https://www.whitehouse.gov/wp-content/uploads/2021/09/FAR-Council-Guidance-on-Agency-Issuance-of-Deviations- to-Implement-EO-14042.pdf.

[148] *See, e.g.*, Florida v. Nelson, No. 8:21-cv-2524 (M.D. Fla. filed Oct. 28, 2021); Kentucky v. Biden, No. 3:21-cv-00055, 2021 WL 5587446 (E.D. Ky. Nov. 30, 2021); Georgia v. Biden, No. 1:21-cv-00163 2021 WL 5779939 (S.D. Ga. Dec. 7, 2021).

[149] *Kentucky*, 2021 WL5587446, at *13–14.

Georgia v. Biden, a challenge filed by Georgia and six other states—granted the states' motion and issued a nationwide injunction.[150] Among other determinations, both district courts concluded that the President likely exceeded his statutory authority under the Procurement Act in imposing the vaccination requirement.[151]

The government has appealed the district courts' orders in both cases. On January 5, 2022, the Sixth Circuit denied the government's application to stay the injunction in *Kentucky*.[152] Among other determinations, the Sixth Circuit agreed with the district court that the federal contractor mandate likely exceeded the President's statutory authority.[153] In the Sixth Circuit's view, the relevant Procurement Act provisions authorize the President "to implement an 'economical and efficient' method of contracting . . . to obtain nonpersonal services," and this authority does not permit the President to "impose whatever medical procedure deemed 'necessary' on the relevant services personnel" *after* those services have been acquired.[154] The government's appeal in *Georgia* is pending before the U.S. Court of Appeals for the Eleventh Circuit (Eleventh Circuit).[155]

CMS's Medicare/Medicaid Provider Mandate

On November 4, 2021, CMS released an Interim Final Rule (IFR), effective November 5, 2021, that requires specified Medicare- and Medicaid-certified providers and suppliers to establish a policy that requires all eligible staff (subject to legally required exceptions) to receive the first dose of a two-dose COVID-19 vaccine or a one-dose COVID-19 vaccine by December 6, 2021, and to complete their vaccination series by January 4, 2022.[156] This mandate applies to 15 provider and supplier types that participate in Medicare and Medicaid, including hospitals, long- term-care facilities, and rural health clinics.[157] The mandate does not apply to other health care entities such as physician offices, organ procurement organizations, and portable X-Ray suppliers.[158]

For providers and suppliers subject to the IFR, their vaccination policy must apply to all staff who directly provide any care, treatment, or other services for the facility and/or its patients, including employees (including administrative staff as well as facility leadership); (2) licensed practitioners; (3) students, trainees, and volunteers; and (4) individuals who provide care, treatment, or other services for the facility and/or its patients under contract or other arrangements (including housekeeping and food services).[159] Individuals who provide services 100% remotely from sites of patient care and away from staff who work at sites of care—such as fully remote telehealth or payroll services—are not subject to the vaccination requirements.[160] CMS states that noncompliant providers and suppliers will be subject to enforcement remedies based on the level of noncompliance and available

---

[150] *Georgia*, 2021 WL 5779939, at *12.
[151] *Kentucky*, 2021 WL5587446, at *6–7; *Georgia*, 2021 WL 5779939, at *10.
[152] Kentucky v. Biden, No. 21-6147, 2022 WL 43178, at *1 (6th Cir. Jan. 5, 2022).
[153] *Id.* at *11–16.
[154] *Id.* at *12.
[155] *See* Georgia v. Biden, No. 21-14269 (11th Cir. filed Dec. 10, 2021).
[156] 86 Fed. Reg. 61,555, 61,563, 61,573 (Nov. 5, 2021).
[157] *Id.* at 61,556.
[158] *Id.*
[159] *Id.* at 61,570–61,571.
[160] *Id.* at 61,571.

remedies, which may include civil monetary penalties, denial of payment for new admissions, and termination of the Medicare/Medicaid provider agreement.[161]

According to CMS, the Medicare/Medicaid provider mandate is based on its determination that a vaccination mandate for health care workers is an essential component of the nation's COVID-19 pandemic response, particularly in light of several factors, including (1) the failure to achieve sufficiently high levels of vaccination based on voluntary efforts and patchwork requirements; (2) potential harm to patients from unvaccinated health care workers; (3) continuing strain on the health care system; and (4) known efficacy and safety of available vaccines.[162] The agency found "good cause" to waive the notice-and-comment rulemaking procedures under the APA and Section 1871(b) of the Social Security Act (SSA).[163] The agency based that determination on several considerations, including (1) that Delta-variant outbreaks showed that current levels of COVID-19 vaccination coverage have been inadequate to protect health care consumers and staff; the pandemic's strain on the health care system; (3) that respiratory infections typically circulate more frequently during the winter months; and (4) the onset of the 2021-2022 influenza season.[164]

CMS relied on several layers of statutory authorities in issuing the IFR.[165] Across all providers and suppliers, CMS invokes SSA Section 1102, a provision that grants the Secretary of HHS general authority to issue rules "as may be necessary to the efficient administration of the functions" with which the Secretary is charged under the SSA.[166] For Medicare providers and suppliers, CMS additionally relies on SSA Section 1871, which authorizes the Secretary to prescribe regulations "as may be necessary to carry out the administration" of the Medicare programs.[167] Finally, for each provider and supplier, CMS also relies on certain provider- and supplier-specific provisions, many of which authorize the Secretary to impose requirements he finds necessary to protect the health and safety of individuals who receive services from the relevant entities.[168]

At least 25 states, on behalf of certain state-run health care facilities that may be subject to the vaccination requirements, filed four separate suits to challenge the IFR shortly after its issuance.[169] Plaintiffs in each case filed a motion for preliminary injunction seeking to enjoin the IFR while the litigation proceeds. In November 2021, one district court, in *Florida v. Department of Health & Human Services*, declined to enjoin the IFR, concluding the state had not shown "irreparable harm" to justify an injunction.[170] In the court's view, the state had not provided sufficient factual evidence to demonstrate that the vaccination requirements' alleged

---

[161] *Id.* at 61,574.
[162] *Id.* at 61,586.
[163] *Id.*
[164] *Id.* at 61,583–61,584, 61,586.
[165] *Id.* at 61,567.
[166] 42 U.S.C. § 1302(a).
[167] *Id.* § 1395hh(a).
[168] *See, e.g.*, 42 U.S.C. §§ 1395x(e)(9) (authorizing the Secretary to impose requirements on hospitals that he "finds necessary in the interest of the health and safety of individuals" who receive service from the hospitals), 1395x(dd) (similar for hospices), 1395x(aa) (rural health clinics), 1395i-3(d)(4)(B) (long-term care facilities).
[169] *See* Florida v. Dep't of Health & Human Servs., No. 3:21-cv-2722, 2021 WL 5416122 (N.D. Fla. Nov. 20, 2021); Missouri v. Biden, No. 4:21-cv-1329, 2021 WL 5564501 (E.D. Mo. Nov. 29, 2021); Louisiana v. Becerra, No. 3:32-cv- 3970, 2021 WL 5609846 (W.D. La. Nov. 30, 2021); Texas v. Becerra, No. 2:21-cv-229, 2021 WL 5964687 (N.D. Tex. filed Nov. 15, 2021).
[170] *Florida*, 2021 WL 5416122, at *1.

likely adverse impact, such as potential staffing shortages, would result if the requirements were not halted.[171]

Later in the same month, however, two district courts—in *Missouri v. Biden* and *Louisiana v. Becerra*—granted the plaintiffs' motions in each respective case.[172] The *Missouri* court enjoined the IFR in 10 plaintiff states, while the *Louisiana* court enjoined the rule in the remaining states.[173] Among other determinations, both courts concluded that CMS likely exceeded its statutory authority in issuing the IFR because the applicable provisions do not specifically authorize the agency to mandate vaccination;[174] the agency likely lacked "good cause" to waive notice-and-comment rulemaking procedures;[175] and the plaintiffs sufficiently demonstrated they would suffer irreparable harm—including in the form of significant staffing shortages—if the IFR was not enjoined.[176] The U.S. Court of Appeals for the Fifth Circuit (Fifth Circuit), in considering the government's motion to stay the preliminary injunction in *Louisiana*, narrowed the scope of the injunction to the 14 plaintiff states.[177] Since the Fifth Circuit's order, the U.S. District Court for the Northern District of Texas, in *Texas v. Becerra*, issued a preliminary injunction order enjoining the IFR's enforcement in that state.[178] As of December 31, 2021, CMS is enjoinedfrom enforcing the IFR in the 25 states that are plaintiffs in *Missouri*, *Louisiana*, or *Texas*.

As noted by the Fifth Circuit in *Louisiana*, one key legal question on the merits concerning the Medicare/Medicaid provider mandate litigation is whether the rule exceeds the agency's statutory authority because the relevant provisions do not explicitly authorize the agency to mandate vaccination. Characterizing this issue as a "close call," the Fifth Circuit—in upholding the preliminary injunction in the 14 plaintiff states—concluded that the government had not sufficiently demonstrated that the rule fell within the agency's statutory authority.[179]

On this issue, a divided panel of the Eleventh Circuit, in considering Florida's motion for an injunction pending its appeal of the district court's order in *Florida*, concluded that the relevant Medicare and Medicaid provisions "plainly encompass[]" the IFR's vaccination requirement.[180] In the Eleventh Circuit's view, the relevant Medicare and Medicaid statutes expressly "authorized the Secretary to set standards to protect the health and safety of patients" served by Medicare and Medicaid facilities.[181] The IFR's vaccination requirements, according to the Eleventh Circuit, fell squarely within this grant of authority, given that COVID-19 is a deadly, highly transmissible disease, health care workers have long been required to obtain inoculations for infectious diseases, and required vaccination is "a common-sense measure designed to prevent healthcare workers . . . from making [patients] sicker."[182] Thus, in the Eleventh Circuit's view, "when it comes to vaccination mandates, there was no reason for Congress to be more specific than authorizing the Secretary to make regulations for the 'health

---

[171] *Id.* at *3–4.
[172] *Missouri*, 2021 WL 5564501, at *15; *Louisiana*, 2021 WL 5609846, at *17.
[173] *Missouri*, 2021 WL 5564501, at *15; *Louisiana*, 2021 WL 5609846, at *17.
[174] *See Missouri*, 2021 WL 5564501, at *3; *Louisiana*, 2021 WL 5609846, at *10-11.
[175] *See Missouri*, 2021 WL 5564501, at *5–6; *Louisiana*, 2021 WL 5609846, at *8–9.
[176] *See Missouri*, 2021 WL 5564501, at *12–13; *Louisiana*, 2021 WL 5609846, at *16.
[177] Louisiana v. Becerra, 2021 WL 5913302, at *2–3 (5th Cir. Dec. 15, 2021).
[178] Texas v. Becerra, 2021 WL 5964687, at *16.
[179] *See Louisiana*, 2021 WL 5913302, at *1.
[180] Florida v. Dep't of Health & Human Servs., 2021 WL 5768796, at *12.
[181] *Id.*
[182] *Id.*

and safety' of Medicare and Medicaid recipients."[183] To suggest otherwise, the court continued, "would mean that Congress had to have anticipated both the unprecedented COVID-19 pandemic and the unprecedented politicization of the disease to regulate vaccination against it."[184] The dissent's analysis, on the other hand, largely echoes that of the district courts in *Missouri* and *Louisiana*.[185]

On December 30, 2021, CMS announced that the IFR will be implemented and enforced, on a modified timeline, in the jurisdictions *not* subject to the preliminary injunctions in *Missouri*, *Louisiana*, and *Texas*.[186] The deadline to receive the first dose of a vaccine is extended to January 27, 2022, and the deadline to complete the vaccination series is extended to February 28, 2022.[187]

The government filed an application with the Supreme Court seeking to stay the preliminary injunctions in both *Louisiana* and *Missouri*. On January 13, 2022, the Supreme Court granted the application.[188] Among other determinations, the Court concluded that the IFR "fits neatly" within the Secretary's statutory authority to impose necessary conditions to protect the "health and safety" of patients served by the relevant providers and suppliers, particularly given that the Secretary routinely imposes conditions of participation that relate to the qualification and duties of health care workers and the fact that vaccination requirements for health care workers are "a common feature of the provision of healthcare in America."[189]

Following the Court's decision, CMS issued an updated guidance on the IFR for the 24 states previously subject to the preliminary injunctions in *Missouri* and *Louisiana*.[190] In these states, the deadline to receive the first dose of a vaccine is February 14, 2022, and the deadline to complete the vaccination series is March 15, 2022.[191]

OSHA's Large-Employer Vaccination and Testing Mandate

On November 4, 2021, OSHA released an emergency temporary standard (ETS) that generally requires private employers with 100 or more employees to establish and enforce a policy that either (1) requires all employees to receive a COVID-19 vaccination, subject to legally required exceptions; or (2) requires employees to receive either a COVID-19 vaccination or provide proof of regular COVID-19 testing and wear a face covering when indoors or occupying a vehicle with another person.[192] For the 26 states, Puerto Rico, and the U.S. Virgin Islands that

---

[183] *Id.*

[184] *Id.*

[185] *Id.* at 24.

[186] *See Current Emergencies*, CTRS. FOR MEDICARE & MEDICAID SERVS., https://www.cms.gov/About-CMS/Agency-Information/Emergency/EPRO/Current-Emergencies/Current-Emergencies-page (last accessed Dec. 30, 2021).

[187] *Id.*

[188] Biden v. Missouri, No. 21A240, 2022 WL 120950, *1 (Jan. 13, 2022) (per curiam).

[189] *Id.* at *3. The Court acknowledged that not all statutory provisions invoked by CMS contain the "health and safety" statutory language. *See id.* at *2 n.*. Noting, however, that facilities not subject to the statutory language represent less than 3% of the workers covered by the rule, and that the pertinent statutory language "may be read as incorporating the 'health and safety' authorities applicable to the other 97%," the Court saw no reason to let the 3% "wag the . . . dog." *Id.*

[190] CTRS. FOR MEDICARE & MEDICAID SERVS., CTRS. FOR CLINICAL STANDARDS AND QUALITY/QUALITY, SAFETY & OVERSIGHT GRP., GUIDANCE FOR THE INTERIM FINAL RULE – MEDICARE AND MEDICAID PROGRAMS; OMNIBUS COVID-19 HEALTH CARE STAFF VACCINATION (Jan. 14, 2022), https://www.cms.gov/files/document/qso-22-09-all-injunction- lifted.pdf.

[191] *Id.* at 3.

[192] 86 Fed. Reg. 61,402, 61,552 (Nov. 5, 2021) (adding 29 C.F.R. § 1910.501(d)).

have opted to adopt their own OSHA-approved state plans, the ETS also applies to state agency and local government employers.[193] To the extent a workplace is subject to both the ETS and one of the preceding mandates, the non-OSHA-ETS mandate generally applies. For those workplaces, OSHA specifically states either that the ETS does not apply (in the case of federal contractors or health care providers and suppliers)[194] or that compliance with the other mandate is deemed sufficient to meet the employers' obligations under the ETS (in the case of executive agencies).[195]

Under the large-employer vaccination and testing mandate, employees who are not fully vaccinated—including those who have been granted exceptions—generally must be tested at least once every seven days if they report at least once every seven days to a work site where others are present.[196] Employees who do not report to such a workplace during a period of seven or more days must be tested within seven days prior to returning to the workplace.[197] Employees exempt from the ETS's requirements include (1) employees who work remotely or at a site where other people are not present; and (2) employees who work exclusively outside.[198] Covered employers can, but are not required to, pay for any costs associated with testing,[199] but they must provide employees with paid leave to receive and recover from the vaccination.[200] Covered employers must establish and begin to implement the relevant vaccination policy by December 6, 2021, and ensure their employees have completed a one-dose vaccine or a two-dose vaccine series by January 4, 2022.[201] After that, all covered employers must ensure that employees who are not fully vaccinated are subject to regular COVID-19 testing.[202] Noncompliant covered employers could face OSHA citations and civil monetary penalties.[203]

The large-employer vaccination and testing mandate is based on OSHA's authority under Section 6(c) of the Occupational Safety and Health Act of 1970 (29 U.S.C. § 655(c)).[204] The provision authorizes the agency to issue an ETS that takes effect immediately upon publication in the *Federal Register*, without undergoing the APA's rulemaking proceedings, if it determines "(A) that employees are exposed to grave danger from exposure to substances or agents determined to be toxic or physically harmful or from new hazards, and (B) that such

---

193 Section 18 of the Occupational Safety and Health Act of 1970 (29 U.S.C. § 667) authorizes states, subject to OSHA's approval, to develop and enforce their own state plans of occupational safety and health standards that are "at least as effective" as OSHA's federal standards and enforcement. Whereas OSHA's jurisdiction does not extend to state agency and local government as employers, *see* 29 U.S.C. § 652(5), OSHA-approved state plans must provide coverage for state agencies and local government entities as employers, *see* 29 U.S.C. § 667. For more information about OSHA's jurisdiction and coverage of OSHA-approved state plans, see CRS In Focus IF11619, *OSHA Jurisdiction Over Public Schools and Other State and Local Government Entities: COVID-19 Issues*, by Scott D. Szymendera.

194 *See* 86 Fed. Reg. 61,402, 61,447 (Nov. 5, 2021).

195 *See id.* at 61,402.

196 *See id.* at 61,553 (adding 29 C.F.R. § 1910.501(g)).

197 *See id.* at 61,553 (adding 29 C.F.R. § 1910.501(g)(ii)).

198 *See id.* at 61,419.

199 *See id.* at 61,553 (Note 1 to paragraph (g)(1)).

200 *See id.* at 61,553 (adding § 1910.501(f)).

201 *See id.* at 61,554 (adding § 1910.501(m)(2)).

202 *See id.*

203 *See id.* at 61,443; *see also OSHA Penalties*, OCCUPATIONAL SAFETY & HEALTH ADMIN., https://www.osha.gov/ penalties (last accessed Dec. 13, 2021). For more information about the ETS's requirements, see CRS Report R46288, *Occupational Safety and Health Administration (OSHA): COVID-19 Emergency Temporary Standards (ETS) on Health Care Employment and Vaccinations and Testing for Large Employers*, by Scott D. Szymendera; and CRS Legal Sidebar LSB10658, *Fifth Circuit Stays OSHA Vaccination and Testing Standard*, by Jon O. Shimabukuro.

204 86 Fed. Reg. 61,402, 61,402 (Nov. 5, 2021).

emergency standard is necessary to protect employees from such danger."[205] OSHA issued the ETS upon its determination that unvaccinated workers face a grave danger from exposure to SARS-CoV-2 in the workplace, given that COVID-19 has killed more than 725,000 people in the United States in fewer than two years; that unvaccinated individuals remain at much higher risk of severe health outcomes; and that evidence demonstrates the virus's transmissibility in the workplace and the prevalence of infections in employee populations.[206] OSHA further determined that the ETS is necessary to protect unvaccinated workers from the risk of contracting COVID-19 given the potential severe health consequences from occupational exposure to COVID-19 and the fact that vaccination provides the most effective and efficient control available, with the use of other mitigation measures further protecting workers who remain unvaccinated.[207]

On the same day the ETS was issued, numerous petitioners—including covered employers, states, and religious groups—moved to stay and permanently enjoin the mandate in several federal courts of appeals.[208] In response to a petition and motion to stay filed by several covered employers and four states, the Fifth Circuit stayed the enforcement of the ETS the day after it was issued.[209]

On November 12, 2021, the Fifth Circuit affirmed the stay, largely based on its conclusion that the ETS "grossly exceeds OSHA's statutory authority."[210] In the Fifth Circuit's view, an airborne virus like SARS-CoV-2 likely falls outside the scope of a "new hazard" within the meaning of Section 6(c) under a canon of statutory construction known as *noscitur a sociis*, which counsels that the more precise meaning of a word should be determined by the neighboring words with which it is associated.[211] Because "new hazard" is neighbored by "substances or agents" and "toxic or physically harmful"—phrases that, in the court's view, connote toxicity and poisonousness—the term likely does not encompass an airborne virus that is both widely present in society and "non-life-threatening to a vast majority of employees."[212] Moreover, the court concluded that COVID-19 does not pose the required "grave danger" for purposes of Section 6(c), given that the agency cannot demonstrate that all covered workplaces are in fact exposed to COVID-19, the effects of COVID-19 could be mild, and the status of the virus's spread has changed over time.[213] The ETS, in the court's view, was also not "necessary" to protect unvaccinated workers given its "staggering[] overb[readth]," such that it was both overinclusive—applying to employers and employees in virtually all industries and workplaces in America without an attempt to account for differences in COVID-19 exposure—and underinclusive—disregarding workplaces with 99 or fewer employees.[214]

---

205 29 U.S.C. § 655(c)(1).

206 *See* 86 Fed. Reg. 61,402, 61,402–61,403 (Nov. 5, 2021).

207 *See id.* at 61,403. Under 29 U.S.C. § 655(f), any person adversely affected by an ETS may file a petition to challenge the validity of the standard in the federal court of appeals in which the person resides.

208 *See* BST Holdings, LLC v. Occupational Safety & Health Admin., 17 F. 4th 604, 610 (5th Cir. 2021).

209 *See id.*

210 *Id.* at 612.

211 *Id.* at 613.

212 *Id.*

213 *Id.* at 613–14.

214 *Id.* at 611, 615. In addition to its statutory analysis, the court commented that the ETS likely exceeds the federal government's authority under the Constitution's Commerce Clause. *Id.* Characterizing the relevant regulated activity as compulsory vaccination, the Fifth Circuit expressed the view that the ETS impermissibly "regulates noneconomic inactivity that falls squarely within the States' police power." *Id.* As discussed *infra* in note 228, the Sixth Circuit disagreed with this conclusion.

Pursuant to 28 U.S.C. § 2112, which specifies the procedures for review when an agency order is challenged in more than one federal appellate court, the Judicial Panel on Multistate Litigation, on November 16, 2021, randomly selected the Sixth Circuit as the court in which all of the pending petitions will be consolidated for review. Under § 2112(a)(4), the Sixth Circuit may modify, revoke, or extend the Fifth Circuit's stay.[215]

On December 17, 2021, a divided panel of the Sixth Circuit, in *In re: MCP No. 165, Occupational Safety and Health Administration, Interim Final Rule: COVID-19 Vaccination and Testing*, granted the government's motion to dissolve the stay issued by the Fifth Circuit.[216] In the Sixth Circuit's view, based on the OSH Act's language, structure, and direct instances of congressional approval following the law's enactment, OSHA has a "clear and exercised authority to regulate viruses" and wide discretion under this authority "to form and implement the best possible solution to ensure the health and safety of all workers" under the OSHAct.[217]

According to the Sixth Circuit, the text of Section 6(c) expressly encompasses the authority to regulate viruses because a virus is an "agent" (i.e., a biologically active principle) that is physically harmful (i.e., causes bodily harm) within the meaning of the provision.[218] This authority to regulate viruses and infectious diseases, the court continued, is reinforced by other provisions of the OSH Act that reference "illnesses arising out of work situations" and "health hazards," as well as a provision that contemplates "medical examination, immunization, or treatment" as possible measures the agency may employ.[219] This interpretation, in the court's view, is further consistent with several instances of Congress's approval of OSHA's authority to regulate bloodborne pathogens and viruses such as HIV, hepatitis B, and hepatitis C.[220] According to the Sixth Circuit, this clear authority to regulate viruses necessarily encompasses "the authority to regulate infectious diseases that are not unique to the workplace."[221] Because "no virus—HIV, [hepatitis B], COVID-19—is unique to the workplace and affects only workers," the court reasoned, OSHA's authority to regulate hazards extends to those that "co-exist in the workplace and in society but are at heightened risk in the workplace."[222] In the court's view, OSHA's issuance of the ETS "[was] not a novel expansion of OSHA's power; it [was] an existing application of authority to a novel and dangerous worldwide pandemic."[223]

After concluding that OSHA did not exceed its statutory authority, the Sixth Circuit further concluded that the agency's determination that the ETS was warranted was supported by substantial evidence, including the agency's determination that employees were exposed to "grave danger" from COVID-19 and that the ETS was "necessary to protect employees from such danger."[224] Under Section 6(f) of the OSH Act, the Secretary's determinations are "conclusive if supported by substantial evidence in the record considered as a whole."[225]

As to the existence of "grave danger," the Sixth Circuit found, for instance, that OSHA has demonstrated "the pervasive danger that COVID-19 poses to workers—unvaccinated workers

---

[215] 28 U.S.C. § 2112(a)(4).
[216] 2021 WL 5989357, at *1 (6th Cir. Dec. 17, 2021).
[217] *Id.* at *5–6.
[218] *Id.* at *4.
[219] *Id.* (citing, for instance, 29 U.S.C. §§ 651(a), 651(b)(1), 669(a)(5)).
[220] *Id.* at *5.
[221] *Id.* at *6.
[222] *Id.*
[223] *Id.* at *7.
[224] *Id.* at *8, 10–16.
[225] 29 U.S.C. § 655(f).

in particular—in their workplaces," explaining why traditional indoor workplaces place workers at heightened risk of contracting COVID-19; evidence of the severity of the harm from COVID-19; the likelihood that the ETS would save over 6,500 worker lives and prevent more than 250,000 hospitalizations over the next six months; and that voluntary guidance on vaccination proved inadequate, particularly in the face of the Delta variant.[226] As to the necessity of the ETS, the court found, for instance, that OSHA sufficiently demonstrated that the evolving course of the pandemic—and in particular, the emergence of the Delta variant—necessitated an ETS at this time and that extensive evidence cited by the agency showed that vaccination reduces the presence and severity of COVID-19 cases in the workplace.[227] The choice to limit the ETS to employers with 100 or more employees, in the court's view, did not undermine the standard's necessity because the agency demonstrated the relationship between this chosen threshold and the underlying regulatory problem, given that "larger employers are better able to implement the policies, are at heightened risk, and regulating them will be a significant step in protecting the entire workforce from COVID-19 transmission."[228]

In the dissent's view, OSHA lacked statutory authority to issue the ETS because the agency did not appropriately establish the standard's "necessity" or the existence of a "grave danger" in the workplace. According to the dissent, an ETS is "necessary" within the meaning of Section 6(c) only if it is an "indispensable" means of addressing COVID-19 in the workplace.[229] Because OSHA "failed to explore whether other feasible alternatives would have allowed [it] to tackle the problem," the dissent reasoned that the agency cannot show the ETS was "necessary" for purposes of Section 6(c).[230] Additionally, the dissent found that OSHA had not provided substantial evidence that all covered employees faced a "grave danger" from COVID-19 because not all employees have a high risk both of contracting COVID-19 and suffering severe consequences from it.[231] Finally, in the dissent's view, OSHA's authority under the OSH Act is limited to "the workplace walls," and thus, such authority does not extend to the regulation of a virus that is not uniquely a workplace condition, particularly when the agency "cannot state with precision the total number of workers in our nation who have contracted COVID-19 at work."[232] The authority to protect "employees" from a "grave danger" under Section 6(c), in the dissent's view, is limited to regulating "workplace hazards with workplace solutions."[233] Thus, the dissent reasoned, this authority does not encompass the authority to mandate safety measures beyond the workplace boundary, "even if taking such precautions would save many 'employee' lives."[234]

---

[226] *In re MCP No. 165*, 2021 WL 5989357, at *10–13.

[227] *Id.* at *14.

[228] *Id.* at *15. The Sixth Circuit also found that OSHA sufficiently determined that the ETS is economically feasible, including considering the Standard's costs in relation to the financial health of the affected industries and its impact on consumer prices. *Id.* at *15–16. The Sixth Circuit also disagreed with the Fifth Circuit's view that the ETS likely exceeded the federal government's Commerce Clause authority because it regulates noneconomic inactivity. *Id.* at *16. In the Sixth Circuit's view, the ETS regulates employers that are "indisputabl[y] . . . engag[ing] in commercial activity that Congress has the power to regulate." To hold otherwise, according to the Sixth Circuit, "would upend nearly a century of precedent upholding laws that regulate employers to effectuate a myriad of employee workplace policies." *Id.*

[229] *See id.* at 22.

[230] *Id.* at *23–24.

[231] *Id.* at *25.

[232] *Id.* at *26 (quoting 86 Fed. Reg. at 61,424).

[233] *Id.* at *27.

[234] *Id.*

Following the Sixth Circuit's dissolution of the stay, several petitioners filed an application with the Supreme Court seeking to stay the ETS. On January 13, 2022, the Supreme Court granted the application and stayed the enforcement of the ETS.[235] The Court concluded that a stay was warranted because the applicants were likely to succeed on the merits of their claim that the ETS exceeded OSHA's statutory authority, which authorizes the agency "to set *workplace* safety standards, not broad public health measures."[236] Because the ETS does not distinguish between workplaces that pose a heightened risk of COVID-19 exposure because of the particular features of an employee's job or the nature of the workplace, and workplaces that pose a generalized risk of exposure from COVID-19 that is not different in kind from the risk presented by other nonwork settings in which people gather, it is, in the Court's view, an impermissible general public health measure rather than a permissible occupational safety or health standard.[237] The Court suggested, for instance, that targeted regulations that address workplaces that face a heightened risk of contracting COVID-19 beyond the everyday risk that all face "are plainly permissible."[238] As examples, the Court stated that "OSHA could regulate researchers who work with the COVID-19 virus" or "regulate risks associated with working in particularly crowded or cramped environments."[239]

The Court's decision stays enforcement of the ETS while the consolidated cases proceed before the Sixth Circuit. In the meantime, the comment period for the ETS, which also acts a notice of proposed rulemaking for a permanent standard, remains open through January 19, 2022.[240] As part of this notice-and-comment rulemaking process, OSHA may consider the comments as well as the Court's decision and issue a more narrowly tailored permanent rule. OSHA may also opt to withdraw the ETS in its entirety.

Table 1. Summary of Federal Nonmilitary COVID-19 vaccination mandates

As of January 18, 2022

Federal Mandate	*Statutory Authority*	*Covered Individuals/ Entities*	*Vaccination Requirement*	*Compliance Deadline(s)*	*Status*
Federal Employee Mandate (Executive Order 14,043)	5 U.S.C. §§ 3301, 3302, 7301	Federal executive branch employees	Employees must be fully vaccinated,[a] unless granted a legally required exception based on a disability/ medical condition or a sincerely held religious belief. Remote-working employees are subject to requirement.	Receive a one- dose vaccine or two-dose vaccine series by November 8, 2021. Be fully vaccinated by November 22, 2021.	In effect

[235] Nat'l Fed. of Ind. Bus. v. Dep't of Labor, No. 21A244, 2022 WL 120952, at *1 (Jan. 13, 2022) (per curiam).
[236] *Id.* at *3.
[237] *Id.*
[238] *Id.* at *4.
[239] *Id.*
[240] *See Covid-19 Vaccination and Testing ETS*, OCCUPATIONAL SAFETY & HEALTH ADMIN. (Jan. 13, 2022), https://www.osha.gov/coronavirus/ets2.

Federal Mandate	*Statutory Authority*	*Covered Individuals/ Entities*	*Vaccination Requirement*	*Compliance Deadline(s)*	*Status*
Federal Contractor (Executive Order 14,042)	40 U.S.C. § 101 et seq.; 3 U.S.C. § 301	Federal contractors/ subcontractors that have a covered contract with executive departments and agencies	Covered contractors must ensure covered contractor-employees are fully vaccinated, except in circumstances where an employee is legally entitled to an exemption based on a disability/medical condition or a sincerely held religious belief. Remote-working covered contractor-employees are subject to requirement.	As of January 18, 2022, covered contractor-employees must be fully vaccinated on the first day of performance on a new contract or the renewal, extension, or exercised option of an existing contract.	Enjoined by courts: Kentucky v. Biden, No. 21-6147), 2022 WL 43178 (6th Cir. Jan. 5, 2022) (declining to stay the district court's preliminary injunction in KY, OH, and TN); Georgia v. Biden, No. 1:21-cv-00163 2021 WL 5779939 (S.D. Ga. Dec. 7, 2021) (enjoined the vaccination requirement nationwide).
CMS's Medicare/ Medicaid Provider Mandate (CMS IFR)	42 U.S.C. §§ 1302, 1395hh, and other provider- or supplier-specific provisions	Specified provider and supplier types that participate in Medicare and Medicaid	Covered providers and suppliers must ensure covered staff who directly provide care or other services for their facilities and/or patients are fully vaccinated, except in circumstances where a staff member is legally entitled to an exemption based on a disability/medical condition or a sincerely held religious belief.	By January 27, 2022, covered providers and suppliers must establish and begin to implement the vaccination policies and covered staff must receive first dose of a two-dose vaccine or a one-dose vaccine.	In effect in all jurisdictions except TX. (Preliminary injunctions in 24 states stayed by the U.S. Supreme Court in Biden v. Missouri, No. 21A240, 2022 WL 120950 (Jan. 13, 2022))[b]

Table 1. (Continued)

Federal Mandate	*Statutory Authority*	*Covered Individuals/ Entities*	*Vaccination Requirement*	*Compliance Deadline(s)*	*Status*
			Staff who work 100% remotely from sites of patient care or away from onsite staff are not subject to the requirement.	Covered staff must complete two-dose vaccine series by February 28, 2022.	
OSHA's Large-Employer Vaccination and Testing Mandate (OSHA ETS)	29 U.S.C. § 655(c)	In all jurisdictions, private employers with 100 or more employees. In 26 states, Puerto Rico, and the U.S. Virgin Islands with OSHA-approved state plans, state and local government employers with 100 or more employees.	A covered employer must establish and enforce a policy that either (1) ensures employees are fully vaccinated, except in circumstances where an employee is legally entitled to an exemption based on a disability/medical condition or sincerely held religious belief; or (2) requires employees to be fully vaccinated or provide proof of regular COVID-19 testing and wear a face covering when indoors. Employees who work remotely, at a site where other people are not present, or exclusively outside are not subject to the requirements.	Covered employers must establish and begin to implement the vaccination policies by January 10, 2022. Covered employees must receive either a one-dose vaccine or a two-dose vaccine series, or begin regular testing by February 9, 2022.	Stayed by the U.S. Supreme Court. (See Nat'l Fed. of Indep. Bus. v. Dep't of Labor, No. 21A244, ---S. Ct.---, 2022 WL 120952 (Jan. 13, 2022))

Source: CRS analysis of the relevant Executive Orders, CMS IFR, and OSHA ETS, as well as related litigation.

[a] For purposes of the relevant Executive Orders, CMS IFR, and OSHA ETS, individuals are considered "fully vaccinated" for COVID-19 two weeks after they have received either a one-dose vaccine or a two-dose vaccine series.

[b] As of January 18, 2022, the IFR remains enjoined in Texas, where a district court issued a separate preliminary injunction that was not before the Supreme Court. The government's motion to stay the preliminary injunction, based on the Supreme Court's order in Biden v. Missouri, is pending before the district court.

Congress's Constitutional Authority to Mandate Vaccination

Although states have traditionally exercised the bulk of authority over public health matters, including vaccination, Congress shares certain concurrent authority in this area emanating from its enumerated powers in the Constitution.[241] This authority derives from, among other sources, the Constitution's Spending and Commerce Clauses, which may be used by Congress to clarify existing statutory authorities as they relate to vaccination requirements, or create additional sources of authority for or limitations on such requirements.[242]

The Spending Clause empowers Congress to tax and spend money for the general welfare.[243] Under this authority, which is subject to several limitations, Congress may offer federal funds to nonfederal entities and prescribe the terms and conditions under which the funds are accepted and used by recipients.[244] Over the past century, Congress has frequently invoked this authority in the public health context, including for purposes of controlling specified diseases, establishing neighborhood or community health centers, and creating federal health insurance programs, including Medicare and Medicaid.[245]

Applying its spending authority in the context of a vaccination mandate, Congress could, for instance, encourage states to enact a vaccination mandate meeting certain federal requirements by imposing it as a condition of receiving certain federal funds.[246] This use of Spending Clause authority, assuming it falls within the broad parameters of being for the "general welfare," would be permissible so long as (1) Congress provides clear notice of the vaccination mandate that states (or other funding recipients) must enact or implement; (2) the mandate is related to the purpose of the federal funds; (3) this conditional grant of funds is not otherwise barred by the Constitution; and (4) the amount of federal funds offered is not "so coercive as to pass the pointat which pressure turns into compulsion."[247]

In addition, the Commerce Clause grants Congress the power "[t]o regulate Commerce with foreign Nations, and among the several States, and with the Indian Tribes."[248] This authority empowers Congress to regulate "three broad categories of activities": (1) "channels of interstate commerce," like roads and canals; (2) instrumentalities of, or persons or things in, interstate commerce; and (3) activities that substantially affect interstate commerce.[249] Congress relied on the Commerce Clause to enact some of the earliest federal health laws aimed

---

[241] McCuskey, *supra* note 16, at 113–20. For instance, while the Supreme Court has long recognized the states' central role in regulating public health, the Court has also recognized, for equally as long albeit in dicta, Congress's power over infectious disease control under its Commerce Clause authority. Commenting in 1913 on quarantine laws used to prevent the introduction or spread of disease, for example, the Supreme Court stated that "[s]uch laws undoubtedly operate upon interstate and foreign commerce" and "could not be effective otherwise." Minnesota Rate Cases, 230 U.S. 352, 406 (1913).

[242] *See id.* at 116–19.

[243] U.S. CONST. art. I, § 8, cl. 1.

[244] *See* Nolan & Lewis, *supra* note 18, at 29–31 (discussing South Dakota v. Dole, 483 U.S. 203, 207–08 (1987)).

[245] *See* James G. Hodge, Jr., *The Role of New Federalism and Public Health Law*, 12 J.L. & HEALTH 309, 335–37 (1998); McCuskey, *supra* note 16, at 118–19.

[246] *See Dole*, 483 U.S. at 211–12 (holding that 23 U.S.C. § 158, which conditioned the provision of certain federal highway funds upon a state's enactment of a minimum drinking age of 21, was a valid exercise of Congress's spending clause authority).

[247] *See id.* at 207–08, 211 (internal quotations omitted).

[248] U.S. CONST. art. I, § 8, cl. 3.

[249] United States v. Lopez, 514 U.S. 549, 558–59 (1995).

at protecting the public from contagion and products posing health concerns.[250] As the federal government increased its role in public health, Congress relied on the Commerce Clause to pass more comprehensive national health regulations, beginning with the Food and Drug Act of 1906.[251]

While Congress's authority under the Commerce Clause is expansive, a majority of the Supreme Court in *National Federation of Independent Business (NFIB) v. Sebelius* agreed that there is a discrete limit to this authority—it cannot *compel* individuals to engage in commercial activity.[252] According to Chief Justice John Roberts, in a portion of the opinion not joined by other Justices but largely echoed in the view of the four dissenting Justices, the Commerce Clause did not empower Congress "to regulate individuals precisely because they are doing nothing."[253] While it is uncertain whether this conclusion constitutes binding precedent,[254] it suggests that a direct federal mandate on individuals to receive a vaccine may be susceptible to challenge because such mandates could be construed as compelling individuals who are "doing nothing" to engage in the commercial activity of receiving a specified health care service.[255] On the other hand, a federal mandate that requires vaccination as a condition to engage in existing economic activities, such as employment or interstate travel, may raise fewer constitutional concerns.[256]

Even if a vaccine mandate falls within Congress's enumerated powers, other constitutional provisions may constrain the government's action.[257] In the context of public health regulations, the key constraints are those grounded in federalism and the protection of individual rights.[258] For example, the Supreme Court has interpreted the Tenth Amendment to prevent the federal government from commandeering or requiring states or localities to adopt or enforce federal policies.[259] In the context of vaccination, this principle prevents Congress from directly requiring states or localities to pass mandatory vaccination laws or implement federal vaccination laws.[260] It does not, however, impede Congress from using its Spending

---

250 McCuskey, *supra* note 16, at 116–19 (noting that the Commerce Clause enabled several early federal health laws, including a law that authorized the quarantine of diseased livestock and people, and a law that regulated certain drugs and food products posing health concerns).

251 *See id.*; *see also* Medtronic, Inc. v. Lohr, 518 U.S. 470, 475 (1996); Hodge, *supra* note 245, at 335–36 (noting that "[f]ederal regulation now reaches broad aspects of public health such as air and water quality, food and drug safety, tobacco advertising, pesticide production and sales, consumer product safety, occupational health and safety, and medical care").

252 *See* Nolan & Lewis, *supra* note 18, at 10.

253 *See id.* at 10–11 (quoting NFIB v. Sebelius, 567 U.S. 519, 551 (2012) (opinion of Roberts, C.J.)).

254 See *id.* at 11.

255 *See NFIB*, 567 U.S. at 551.

256 *See In re* MCP No. 165, Occupational Safety & Health Admin., Interim Final Rule: COVID-19 Vaccination and Testing, 2021 WL 5989357, at *16 (6th Cir. 2021) (commenting that OSHA's large-employer vaccination and testing mandate regulates employers that are "indisputabl[y] . . . engag[ing] in commercial activity that Congress has the power to regulate," and stating that holding otherwise "would upend nearly a century of precedent upholding laws that regulate employers to effectuate a myriad of employee workplace policies"); *see also* Liberty Univ., Inc. v. Lew, 773 F.3d 72, 93 (4th Cir. 2013) (rejecting a Commerce Clause challenge to an Affordable Care Act requirement that certain employers offer a minimum level of health insurance coverage to their employees and dependents on the grounds that the requirement merely regulates an existing commercial activity). *But see* BST Holdings, LLC v. Occupational Safety & Health Admin., 17 F. 4th 604, 615 (5th Cir. 2021) (commenting that OSHA's large-employer vaccination and testing mandate impermissibly "regulates noneconomic inactivity that falls squarely within the States' police power").

257 *See* Nolan & Lewis, *supra* note 18, at 24–25.

258 *See id.* at 19, 24–25.

259 *Id.* at 25.

260 *See id.*

Clause authority to incentivize states to do so, as long as the amount offered is not so significant as to effectively coerce, or functionally commandeer, states into enacting the mandate.[261]

As to protection of individual rights, courts have recognized few rights-based constraints on the ability to impose mandatory vaccination requirements.[262] As explained above, courts have largely rejected due process and equal protection challenges to compulsory vaccination under *Jacobson* and *Zucht*. As with state vaccination requirements, the principal area of legal uncertainty as to rights-based constraints on federal requirements is whether and under what circumstances states must provide religious exemptions to a vaccination requirement.[263]

Emergency Use Authorization and Vaccination Mandates

Prior to the COVID-19 pandemic, all vaccines subject to governmental mandates were licensed under a biological license application (BLA), the standard regulatory framework under which vaccines are typically introduced into interstate commerce.[264] By contrast, as of December 2021, only one COVID-19 vaccine—Pfizer's Comirnaty—is licensed by FDA under a BLA.[265] Several other COVID-19 vaccines are authorized for emergency use under the FD&C Act's EUA provision, which allows the Secretary of HHS to permit patient access to an unlicensed vaccine for emergency use under specified conditions, including during a public health emergency.[266]

Before FDA licensed Pfizer's COVID-19 vaccine, some commentators raised a legal issue unique to COVID-19 vaccination mandates. Specifically, they argued that Section 564(e)(1) of the EUA provision precludes entities—including governmental entities—from mandating the COVID-19 vaccines.[267] Section 564(e)(1) directs the Secretary of HHS, when issuing an EUA for a medical product, to impose such necessary conditions to protect the public health, including appropriate conditions designed to inform individuals "of the option to accept or refuse administration of the product, of the consequences, if any, of refusing administration of the product, and of the alternatives to the product that are available and of their benefits and risks."[268] Because each individual must be provided with "the option to accept or refuse," some commentators asserted that this provision "suggests that mandates are categorically prohibited."[269]

After some state and private entities began mandating COVID-19 vaccinations in 2021, some litigants advanced this argument in court, asserting that COVID-19 vaccination requirements violated Section 564(e) of the FD&C Act. Courts have generally rejected this claim, holding that Section 564(e) imposes only an informed consent requirement on medical

---

[261] *See id.*

[262] *See supra* notes 39–47 and accompanying text.

[263] *See supra* "State COVID-19 Vaccination Mandates and Related Litigation."

[264] *See, e.g.*, CRS Report R46593, *Vaccine Safety in the United States: Overview and Considerations for COVID-19 Vaccines*, by Kavya Sekar and Agata Bodie, at 15, 34–35.

[265] For more information about FDA's approval of Comirnaty, the Pfizer-BioNTech COVID-19 vaccine, see Hickey, Ward & Bodie, *supra* note 7.

[266] *See id.*; *see also* Hickey et al., *supra* note 2, at 12–14.

[267] *See* Efthimios Parasidis & Aaron S. Kesselheim, *Assessing the Legality of Mandates for Vaccines Authorized Via an Emergency Use Authorization*, HEALTH AFFAIRS (Feb. 16, 2021), https://www.healthaffairs.org/do/10.1377/hblog20210212.410237/full/.

[268] 21 U.S.C. § 360bbb-3(e)(1)(A)(ii)(III).

[269] Parasidis & Kesselheim, *supra* note 267.

providers administering the vaccines to inform would-be recipients of the vaccines' risks and their right to refuse it.[270] As a result, courts generally have concluded that the provision does not prohibit entities from requiring individuals, duly informed by their medical providers, to be vaccinated.[271] Now that FDA has fully licensed Comirnaty, a COVID-19 vaccine, legal challenges to COVID- 19 vaccination requirements based on the EUA statute are largely moot.[272]

Considerations for Congress

A vaccination mandate is one available legal tool that governments could use to increase COVID- 19 vaccine uptake. Whether the federal government has existing statutory authority to mandate COVID-19 vaccination in certain contexts is an issue in several pending lawsuits.[273] Depending on whether Congress determines that the executive branch's use of these authorities, including provisions of the Procurement Act, the SSA, and the OSH Act, appropriately reflects congressional intent, Congress—subject to constitutional limits—can generally clarify the scope of these statutory provisions as they apply to vaccination requirements.

To the extent Congress determines that a federal vaccination mandate may be necessary to address the evolving pandemic, Congress could also impose a mandate through other legislative actions. Any such legislation, however, must be grounded in Congress's enumerated constitutional authority and structured consistently with constitutional due process and religious freedom guarantees.

---

[270] *See, e.g.*, Valdez v. Grisham, No. 21-cv-783, 2021 WL 4145746, at *4–5 (D.N.M. Sept. 13, 2021); Norris v. Stanley, No. 1:21-cv-756, 2021 WL 4738827, at *3 n.2 (W.D. Mich. Oct. 8, 2021) (rejecting plaintiffs' argument that a university's vaccination requirement is preempted by Section 564(e) because the policy "does not preclude Plaintiff from receiving informed consent, nor does it prevent her from accepting or refusing administration of the vaccine"); Johnson v. Brown, 3:21-cv-1494, 2021 WL 4846060, at *18 (D. Ore. Oct. 18, 2021) (holding that Section 564(e)'s "conditions of informed consent only relate to . . . the medical providers who administer the vaccine, not those who issue vaccine mandates").

[271] *See Valdez*, 2021 WL 4145746, at *4–5; *Norris*, 2021 WL 4738827, at *3 n.2; *Johnson*, 2021 WL 4846060, at *18; *see also* Bridges v. Houston Methodist Hosp., No. H-21-1774, 2021 WL 2399994, at *2 (S.D. Tex. Jun 12, 2021) (holding that Section 546(e) "confers certain powers and responsibilities to the Secretary of Health and Human Services in an emergency," such that "[i]t neither expands nor restricts the responsibilities of private employers"); *see also* U.S. DEP'T OF JUSTICE, OFF. OF LEGAL COUNS., WHETHER SECTION 564 OF THE FOOD, DRUG, AND COSMETIC ACT PROHIBITS ENTITIES FROM REQUIRING THE USE OF A VACCINE SUBJECT TO AN EMERGENCY USE AUTHORIZATION, 45 Op.O.L.C. , 2021 WL 3418599 (July 6, 2021) (concluding that "section 564 specifies only that certain information be provided to potential vaccine recipients and does not prohibit entities from imposing vaccination requirements"). In addition, courts have emphasized that at least one COVID-19 vaccine has received full FDA approval and is therefore no longer being distributed under an EUA, rendering this claim moot as to that vaccine. *See, e.g.*, *Valdez*, 2021 WL 4145746, at *4.

[272] *See, e.g.*, Norris v. Stanley, No. 1:21-CV-756, 2021 WL 3891615, at p. *2 (W.D. Mich. Aug. 31, 2021) ("[S]hould Plaintiff be offered the FDA-approved Pfizer Comirnaty vaccine, her argument under the EUA statute would be moot. . . ."). The legal issue may remain open with respect to vaccine mandates imposed on individuals 12 to 15 years old, however, as no vaccine is licensed under a BLA for use in this age group, as of the time of this writing.

[273] *See supra* "Executive Branch Authority to Mandate Vaccination."

Chapter 14

Status of Federal COVID-19 Vaccination Mandate Litigation*

Wen W. Shen

In 2021, various federal, state, and private entities instituted Coronavirus Disease 2019 (COVID-19) vaccination requirements to address the pandemic, particularly as the Delta variant—a highly contagious strain of SARS-CoV-2 (the virus that causes COVID-19)—spread in the United States. The federal COVID-19 vaccination requirements issued to date by the President or executive agencies include those directed at (1) federal executive agency civilian employees (federal employee mandate); (2) federal contractors for executive departments, agencies, and offices (federal contractor mandate); (3) most Medicare- and Medicaid-certified providers and suppliers (Centers for Medicare and Medicaid Services' [CMS's] Medicare/Medicaid provider mandate); and (4) employers with 100 or more employees (Occupational Safety and Health Administration's [OSHA's] large employer vaccination and testing mandate). These employment- or workforce-based mandates—subject to accommodations required by federal law—either directly require certain employees to receive COVID-19 vaccinations or direct certain employers to impose a vaccination or vaccination-and-testing requirement on their employees or staff.

These federal vaccination mandates have generated numerous legal challenges that have moved quickly through the courts. To date, some of these mandates have been enjoined by courts either on a nationwide basis or only in certain states. *Table 1* below provides a summary of the mandates and their statuses

* This is an edited, reformatted and augmented version of Congressional Research Service Publication No. LSB10681, updated January 18, 2022.

In: COVID-19 Vaccines
Editor: John Schroder
ISBN: 979-8-88697-150-7

Table 1. Summary of federal nonmilitary COVID-19 vaccination mandates as of January 18, 2022

Federal Mandate	*Statutory Authority*	*Covered Individuals/ Entities*	*Vaccination Requirement*	*Compliance Deadline(s)*	*Status*
Federal Employee Mandate (Executive Order 14,043)	5 U.S.C. §§ 3301, 3302, 7301	Federal executive branch employees	Employees must be fully vaccinated[a] unless granted a legally required exception based on a disability/medical condition or a sincerely held religious belief. Remote-working employees are subject to requirement.	Receive a one-dose vaccine or two- dose vaccine series by November 8, 2021. Be fully vaccinated by November 22, 2021.	In effect
Federal Contractor (Executive Order 14,042)	40 U.S.C. § 101 *et seq.*; 3 U.S.C. § 301	Federal contractors/ subcontractors that have a covered contract with executive departments and agencies	Covered contractors must ensure covered contractor-employees are fully vaccinated, except in circumstances where an employee is legally entitled to an exemption based on a disability/medical condition or a sincerely held religious belief. Remote-working covered contractor-employees are subject to requirement.	As of January 18, 2022, covered contractor-employees must be fully vaccinated on the first day of performance on a new contract or the renewal, extension, or exercised option of an existing contract.	Enjoined by courts: Kentucky v. Biden, No. 21-6147), 2022 WL 43178 (6th Cir. Jan. 5, 2022) (declining to stay the district court's preliminary injunction in KY, OH, and TN); Georgia v. Biden, No. 1:21-cv-00163 2021 WL 5779939 (S.D. Ga. Dec. 7, 2021) (enjoined the vaccination requirement nationwide).

Table 1. (Continued)

CMS's Medicare/ Medicaid Provider Mandate (CMS IFR)	42 U.S.C. §§ 1302, 1395hh, and other provider- or supplier-specific provisions	Specified provider and supplier types that participate in Medicare and Medicaid	Covered providers and suppliers must ensure covered staff who directly provide care or other services for their facilities and/or patients are fully vaccinated, except in circumstances where a staff member is legally entitled to an exemption based on a disability/ medical condition or a sincerely held religious belief. Staff who work 100% remotely from sites of patient care or away from onsite staff are *not* subject to the requirement.	By January 27, 2022, (1) covered providers and suppliers must establish and begin to implement the vaccination policies and (2) covered staff must receive first dose of a two- dose vaccine or a one-dose vaccine. Covered staff must complete two-dose vaccine series by February 28, 2022.	In effect in all jurisdictions except TX. (Preliminary injunctions in 24 states stayed by the U.S. Supreme Court in Biden v. Missouri, No. 21A240, ---S. Ct.---, 2022 WL 120950 (Jan. 13, 2022))[b]
OSHA's Large Employer Vaccination and Testing Mandate (OSHA ETS)	29 U.S.C. § 655(c)	In all jurisdictions, private employers with 100 or more employees. In 26 states, Puerto Rico, and the U.S. Virgin Islands with OSHA-approved state plans, state and local government employers with 100 or more employees.	A covered employer must establish and enforce a policy that either ensures employees are fully vaccinated, except in circumstances where an employee is legally entitled to an exemption based on a disability/medical condition or sincerely held religious belief; or requires employees to be fully vaccinated or provide proof of regular COVID-19 testing and wear a face covering when indoors. Employees who work remotely, at a site where other people are not present, or exclusively outside are not subject to the requirements.	Covered employers must establish and begin to implement the vaccination policies by January 10, 2022. Covered employees must receive either a one-dose vaccine or a two-dose vaccine series, or begin regular testing by February 9, 2022.	Stayed by the U.S. Supreme Court. (See Nat'l Fed. of Indep. Bus. v. Dep't of Labor, No. 21A244, ---S. Ct.---, 2022 WL 120952 (Jan. 13, 2022))

Source: CRS analysis of the relevant Executive Orders, CMS IFR, and OSHA ETS as well as related litigation.

[a] For purposes of the relevant Executive Orders, CMS IFR, and OSHA ETS, individuals are considered "fully vaccinated" for COVID-19 two weeks after they have received either a one-dose vaccine or a two-dose vaccine series.

[b] As of January 18, 2022, the IFR remains enjoined in Texas, where a district court issued a separate preliminary injunction that was not before the Supreme Court. The government's motion to stay the preliminary injunction, based on the Supreme Court's order in Biden v. Missouri, is pending before the district court.

Chapter 15

Liability Issues Related to COVID-19 Vaccine Manufacturing and Global Distribution*

Sara M. Tharakan and Nina M. Hart

Background

In March 2021, the United States announced efforts to donate Coronavirus Disease 2019 (COVID-19) vaccines abroad. In many high-income countries, vaccines and other medical countermeasures are playing a critical role in controlling the spread of COVID-19. Vaccine distribution efforts in low- and middle-income countries (LMICs) have been comparatively slow for a variety of reasons, raising concerns about how inequities may hinder pandemic control. Some vaccine manufacturers and others willing to donate COVID-19 vaccines are concerned about legal exposure should there be adverse health events arising from COVID-19 vaccination outside of the United States.

In several countries, legal liability issues have slowed or entirely stalled vaccine rollout.

For example, U.S. government vaccine donations to India reportedly remain in a Delhi warehouse because the Indian government has not agreed to indemnify vaccine manufacturers for vaccine-related injuries. Only a relatively small percentage of the Indian population is fully vaccinated against COVID-19; donated doses could potentially increase vaccination rates in the country. This chapter discusses potential liability issues that vaccine manufacturers and donors may face and options Congress might consider while deliberating vaccine distribution and liability issues.

Vaccine Distribution and Liability Concerns

Due to the novelty of the therapeutics used to control the COVID-19 pandemic, liability insurance is generally unavailable for COVID-19 vaccine manufacturers. Many pharmaceutical companies have expressed concern about the costs they may face from vaccine-related injury litigation, with some preventing governments from exporting vaccines to other countries without liability and indemnification agreements in place. In February 2021, the World Health Organization (WHO) and Chubb Limited, an insurance company, signed an agreement on behalf of COVAX—a multilateral initiative for global COVID-19 vaccine distribution—to create a No-Fault

* This is an edited, reformatted and augmented version of Congressional Research Service Publication No. IF11905, dated August 19, 2021.

Compensation Programfor those who suffer serious adverse events associated with a vaccine administered through COVAX.

In May 2021, the Task Force on COVID-19 Vaccines, Therapeutics, and Diagnostics for Developing Countries (the Task Force), composed of the International Monetary Fund, the World Bank Group, WHO, and the World Trade Organization, called for $50 billion in additional funding to support efforts to vaccinate 40% of all eligible people worldwide by the end of 2021. The Task Force cited liability issues and insufficient indemnification schemes as among the primary obstacles to achieving this goal.

According to COVAX, as of July 31, 2021, approximately 5% of COVID-19 vaccines that were pre-purchased by or for LMICs have been delivered to these countries. The Task Force indicated that the resolution of liability issues and negotiation of indemnification agreements through the No- Fault Compensation Program might incentivize additional donations to COVAX and mitigate acute near-termvaccine supply shortages.

Methods of Limiting Liability

Manufacturers may secure legal protection through a variety of means, including legislation and contracts (*Table 1*). Some legislation provides immunity for manufacturers or creates no-fault compensation funds that may apply to injuries related to vaccines. In addition, some governments and manufacturers have negotiated agreements to address distribution of COVID-19 vaccines, which vary by country and manufacturer. The relevant legal regimes involved may also vary depending on how vaccines are acquired and distributed, whether via COVAX or through other channels.

Table 1. Classification of liability regimes

Type	Description	Examples
Immunity	Prevents entities from being held legally liable and generally prevents individuals from receiving compensation	U.S.: Public Readiness and Emergency Preparedness (PREP) Act Philippines: COVID-19 Vaccination Programme Act
Indemnification	Requires a government to compensate entities for damages the entities owe to injured individuals	Contractual provision between the EU and AstraZeneca Contractual provision between the Dominican Republic and Pfizer
No-fault compensation	Individuals apply for compensation to a fund, and no liability attaches to the entities	U.S.: National Vaccine Injury Compensation Program COVAX mechanism

Source: Created by CRS.

Liability Issues for Doses Delivered via COVAX

To address liability and compensation issues related to serious adverse events, COVAX created the No-Fault Compensation Program. Through the program, individuals who sustain qualifying injuries after being vaccinated through COVAX may apply for compensation through a centralized online portal. While their claims are pending, individuals may not file claims in courts or other fora.

Applicants whose claims receive approval may obtain compensation froma centralized fund; if they accept the compensation offered, they must agree not to pursue any other claims in relation to the same vaccine-related injury. If an applicant's claimis rejected, the individual may then file a claim in a court or other forum. The Task Force hopes that the No-Fault Compensation Programmight avert a potentially burdensome caseload of COVID-19 vaccine-related claims, particularly in resource-limited countries.

Although this arrangement seeks to balance concerns about liability and responsibility to injured parties, there remain some concerns within the international community about claims settled outside of the COVAX program. In particular, WHO has raised concerns about whether lower- income countries will be able to pay indemnification costs owed to manufacturers under contracts or other agreements. COVAX is currently involved in ongoing discussions about the potential to provide loans to those countries through entities such as the Multilateral Investment Guarantee Agency, which is a member of the World Bank Group.

Vaccine Distribution in Humanitarian and Conflict Settings. In March 2021, COVAX agreed to set aside 5% of its vaccine doses to the COVAX Buffer for "high-risk groups in humanitarian settings," recognizing these groups may be hard to reach. According to the United Nations, 167 million people are at risk of exclusion from COVID-19 vaccination. The majority of those at risk are in COVAX Advanced Market Commitment (AMC)-eligible economies. AMC is a financial mechanismused by Gavi, the Vaccine Alliance, a multilateral public-private partnership that co-leads COVAX, to leverage high-income countries' large-scale purchases of COVID-19 vaccines to assure LMIC participation. However, roughly one-third of those in the high-riskgroup reside in areas not covered by COVAX's No-Fault Compensation Program. Humanitarian organizations have voiced concernabouttheir ability to administervaccinesbecause theycannot affordto shoulder the cost of indemnification agreements. COVAX is reportedly in discussions with manufacturers to address these issues.

Bilateral Agreements

Outside of COVAX, doses are exported and distributed to recipient countries through several mechanisms. The United States and other countries have donated vaccine doses on a bilateral basis, and governments have purchased doses directly from manufacturers to be imported into their territories.

Unlike distributions made via COVAX, arrangements between governments and manufacturers are not part of a global legal regime that addresses vaccine manufacturers' potential liability. Instead, to limit their legal liability or financial responsibility, pharmaceutical companies generally have to rely on domestic immunity laws, no-fault compensation laws, or contractually negotiated provisions (although not all companies have sought indemnification clauses in their contracts).

Considerations for Congress

Some Members of Congress have raised questions about the variables affecting global distribution efforts for COVID-19 vaccines. Such questions include whether manufacturers can receive liability protection in the United States and abroad and whether liability issues are restricting or delaying vaccine shipments. As described, there are international and bilateral efforts in place to address liability concerns. Some stakeholders remain concerned about whether countries receiving COVID-19 vaccines outside of COVAX will be able to cover future legal costs they may incur under indemnification clauses.

Congress may consider a variety of actions related to these issues, including

- whether to amend the PREP Act to address the scope of immunity provided to manufacturers for claims brought in the United
- whether to authorize funds in future foreign assistance legislation to assist LMICs required to indemnify vaccine manufacturers, or provide technical assistance to governments working on laws or agreements addressing liability concerns;
- whether to encourage the Biden Administration to engage in additional efforts, bilaterally or multilaterally, to mobilize private investments, public-private partnerships, or other such agreements, to help countries cover potential costs associated with indemnification agreements; and
- whether to encourage the Administration to engage with other developed countries about how to contribute collectively to meet the financial needs of countries required to indemnify manufacturers, potentially through the Task Force, World Bank, the Group of 7 (G7), or Group of 20 (G20), to hasten the pace of vaccine distribution.

Chapter 16

Compensation Programs for COVID-19 Vaccine Injuries*

Kevin J. Hickey and Erin H. Ward

Summary

More than 200 million Americans, and billions of people worldwide, have received one or more doses of a vaccine to protect against Coronavirus Disease 2019 (COVID-19). Most common side effects to COVID-19 vaccines are mild and generally resolve in a few days. However, in rare instances, COVID-19 vaccines can cause serious adverse events. For example, roughly one person out of every 200,000 who receives an mRNA-based COVID-19 vaccine experiences a severe allergic reaction. Other reported serious adverse events, such as myocarditis and Guillain- Barré Syndrome, are rare but may be associated with some COVID-19 vaccines.

Individuals who believe they are injured by COVID-19 vaccines may seek compensation for those injuries and other associated harms or costs. Absent an applicable federal law, individuals allegedly injured by a vaccine might seek redress by filing a state tort law claim against the vaccine manufacturer. However, federal law has two distinct compensation regimes that limit legal liability for vaccine manufacturers and provide potential compensation—without requiring a showing of fault—for individuals harmed by adverse reactions to vaccines. For injuries and deaths associated with most vaccines recommended by the Centers for Disease Control and Prevention (CDC) for routine administration in the United States (such as pediatric and seasonal influenza vaccines), the National Vaccine Injury Compensation Program (VICP) may provide compensation. During public health emergencies declared under the Public Readiness and Emergency Preparedness Act (PREP Act), the Countermeasures Injury Compensation Program (CICP) may provide compensation for injuries and deaths resulting from the administration of "covered countermeasures," which may include vaccines.

The VICP and CICP regimes are similar but distinct. Compensation through CICP is generally somewhat more limited than through VICP. CICP is a regulatory process administered by the Health Resources and Services Administration (HRSA), an agency within the U.S. Department of Health and Human Services (HHS). CICP compensation is available only for death or serious injuries resulting from a covered countermeasure that warrant hospitalization or lead to a significant loss of function or disability. A claimant must generally file a request form and associated documentation with HRSA within one year of the date that the covered countermeasure was administered. For injuries not listed by the Secretary of HHS on a Countermeasure Injury Table, the claimant must demonstrate that the injury was a direct result of the countermeasure's administration based on compelling medical and scientific evidence.

* This is an edited, reformatted and augmented version of Congressional Research Service Publication No. R46982, dated December 9, 2021.

Eligibility and compensation decisions are made by HRSA; judicial review is not available. CICP compensation is limited to reasonable medical expenses, loss of employment income, and a death benefit in cases where the claimant's death is a direct result of the administration or use of a covered countermeasure.

Under the Secretary of HHS's current PREP Act Declaration for COVID-19, FDA-authorized or -approved COVID-19 vaccines are covered countermeasures. While a PREP Act declaration is in effect, CICP is the sole remedy available for injuries related to covered countermeasures, including any covered vaccines. As a result, CICP—and not VICP—will apply to injuries resulting from COVID-19 vaccinations while the public health emergency persists and the Declaration remains in force. After the termination of the PREP Act public health emergency for COVID-19, COVID-19 vaccine injuries may be compensated through VICP, contingent on additional regulatory and statutory changes. In order for VICP to apply to a COVID-19 vaccine, (1) the vaccine must be recommended by the CDC for routine administration to children or pregnant women; (2) the vaccine must be made subject by act of Congress to the excise tax that funds VICP; and (3) the Secretary of HHS must add the vaccine to the Vaccine Injury Table, which lists injuries and conditions associated with covered vaccines.

Presuming all of those changes occur, VICP would apply to COVID-19 vaccine injuries. To receive compensation through VICP for a vaccine-related injury or death, the injured person must file a petition with the U.S. Court of Federal Claims, generally within three years of the first symptom or significant aggravation of the injury, or within two years of a death or four years of the first symptom resulting in death. To receive compensation, the injured party must show either that he or she experienced an injury listed for the vaccine in the Vaccine Injury Table within the time frame specified in the Table, or directly prove that the vaccine caused the injury. Eligibility and compensation determinations are made by a special master in a trial-like proceeding, which may be appealed to the U.S. Court of Federal Claims and the U.S. Court of Appeals for the Federal Circuit. Successful petitioners may receive medical expenses, lost income, a set death benefit, and reasonable attorneys' fees. Petitioners who are dissatisfied with the compensation they receive, or whose claims are delayed, may opt to pursue civil actions in court, subject to certain limitations on vaccine manufacturer liability.

More than 200 million Americans have received one or more doses of a Coronavirus Disease 2019 (COVID-19) vaccine,[1] along with billions of people worldwide.[2] The Food and Drug Administration's (FDA's) emergency use authorizations for the Pfizer-BioNTech, Moderna, and Johnson & Johnson COVID-19 vaccines were based on months-long clinical trials (including safety monitoring) of each vaccine, involving tens of thousands of participants.[3] These trials did not identify any safety concerns that would preclude such authorization.[4] (The

---

[1] *COVID-19 Vaccinations in the United States*, CTRS. FOR DISEASE CONTROL & PREVENTION (CDC), https://covid.cdc.gov/covid-data-tracker/#vaccinations_vacc-total-admin-rate-total (last updated Nov. 24, 2021).

[2] *More Than 7.79 Billion Shots Given: Covid-19 Tracker*, BLOOMBERG, https://www.bloomberg.com/graphics/covid-vaccine-tracker-global-distribution/ (last updated Nov. 24, 2021).

[3] Letter from FDA to Pfizer Inc., at 1-2 (May 10, 2021), https://www.fda.gov/media/144412/download [hereinafter Pfizer EUA]; Letter from FDA to ModernaTX, Inc., at 1-2 (Aug. 12, 2021), https://www.fda.gov/media/144636/download [hereinafter Moderna EUA]; Letter from FDA to Janssen Biotech, Inc., at 1-2 (June 10, 2021), https://www.fda.gov/media/146303/download [hereinafter J&J EUA].

[4] Pfizer EUA, *supra* note 3, at 2; Moderna EUA, *supra* note 3, at 2; J&J EUA, *supra* note 3, at 2.

Pfizer-BioNTech COVID-19 vaccine subsequently received full FDA approval for individuals 16 years of age and older.[5]) Post-authorization, the COVID-19 vaccines have been subject to safety monitoring requirements by FDA and the Centers for Disease Control and Prevention (CDC) to track the incidence of side effects and detect long-term, rare, or unexpected adverse health events.[6]

The most common side effects of COVID-19 vaccines are mild—such as local pain around the injection side, fatigue, or fever—and usually resolve within a few days.[7] As with most vaccines, however, a very small percentage of inoculated individuals experience serious adverse reactions to a COVID-19 vaccine.[8] For example, approximately two to five people per million receiving mRNA COVID-19 vaccines experience anaphylaxis, a severe allergic reaction, following vaccination.[9] (For this reason, the CDC recommends that all individuals be monitored for at least 15 minutes following their vaccinations, and that all vaccination sites have epinephrine available for treatment of anaphylaxis.[10]) Other serious adverse events reported following vaccination, such as myocarditis and Guillain-Barré Syndrome (GBS), are similarly rare and may be associated with COVID-19 vaccines.[11]

Federal law has two distinct compensation regimes that may compensate individuals harmed by adverse reactions to vaccines. In general, the National Vaccine Injury Compensation Program (VICP) may provide compensation for injuries or deaths associated with most vaccines routinely administered in the United States (such as pediatric and seasonal influenza vaccines).[12] During certain public health emergencies, the Countermeasures Injury Compensation Program (CICP) may provide compensation for injuries and deaths resulting

---

[5] Letter from FDA to BioNTech Manufacturing GmbH & Pfizer Inc., at 1 (Aug. 23, 2021), https://www.fda.gov/media/151710/download; *see generally* CRS Report R46913, *FDA Approval of the Pfizer-BioNTech COVID-19 Vaccine: Frequently Asked Questions*, by Kevin J. Hickey, Erin H. Ward, and Agata Bodie.

[6] *Ensuring COVID-19 Vaccine Safety in the US*, CDC, https://www.cdc.gov/coronavirus/2019-ncov/vaccines/safety.html (last updated Sept. 28, 2021) ("Millions of people in the United States have received COVID-19 vaccines under the most intense safety monitoring in U.S. history."); *see generally* CRS Report R46593, *Vaccine Safety in the United States: Overview and Considerations for COVID-19 Vaccines*, by Kavya Sekar and Agata Bodie.

[7] *Possible Side Effects After Getting a COVID-19 Vaccine,* CDC, https://www.cdc.gov/coronavirus/2019-ncov/vaccines/expect/after.html (last visited Nov. 17, 2021).

[8] *Selected Adverse Events Reported After COVID-19 Vaccination*, CDC, https://www.cdc.gov/coronavirus/2019-ncov/ vaccines/safety/adverse-events.html (last updated Nov. 16, 2021).

[9] *Id.* ("Anaphylaxis, a severe type of allergic reaction, following administration of COVID-19 vaccination is rare and has occurred in approximately 2 to 5 people per million vaccinated in the United States."); *accord* Tom T. Shimabukuro, Matthew Cole, & John R. Su, *Reports of Anaphylaxis After Receipt of mRNA COVID-19 Vaccines in the US: December 14, 2020–January 18, 2021*, 325 JAMA 1101–02 (Feb. 12, 2021), https://jamanetwork.com/journals/ jama/fullarticle/2776557.

[10] *Interim Considerations: Preparing for the Potential Management of Anaphylaxis After COVID-19 Vaccination*, CDC, https://www.cdc.gov/vaccines/covid-19/clinical-considerations/managing-anaphylaxis.html (last visited Nov. 17, 2021).

[11] *Myocarditis and Pericarditis After mRNA COVID-19 Vaccination*, CDC, https://www.cdc.gov/coronavirus/2019-ncov/vaccines/safety/myocarditis.html (last updated Nov. 12, 2021); *Selected Adverse Events Reported After COVID- 19 Vaccination*, CDC, https://www.cdc.gov/coronavirus/2019-ncov/vaccines/safety/adverse-events.html (last updated Nov. 16, 2021); Hannah G. Rosenblum et al., *Use of COVID-19 Vaccines After Reports of Adverse Events Among Adult Recipients of Janssen (Johnson & Johnson) and mRNA COVID-19 Vaccines (Pfizer-BioNTech and Moderna): Update from the Advisory Committee on Immunization Practices—United States, July 2021*, 70 MMWR 1094–99 (Aug. 13, 2021), https://www.cdc.gov/mmwr/volumes/70/wr/ mm7032e4.htm (estimating rates of GBS, myocarditis, and other serious adverse events per million vaccine doses administered).

[12] *National Vaccine Injury Compensation Program*, HEALTH RES. & SERVS. ADMIN. (HRSA), https://www.hrsa.gov/vaccine-compensation/index.html (last updated Nov. 2021); *Covered Vaccines*, HRSA, https://www.hrsa.gov/vaccine- compensation/covered-vaccines/index.html (last updated Nov. 2021) ("The National Vaccine Injury Compensation Program (VICP) covers most vaccines routinely given in the U.S.").

from the administration of "covered countermeasures," which may include vaccines, under the Public Readiness and Emergency Preparedness Act (PREP Act).[13]

Under the Secretary of Health and Human Services' (HHS's) PREP Act Declaration for COVID- 19 (and its amendments), COVID-19 vaccines are covered countermeasures within the PREP Act's scope.[14] As a result, CICP—and not VICP—will apply to injuries resulting from COVID-19 vaccinations while the public health emergency persists and the Declaration remains in force.[15] Compensation through CICP is generally somewhat more limited than through VICP.[16]

The Countermeasures Injury Compensation Program (CICP)

To encourage expeditious development and deployment of medical countermeasures during a public health emergency, the PREP Act authorizes the Secretary of HHS (the Secretary) to limit legal liability for losses resulting from the administration of medical countermeasures such as diagnostics, treatments, and vaccines.[17] In a declaration effective February 4, 2020 (the PREP Act Declaration), the Secretary invoked the PREP Act and declared COVID-19 to be a public health emergency warranting liability protections for covered countermeasures.[18] Pursuant to the PREP Act Declaration and its subsequent amendments,[19] manufacturers, distributors, and health care providers are generally immune from legal liability (i.e., they cannot be sued for money damages in court) for losses related to the administration or use of covered countermeasures against COVID-19.[20]

In addition to providing immunity from liability, the PREP Act established CICP, a compensation program for individuals seriously injured or killed as a direct result of the administration or use of a covered countermeasure.[21] CICP is a regulatory process administered

[13] *See Countermeasures Injury Compensation Program (CICP)*, HRSA, https://www.hrsa.gov/cicp/ (last updated Nov. 2020); Public Readiness and Emergency Preparedness Act, Pub. L. No. 109-148, div. C, 119 Stat. 2818 (2005).

[14] Fourth Amendment to the Declaration under the Public Readiness and Emergency Preparedness Act for Medical Countermeasures Against COVID-19 and Republication of the Declaration, 85 Fed. Reg. 79,190, 79,196 (Dec. 9, 2020) ("Covered countermeasures [include] any vaccine [used to] prevent, treat, or cure COVID-19."); *Public Readiness and Emergency Preparedness Act*, U.S. DEP'T OF HEALTH & HUMAN SERVS. HHS OFF. OF THE ASST. SEC. FOR PREPAREDNESS & RESPONSE (HHS ASPR), https://www.phe.gov/Preparedness/legal/prepact/Pages/default.aspx (last updated Oct. 8, 2021) (links to the PREP Act Declaration and amendments).

[15] *Frequently Asked Questions*, HRSA, https://www.hrsa.gov/cicp/faq (last updated Jan. 2021) ("COVID-19 vaccines are covered countermeasures under the Countermeasures Injury Compensation Program (CICP), not the National Vaccine Injury Compensation Program (VICP).").

[16] *See Comparison of Countermeasures Injury Compensation Program (CICP) to the National Vaccine Injury Compensation Program (VICP)*, HRSA, https://www.hrsa.gov/cicp/cicp-vicp (last updated Apr. 2021); *see also infra Appendix.*

[17] 42 U.S.C. § 247-6d(a)–(b).

[18] Declaration Under the Public Readiness and Emergency Preparedness Act for Medical Countermeasures Against COVID-19, 85 Fed. Reg. 15,198 (Mar. 17, 2020).

[19] *See Public Readiness and Emergency Preparedness Act*, HHS ASPR, https://www.phe.gov/Preparedness/legal/prepact/Pages/default.aspx (last updated Oct. 8, 2021) (linking to the PREP Act Declaration amendments).

[20] *See* 42 U.S.C. § 247d-6d(a); *see generally PREP Act Q&As*, HHS ASPR, https://www.phe.gov/Preparedness/legal/prepact/Pages/prepqa.aspx. For a detailed discussion of the scope of liability immunity under the PREP Act, see CRS Legal Sidebar LSB10443, *The PREP Act and COVID-19: Limiting Liability for Medical Countermeasures*, by Kevin J. Hickey.

[21] 42 U.S.C. § 247d-6e; *Countermeasures Injury Compensation Program (CICP)*, HRSA, https://www.hrsa.gov/cicp/ (last updated Nov. 2020).

by HHS's Health Resources and Services Administration (HRSA).[22] HRSA regulations govern CICP's procedures and eligibility determinations.[23]

Covered Vaccines and Injuries

Under the PREP Act and the amended Declaration, covered countermeasures for COVID-19 may include drugs, biological products, and medical devices that the FDA approves, licenses, or authorizes for emergency use "to diagnose, mitigate, prevent, treat, or cure" COVID-19, or used "to limit the harm that COVID-19 . . . might otherwise cause."[24] For example, personal protective equipment (PPE) (e.g., respirators), ventilators, therapeutic drugs (e.g., remdesivir), and monoclonal antibody treatments approved or authorized by FDA to treat or prevent COVID-19 are covered countermeasures under the PREP Act.[25] Notably, FDA-authorized or -approved COVID-19 vaccines—such as those produced by Pfizer, Moderna, and Johnson & Johnson—are covered countermeasures under the PREP Act Declaration.

Under the PREP Act, CICP remedies "shall be exclusive of any other civil action or proceeding" for injuries directly caused by administering covered countermeasures, with limited exceptions.[26] Thus, while the current PREP Act Declaration and public health emergency remain in effect, CICP is the exclusive remedy for claims within the PREP Act's scope, including injuries resultingfrom COVID-19 vaccinations.[27] (As discussed in detail below, VICP may eventually apply to COVID-19-vaccine injuries after the public health emergency terminates, contingent on certain statutory and regulatory changes.)

CICP compensation is limited to eligible individuals, such as persons injured by countermeasures or their survivors.[28] CICP provides compensation only for death or "serious physical injuries"— that is, injuries that warrant hospitalization or lead to a significant loss of function or disability.[29] Thus, individuals who experience only minor, short-term side effects from a COVID-19 vaccine—such as mild soreness, headache, or fatigue—would not be eligible for CICP compensation.[30]

---

[22] *See CICP Frequently Asked Questions*, HRSA, https://www.hrsa.gov/cicp/faq/index.html (last updated Jan. 2021).

[23] *See* 42 C.F.R. pt. 110.

[24] Fourth Amendment to the Declaration under the Public Readiness and Emergency Preparedness Act for Medical Countermeasures Against COVID-19 and Republication of the Declaration, 85 Fed. Reg. 79,190, 79,196 (Dec. 9, 2020); 42 U.S.C. § 2476d-6d(i)(7).

[25] *Emergency Use Authorization*, FDA, https://www.fda.gov/emergency-preparedness-and-response/mcm-legal-regulatory-and-policy-framework/emergency-use-authorization#2019-ncov (last updated Nov. 18, 2021) (listing FDA emergency use authorizations for vaccines, drugs, biologics, and medical devices used against COVID-19).

[26] 42 U.S.C. § 247d-6e(d)(4).

[27] *See id.*; *see also CICP Frequently Asked Questions*, HRSA, https://www.hrsa.gov/cicp/faq/index.html (last updated Jan. 2021) ("COVID-19 vaccines are covered countermeasures under the Countermeasures Injury Compensation Program (CICP), not the National Vaccine Injury Compensation Program (VICP)."). The "sole exception" is a claim for willful misconduct. 42 U.S.C. §§ 247d-6d(d)(1), 247d-6e(d)(4).

[28] *See* 42 C.F.R. § 110.10.

[29] *See id.* § 110.3(z); 42 U.S.C. § 247d-6e(e)(3).

[30] *Possible Side Effects After Getting a COVID-19 Vaccine,* CDC, https://www.cdc.gov/coronavirus/2019-ncov/vaccines/expect/after.html (last visited Nov. 17, 2021) (describing temporary arm pain, tiredness, muscle pain, fever, and other "common side effects" of COVID-19 vaccines).

Procedure for Obtaining Compensation

To apply for CICP compensation, a claimant must file a request for benefits within one year of the date the countermeasure was administered.[31] (If the Secretary publishes a new Countermeasure Injury Table, a newly eligible claimant may file within one year after the new table is established.[32]) In addition to the request form, claimants may need to submit medical records and other evidence to establish eligibility.[33] If determined to be eligible, claimants may submit additional documentation to demonstrate the compensation amount.[34] Eligibility and compensation determinations are made by CICP as the Secretary's delegate.[35] Claimants may seek reconsideration of an adverse eligibility decision by CICP, but the ultimate decisionmaking authority lies with the Secretary.[36] The PREP Act precludes judicial review of the Secretary's eligibility and compensation decisions.[37]

CICP claimants can prove eligibility for compensation in one of two ways.[38] The first applies only to injuries listed on a Countermeasure Injury Table, which the Secretary must establish by regulation when compelling medical and scientific evidence shows that administration or use of a covered countermeasure directly causes particular injuries.[39] (The table established for the H1N1 pandemic influenza vaccine is one example;[40] no such table has yet been promulgated for COVID-19 countermeasures, including vaccines.) For injuries listed on a Countermeasure Injury Table, if the claimant can show that the countermeasure recipient's injury is listed on the table and was sustained within the relevant time interval (and meets any other requirements set forth in the table), CICP will presume the injury was a direct result of the covered countermeasure.[41] For injuries not on a Countermeasure Injury Table (or outside its scope), the claimant must prove the non-table injury was the "direct result" of the countermeasure's administration based on "compelling, reliable, valid, medical and scientific evidence" beyond mere temporal association.[42]

Available Compensation

Compensation under CICP is limited to (1) reasonable medical expenses (e.g., unreimbursed hospitalization costs); (2) loss of employment income (e.g., income lost from inability to work

---

[31] 42 C.F.R. § 110.42(a).

[32] *Id.* § 110.42(f).

[33] *See id.* § 110.50–110.53; *see also Criteria to Demonstrate that a Covered Injury Occurred*, HRSA, https://www.hrsa.gov/cicp/injury-occurred (last updated Nov. 2020).

[34] *See* 42 C.F.R. § 110.60–110.63; *see also Filing for Benefits*, HRSA, https://www.hrsa.gov/cicp/filing-benefits (last updated Oct. 2021) ("If the requester is determined to be eligible for program benefits, the requester is asked to submit additional documentation to determine the type and amount of compensation the requester may be entitled to receive.").

[35] *See* 42 C.F.R. § 110.72–110.74.

[36] *See id.* §§ 110.90 (process to request reconsideration of eligibility determinations), 110.91 ("[T]he Secretary may, at any time, on her own motion or on application, review any determination made under this part [and] may affirm, vacate, or modify the determination in any manner the Secretary deems appropriate.").

[37] *See* 42 U.S.C. § 247d-6e(b)(4) (incorporating 42 U.S.C. § 239a(f)(2)); 42 C.F.R. § 110.92 ("[N]o judicial review of the Secretary's actions concerning eligibility and benefits determinations under [CICP] is permitted.").

[38] *See* 42 C.F.R. § 110.20(b)–(c).

[39] 42 U.S.C. § 247d-6e(5)(A).

[40] 42 C.F.R. § 110.100.

[41] *See id.* § 110.20(b).

[42] *See id.* § 110.20(c).

due to disability); and (3) a set death benefit where the death is a direct result of the administration or use of a covered countermeasure.[43] Attorneys' fees and pain-and-suffering damages are not available under CICP.[44] CICP awards are also subject to various annual and lifetime limits. For example, annual lost employment income awards are capped at $50,000 per year,[45] and the standard maximum death benefit is the same as that under the Public Safety Officers' Benefits program (currently $389,825.45).[46]

Given the limited number and scope of past PREP Act declarations, CICP has been used relatively infrequently since the PREP Act's 2005 enactment.[47] The majority of these non-COVID-19 claims were related to the H1N1 pandemic influenza vaccine.[48] According to HRSA, for FY2010 through FY2021, CICP received 491 claims unrelated to COVID-19, of which at least 408 (83%) appear to relate to the H1N1 vaccine. Of these, 39 (8%) were determined to be eligible for compensation and 29 (6%) have been paid out by CICP, amounting to $6 million in awards.[49] (Ten of the claims determined to be eligible for compensation had no eligible reported medical expenses or lost employment income.)

In light of the COVID-19 pandemic, HRSA has received a larger number of CICP claims than it has received historically. As of October 1, 2021, CICP has received 3,158 claims alleging injury or death relating to COVID-19 countermeasures, of which 1,357 claims (43%) relate to COVID- 19 vaccines.[50] CICP has not yet compensated any claims relating to COVID-19 countermeasures; it has denied three claims because the standard of proof for causation was not met and/or a covered injury was not sustained, and determined one claim to be eligible for compensation, pending a review of the eligible expenses.[51] The remainder of the COVID-19 countermeasure claims (99.9%) are in review or pending CICP review.[52]

Several COVID-19 emergency appropriations allow the Secretary to transfer funds to the Covered Countermeasure Process Fund.[53] Such funds, in addition to prior-year fund balances, can be used for CICP compensation awards.

---

[43] *Id.* § 110.2(a).

[44] *See Comparison of Countermeasures Injury Compensation Program (CICP) to the National Vaccine Injury Compensation Program (VICP)*, HRSA, https://www.hrsa.gov/cicp/cicp-vicp (last updated Apr. 2021) ("Attorneys' fees and costs are not paid by [CICP]."); Nicholas M. Pace, Lloyd Dixon, Bethany Saunders-Medina, *The Compensation System for Potential Side Effects Is an Important Part of a COVID-19 Vaccine Campaign,* THERANDBLOG (Dec. 18, 2020), https://www.rand.org/blog/2020/12/the-compensation-system-for-potential-side- effects.html ("The CICP does not provide any compensation for pain, suffering, emotional distress, or similar damages . . . .").

[45] 42 C.F.R. § 110.81(c)(2).

[46] *Id.* § 110.82(b)(1); *Benefits by Year: Public Safety Officers' Benefits Program*, U.S. DEP'T OF JUSTICE BUR. OF JUST. ASSISTANCE, https://psob.bja.ojp.gov/knowledge-base/benefits-by-year/ (last visited Nov. 18, 2021).

[47] *See* Pace et al., *supra* note 44 ("The NVICP has handled more than 20,000 vaccine injury claims since its inception, while the CICP, as far as can be determined, has processed about 500 since the law that created the program was enacted in 2005 [and prior to COVID-19].").

[48] *See* Bernard Condon & Matt Sedensky, *How U.S. Government Will Handle COVID-19 Vaccine Injury Claims Is Largely a Secret,* INS. J., https://www.insurancejournal.com/news/national/2020/12/29/595414.htm (Dec. 29, 2020) ("[Prior to COVID-19], the vast majority of the claims under [CICP] have stemmed from the H1N1 swine flu vaccine a decade ago.").

[49] *See Countermeasures Injury Compensation Program (CICP) Data,* HRSA, https://www.hrsa.gov/cicp/cicp-data (last updated Oct. 1, 2021) (listing 3,649 total claims, of which 3,158 relate to COVID-19 countermeasures, 408 relate to the H1N1 vaccine, 39 were eligible for compensation, and 29 were compensated).

[50] *See id.* at tbl. 1.

[51] *Id.* at "Has the CICP made any decisions regarding COVID-19 Claims?"

[52] *See id.* at tbl. 1 (listing 3,158 COVID-19 countermeasure claims, of which 4 have an eligibility determination).

[53] *See, e.g.*, Coronavirus Aid, Relief, and Economic Security (CARES) Act, Pub. L. No. 116-136, div. B, tit. VIII, 134 Stat. 281, 560–61 (Mar. 27, 2020).

The National Vaccine Injury Compensation Program (VICP)

After the Secretary terminates the PREP Act Declaration for the COVID-19 pandemic, any injuries or death from COVID-19 vaccines administered after the Declaration ends would be addressed in court under tort law unless the COVID-19 vaccines are added to VICP.[54] VICP provides compensation for injuries and deaths caused by certain vaccines that are subject to an excise tax and listed on the Vaccine Injury Table.[55]

VICP was created by the National Childhood Vaccine Injury Act of 1986 (NCVIA) amid concerns that lawsuits against vaccine manufacturers and health care providers alleging vaccine injuries could lead to vaccine shortages and lower immunization rates.[56] Under a typical state tort law framework, an injured person must generally prove that a vaccine caused the injury and that either the vaccine manufacturer is at fault (e.g., negligent, failed to warn adequately) or, under products liability doctrines, that the vaccine was defective.[57] If the person cannot prove one of these elements—for example, if the manufacturer adequately warned of side effects or it is unclear whether the vaccine caused the injury—the claimant receives no compensation. If the vaccine manufacturer is found liable, however, it may be responsible for compensatory damages and potentially punitive damages as determined by a jury.[58] Regardless of the outcome, both sides generally would be responsible for litigation costs.[59]

The NCVIA created a no-fault alternative compensation program for deaths and injuries caused by certain vaccines that are recommended by the CDC for routine administration in children or pregnant women.[60] The program shields manufacturers of certain vaccines from most liability for vaccine-related injuries and deaths, while providing compensation to those injured by vaccines from a trust fund funded by excise taxes paid by the vaccine manufacturers.[61] By limiting liability exposure for vaccine manufacturers, expanding the availability of compensation for injured parties, and lowering the burden of proof, the program reduces uncertainty for both injured persons and vaccine manufacturers. From implementation of the program in 1988 through November 1, 2021, more than 24,538 petitions for compensation have been filed, of which 20,400 have been adjudicated, and 8,439 determined to merit compensation.[62] The program has paid out more than $4.6 billion in compensation since its inception.[63]

---

[54] 42 U.S.C. §§ 300aa-10–300aa-44; 26 U.S.C. §§ 4131, 4132, 9510. *See also National Vaccine Injury Compensation Program*, HRSA, https://www.hrsa.gov/vaccine-compensation/index.html (last updated November 2021).

[55] 42 U.S.C. §§ 300aaa-11–300aa-15; 26 U.S.C. §§ 4131, 4132, 9510; 42 C.F.R. § 100.3; *Vaccine Injury Table*, HRSA, https://www.hrsa.gov/sites/default/files/hrsa/vaccine-compensation/vaccine-injury-table.pdf.

[56] Pub. L. No. 99-660, § 311, 100 Stat. 3758 (1986); *see, e.g.*, S. REP. NO. 99-483, at 2–6 (1986); H. REP. NO. 99-908, at 4–7 (1986).

[57] RESTATEMENT (SECOND) OF TORTS § 281; RESTATEMENT (THIRD) OF TORTS: PRODUCTS LIABILITY §§ 1, 10. *See also* CRS In Focus IF11291, *Introduction to Tort Law*, by Kevin M. Lewis.

[58] RESTATEMENT (SECOND) OF TORTS §§ 901–917.

[59] Alyeska Pipeline Serv. Co. v. Wilderness Soc'y, 421 U.S. 240, 247 (1975).

[60] 42 U.S.C. §§ 300aa-13–300aa-15.

[61] *Id.* §§ 300aa-13–300aa-15, 300aa-21–300aa-22; 26 U.S.C. §§ 4131, 4132, 9510.

[62] *Data & Statistics*, HRSA, https://www.hrsa.gov/sites/default/files/hrsa/vaccine-compensation/data/ vicpmonthly reporttemplate%2011-01-21.pdf (last updated Nov. 1, 2021).

[63] *Id.*

Covered Vaccines and Injuries

To receive compensation, an injured party must show he or she received a "covered vaccine."[64] Not every FDA-approved vaccine is covered by VICP. The NCVIA included an initial Vaccine Injury Table listing vaccines covered by the program.[65] Under the Act, the Secretary can add vaccines to the program by amending the Vaccine Injury Table to add vaccines recommended by the CDC for routine administration to children or pregnant women within two years of such a recommendation.[66]

To receive compensation through VICP, the injured person must have received a vaccine that is

1) recommended by the CDC for routine administration to children or pregnant women,
2) listed by the Secretary on the Vaccine Injury Table, and (3) subject to an excise tax that funds the Vaccine Injury Compensation Trust Fund from which compensation is paid.[67] The types of vaccines subject to the excise tax are specified in statute and therefore can be amended only by an act of Congress.[68]

In addition to having received a covered vaccine, the injured party must show either that (1) he or she experienced an injury listed for the vaccine in the Vaccine Injury Table and the first symptom of the onset or significant aggravation of the injury occurred within the time frame specified in the table, or (2) the vaccine caused the injury.[69] The Vaccine Injury Table accordingly allows injured persons to avoid having to prove a vaccine caused their injuries by allowing them instead to show they received an injury that has been associated with the vaccine soon after receiving the vaccine.[70] Nonetheless, injured persons still have the option of directly proving that a vaccine caused their injuries if they experience an injury not listed in the Vaccine Injury Table or the onset or aggravation of the injury is delayed.[71]

Procedure for Obtaining Compensation

To receive compensation through VICP for a vaccine-related injury or death, the injured person (or the estate in the case of a death) files a petition with the U.S. Court of Federal Claims (Claims Court).[72] The petition must generally contain an affidavit and supporting documentation, including relevant medical records, showing the person

- received a vaccine listed in the Vaccine Injury Table;
- sustained an illness, disability, injury, or condition either

[64] 42 U.S.C. §§ 300aa-11(c), 300aa-33(5).
[65] *Id.* § 300aa-14(a).
[66] *Id.* § 300aa-14(e).
[67] *Id.* § 300aa-14; 26 U.S.C. §§ 4132, 9510.
[68] 26 U.S.C. § 4132.
[69] 42 U.S.C. § 300aa-11(c).
[70] *Id.* §§ 300a-11, 300aa-14.
[71] *Id.* § 300a-11(c)(1)(C)(ii).
[72] *Id.* § 300aa-11.

- set forth in the Vaccine Injury Table for the particular vaccine, and the first symptom or manifestation occurred within the required time period; or
- caused by the vaccine;
- suffered residual effects or complications that lasted for more than six months or required inpatient hospitalization and surgery, or died; and
- has not collected another award or settlement for the injury or death.[73]

Petitions for vaccine-related injuries must generally be filed within three years of the first symptom or significant aggravation of the injury.[74] Petitions for vaccine-related deaths must be filed within two years of the death and within four years of the first symptom or significant aggravation of the injury from which the death resulted.[75] If the Vaccine Injury Table is amended such that a person qualifies for compensation who previously did not, that person has two years from when the table is revised to seek compensation for injuries or deaths that occurred up to eight years before the table was revised.[76]

When a person files a petition with the Claims Court, the clerk of the court forwards the petition to the chief special master to assign the petition to one of eight special masters.[77] The assigned special master conducts a proceeding to evaluate whether the petition merits compensation under VICP and, if so, how much.[78] The proceedings resemble trials in allowing the presentation of evidence and submission of testimony, but they operate under more flexible, informal procedures to allow for expeditious resolution.[79] Once a petition is filed, the special master has 240 days to issue a decision that includes factual findings and legal conclusions, though the parties may suspend the proceedings by motion for up to 150 days if necessary.[80]

Following the decision, the petitioner has 30 days to appeal a special master's decision to the Claims Court for review.[81] The court then has 120 days to uphold the decision, issue its own decision, or remand to the special master for further proceedings.[82] Once the court issues its judgment, either because the petitioner does not appeal the special master's decision within 30 days or the court issues a decision after review, the petitioner has 60 days to appeal the judgment to the U.S. Court of Appeals for the Federal Circuit (Federal Circuit).[83] If the petitioner chooses not to appeal the decision, the judgment becomes final.[84]

After a final judgment, the petitioner has 90 days to inform the Claims Court whether the petitioner accepts the judgment or will file a separate civil action for damages.[85] A petitioner may also withdraw its petition and file a civil action if the special master fails to act within 240

---

[73] *Id.* § 300aa-11(c).
[74] *Id.* § 300aa-16(a).
[75] *Id.*
[76] *Id.* § 300aa-16(b).
[77] *Id.* §§ 300aa-12(c)(1), 300aa-12(d); *see also Vaccine Claims/Office of Special Masters*, U.S. COURT OF FEDERAL CLAIMS, https://www.uscfc.uscourts.gov/vaccine-programoffice-special-masters (last visited Nov. 24, 2021).
[78] 42 U.S.C. § 300aa-12.
[79] *Id.* § 300aa-12(d)(3)(B); *Vaccine Rules, Appendix B, Rules of the United States Court of Federal Claims*, U.S. COURT OF FEDERAL CLAIMS, https://www.uscfc.uscourts.gov/sites/default/files/20.08.03%20FINAL%20Vaccine%20Rules.pdf (last updated Aug. 3, 2020).
[80] 42 U.S.C. § 300aa-12(d)(3).
[81] *Id.* § 300aa-12(e)(1).
[82] *Id.* § 300aa-12(e)(2).
[83] *Id.* § 300aa-12(e)–(f).
[84] *Id.* § 300aa-12(e)(3).
[85] *Id.* § 300aa-21(a).

days or the Claims Court fails to enter the judgment within 420 days, both time frames excluding any suspended time.[86] (Petitioners may opt not to withdraw their petitions if they do not want to risk proceeding in civil court.[87]) Petitioners who neither rejected a judgment nor withdrew their petition due to the court's failure to act in time are barred from filing civil claims.[88]

In addition to limiting the availability of civil actions to parties who have gone through the petition process, VICP imposes certain limitations on vaccine manufacturers' liability.[89] For example, vaccine manufacturers are not liable for injuries or deaths due to unavoidable side effects from properly prepared vaccines accompanied by proper directions and warnings.[90] Any action that proceeds against a vaccine manufacturer is tried in three stages: (1) liability, general damages, and (3) punitive damages.[91] Trifurcating the trial in this manner limits the evidence presented to the jury in the first and second stages to the evidence relevant to each stage of the trial.

Available Compensation

VICP allows individuals to receive compensation for

- actual and reasonably projectable unreimbursable expenses directly related to the vaccine-related injury, including the cost of diagnosis, medical care,
- rehabilitation, counseling, and vocational training, among others;
- actual and anticipated loss of earnings;
- actual and projected pain and suffering and emotional distress, capped at $250,000;
- vaccine-related death, in the amount of $250,000; and
- reasonable attorneys' fees and other costs associated with proceeding onthe petition.[92]

The NCVIA authorized appropriations to compensate individuals injured by vaccines administered before October 1, 1988.[93] Compensation for injuries for vaccines administered after October 1, 1988, is paid out of the Vaccine Injury Compensation Trust Fund (Trust Fund).[94]

Vaccine manufacturers pay into the Trust Fund through excise taxes imposed on covered vaccines.[95] The Trust Fund may be used to pay only for vaccine-related injuries from vaccines subject to the excise tax at the time of payment, and for certain government administrative expenses incurred when administering the program.[96] Consequently, only vaccines subject to the excise tax are included in VICP.

---

86 *Id.* § 300aa-21(b).
87 *Id.*
88 *Id.* § 300aa-11(a)(2)(A).
89 *Id.* § 300aa-22.
90 *Id.* § 300aa-22(b).
91 *Id.* § 300aa-23.
92 *Id.* § 300aa-15(a)–(e).
93 *Id.* § 300aa-15(j).
94 *Id.* § 300aa-15(i)(2); 26 U.S.C. § 9510.
95 26 U.S.C. §§ 4131–4132.
96 *Id.* § 9510(c).

Considerations for Congress

The future of the COVID-19 pandemic, the impact of SARS-CoV-2 variants (such as the Delta and Omicron variants), and the status of vaccines authorized to prevent COVID-19 remain uncertain. The Moderna and Johnson & Johnson COVID-19 vaccines are currently available only pursuant to emergency use authorizations, and certain uses of the Pfizer-BioNTech COVID-19 vaccine are also authorized only by emergency use authorization.[97] The CDC has issued an interim recommendation that children aged 5 to 17 and people who are pregnant receive a COVID-19 vaccine, but it remains to be seen whether inoculations will continue to be recommended for these groups or the general population on a regular basis as the virus evolves.[98] Accordingly, it is unknown whether COVID-19 vaccines will become routinely administered, and whether the CDC will recommend any such vaccine for routine administration to children or pregnant women.

If the CDC does recommend COVID-19 vaccines for routine administration to children or pregnant women, Congress may consider whether to add COVID-19 vaccines to the excise tax list, which would include them in VICP. Alternatively, Congress might consider a broader amendment to the excise tax statute to allow any vaccine recommended for routine administration to children or pregnant women to be automatically subject to the excise tax and therefore eligible for VICP. Or, if Congress decides that COVID-19 injuries should be compensated through VICP even while the public health emergency persists, Congress could amend the PREP Act and NCVIA accordingly.

Congress could also implement an entirely new program specifically addressing compensation for COVID-19 vaccine-related injuries or deaths, should it so choose. Alternatively, Congress could opt to leave COVID-19 vaccines out of VICP and allow the traditional tort system to address any vaccine-related injuries after the public health emergency ends and CICP no longer applies.

Appendix. Comparison of Vaccine-Injury Programs: CICP vs. VICP

	Countermeasures Injury Compensation Program (CICP)	*Vaccine Injury Compensation Program (VICP)*
Scope of Coverage	"Covered countermeasures" under the PREP Act, such as pandemic and epidemic products used to treat, mitigate, prevent, or cure COVID-19 (e.g., vaccines, PPE, treatments)	"Covered Vaccines" are those recommended by CDC for routine administration to children or pregnant women, subject to a federal excise tax, and added to the Vaccine Injury Table

[97] Letter from Dr. Jacqueline A. O'Shaughnessy, Acting Chief Scientist, FDA, to Ruta Walawalkar, Janssen Biotech Inc., Nov. 19, 2021, https://www.fda.gov/media/146303/download; Letter from Dr. Jacqueline A. O'Shaughnessy, Acting Chief Scientist, FDA, to Michelle Olsen, ModernaTX, Inc., Nov. 19, 2021, https://www.fda.gov/media/144636/ download; Letter from Dr. Jacqueline A. O'Shaughnessy, Acting Chief Scientist, FDA, to Amit Patel, Pfizer Inc., Nov. 19, 2021, https://www.fda.gov/media/150386/download.

[98] *COVID-19 Vaccines for Children and Teens*, CDC, www.cdc.gov/coronavirus/2019-ncov/vaccines/ recommendations/children-teens.html (updated Nov. 23, 2021); *COVID-19 Vaccines While Pregnant or Breastfeeding*, CDC, www.cdc.gov/coronavirus/2019-ncov/vaccines/recommendations/pregnancy.html (updated Nov. 19, 2021); *COVID-19 ACIP Vaccine Recommendations*, CDC, https://www.cdc.gov/vaccines/ hcp/acip-recs/vacc-specific/covid- 19.html (updated Nov. 5, 2021).

	Countermeasures Injury Compensation Program (CICP)	*Vaccine Injury Compensation Program (VICP)*
Covered Injuries	Death, or serious physical injury that (1) warrants hospitalization or (2) leads to a significant loss of function or disability	Death or an illness, injury, or condition that lasted more than six months or required inpatient hospitalization and surgical intervention and was associated with one or more vaccines in the Vaccine Injury Table (unless the cause was an adulterant or contaminant that was intentionally added to the vaccine)
Process for Obtaining Compensation	Administrative Process: file request form and supporting documentation with CICP to prove eligibility and compensation amounts	Judicial Process ("vaccine court"): file a petition in the U.S. Court of Federal Claims
Available Benefits	Reasonable medical expenses, lost employment income, and death benefits	Non-reimbursed expenses related to the injury for the diagnosis, medical care, and various rehabilitation and recovery services; lost employment income; pain, suffering, and emotional distress damages; death benefits; attorney's fees
Unavailable Benefits	Attorneys' fees, pain-and-suffering damages, punitive damages	Punitive or exemplary damages
Benefit Caps	\$50,000/year for lost employment income; lifetime cap for lost income (except for permanent disability); and standard death benefit of \$389,825.45 for FY2022	\$250,000 for death; \$250,000 for pain and suffering and emotional distress
Filing Deadlines	Within one year of administration of covered countermeasure (or within one year of the issuance of an amended Countermeasure Injury Table)	For injuries, within three years of the first symptom; for deaths, within two years of the death and four years of the first symptom
Standard of Proof	Must show the injury (1) meets the requirements on a Countermeasure Injury Table; or (2) was a direct result of the administration or use of a covered countermeasure	Must show the person (1) received a vaccine on the Vaccine Injury Table; (2) sustained or significantly aggravated an illness, disability, injury, or condition, or died; (3) the illness, disability, injury, condition, or death is either listed in the Vaccine Injury Table in association with the vaccine and occurred within a set time period as specified in the table or was caused by the vaccine; (4) suffered the effects for more than six months or required inpatient hospitalization and surgery or died; and (5) has not previously collected an award for the injury or death
Initial Decisionmaker	CICP (as delegate of the Secretary of HHS)	U.S. Court of Federal Claims special master
Appeals & Judicial Review	Claimant may seek reconsideration of CICP decision to a qualified independent panel within 60 days; no further judicial or administrative review	Claimant may seek review of special master decision by U.S. Court of Federal Claims within 30 days of decision; claimant may seek review by the U.S. Court of Appeals for the Federal Circuit within 60 days of final judgment; claimant may accept the judgment or reject it and file a tort claim
Funding Source	Emergency appropriations to Covered Countermeasure Process Fund	Vaccine Injury Compensation Trust Fund based on excise tax of \$0.75 per dose on "taxable vaccines"

Appendix. (Continued)

Number of Claims Processed	Non-COVID-19 claims (2010–2021): 491 claims, of which 452 were determined ineligible and 29 compensated (6%) COVID-19 countermeasure claims (as of October 1, 2021): 3,158 claims, of which 1,357 claims (43%) relate to COVID-19 vaccines; most of these claims (99.9%) remain in or are pending review	24,441 petitions as of 10/1/2021, of which 20,300 have been adjudicated: 11,947 were determined ineligible and 8,353 compensated (41%)
Process for Adding New Vaccines	Scope of "covered countermeasures" is determined by Secretary of HHS's PREP Act declarations (within statutory limits)	Secretary of HHS may add vaccines to the Vaccine Injury Table that are (1) subject to the excise tax; and (2) recommended by the CDC for routine administration to children or pregnant women

Source: 42 U.S.C. §§ 300aa-10–300aa-34; 42 U.S.C. § 247d-6d to -6e; 42 C.F.R. pt. 110; HRSA; CRS.

Index

D

E

Index

D

E

N

O

P

R

S

T

U

V

W

Y